Cardiac Surgery: Advances in Operative Techniques

Cardiac Surgery: Advances in Operative Techniques

Editor: Evie Brooks

FOSTER ACADEMICS

www.fosteracademics.com

www.fosteracademics.com

FOSTER ACADEMICS

Cataloging-in-publication Data

Cardiac surgery : advances in operative techniques / edited by Evie Brooks.
p. cm.
Includes bibliographical references and index.
ISBN 978-1-63242-970-4
1. Heart--Surgery. 2. Surgery, Operative. 3. Cardiovascular system--Diseases--Treatment. I. Brooks, Evie.
RD598 .C37 2020
617.412--dc23

Foster Academics,
118-35 Queens Blvd., Suite 400,
Forest Hills, NY 11375, USA

ISBN 978-1-63242-970-4 (Hardback)

Contents

Preface IX

Chapter 1 **Preoperative serum h-FABP concentration is associated with postoperative incidence of acute kidney injury in patients undergoing cardiac surgery** 1
Mehmet Oezkur, Armin Gorski, Jennifer Peltz, Martin Wagner, Maria Lazariotou, Christoph Schimmer, Peter U Heuschmann and Rainer G Leyh

Chapter 2 **Factors associated with length of stay following trans-catheter aortic valve replacement** 7
Yaron Arbel, Nevena Zivkovic, Dhruven Mehta, Sam Radhakrishnan, Stephen E. Fremes, Effat Rezaei, Asim N. Cheema, Sami Al-Nasser, Ariel Finkelstein and Harindra C. Wijeysundera

Chapter 3 **IgG4-positive cell infiltration in various cardiovascular disorders - results from histopathological analysis of surgical samples** 16
Ryoto Hourai, Satomi Kasashima, Koichi Sohmiya, Yohei Yamauchi, Hideki Ozawa, Yoshinobu Hirose, Yasuhiro Ogino, Takahiro Katsumata, Masahiro Daimon, Shu-ichi Fujita, Masaaki Hoshiga and Nobukazu Ishizaka

Chapter 4 **Pre- and post-surgical evaluation of the inflammatory response in patients with aortic stenosis treated with different types of prosthesis** 24
Maria Elena Soto, Jose Luis Salas, Jesus Vargas-Barron, Ricardo Marquez, Alejandra Rodriguez-Hernandez, Rafael Bojalil-Parra, Israel Pérez-Torres and Veronica Guarner-Lans

Chapter 5 **Mapping strategy for multiple atrial tachyarrhythmias in a transplant heart** 32
Qi Jin, Steen Pehrson, Peter Karl Jacobsen and Xu Chen

Chapter 6 **Efficacy and safety of transcatheter aortic valve replacement in aortic stenosis patients at low to moderate surgical risk** 36
Ahmed Elmaraezy, Ammar Ismail, Abdelrahman Ibrahim Abushouk, Moutaz Eltoomy, Soha Saad, Ahmed Negida, Osama Mahmoud Abdelaty, Ahmed Ramadan Abdallah, Ahmed Magdy Aboelfotoh, Hossam Mahmoud Hassan, Aya Gamal Elmaraezy, Mahmoud Morsi, Farah Althaher, Moath Althaher and Ammar M. AlSafadi

Chapter 7 **Clinical outcomes of conventional surgery versus MitraClip® therapy for moderate to severe symptomatic mitral valve regurgitation in the elderly population** 47
Anthony Alozie, Liliya Paranskaya, Bernd Westphal, Alexander Kaminski, Mohammad Sherif, Magnus Sindt, Stephan Kische, Jochen Schubert, Doreen Diedrich, Hüseyin Ince, Gustav Steinhoff and Alper Öner

Chapter 8 **An inappropriate pacing threshold increase after repeated electrical storm in a patient with implantable cardioverter defibrillator** 56
Ye Zhu, Xiang Gu and Chao Xu

Chapter 9 **Alcohol consumption and mortality in patients undergoing coronary artery bypass graft (CABG)-a register-based cohort study** 61
Mads Phillip Kofoed Grabas, Steen Møller Hansen, Christian Torp-Pedersen, Henrik Bøggild, Line Rosenkilde Ullits, Ulrik Deding, Berit Jamie Nielsen, Per Føge Jensen and Charlotte Overgaard

Chapter 10 **Self-rated health is associated with the length of stay at the intensive care unit and hospital following cardiac surgery** 71
Zsuzsanna Cserép, Eszter Losoncz, Roland Tóth, Attila Tóth, Boglárka Juhász, Piroska Balog, Péter Vargha, János Gál, Richard J Contrada, Paul RJ Falger and Andrea Székely

Chapter 11 **Effects of angiotensin receptor blockers on neointimal characteristics in angina patients requiring stent implantation: optical coherence tomography analysis** 80
Jae Young Cho, Soon Jun Hong and Do-Sun Lim

Chapter 12 **Left ventricle remodeling predicts the recurrence of ventricular tachyarrhythmias in implantable cardioverter defibrillator recipients for secondary prevention** 88
Wei-Chieh Lee, Huang-Chung Chen, Yung-Lung Chen, Tzu-Hsien Tsai, Kuo-Li Pan, Yu-Sheng Lin and Mien-Cheng Chen

Chapter 13 **Comparing the effectiveness and safety between triple antiplatelet therapy and dual antiplatelet therapy in type 2 diabetes mellitus patients after coronary stents implantation** 96
Pravesh Kumar Bundhun, Tao Qin and Meng-Hua Chen

Chapter 14 **Investigation of the pathophysiology of cardiopulmonary bypass using rodent extracorporeal life support model** 108
Ru-Wen Chang, Chien-Ming Luo, Hsi-Yu Yu, Yih-Sharng Chen and Chih-Hsien Wang

Chapter 15 **In-hospital resource utilization in surgical and transcatheter aortic valve replacement** 115
Jochen Reinöhl, Klaus Kaier, Anja Gutmann, Stefan Sorg, Constantin von zur Mühlen, Matthias Siepe, Hardy Baumbach, Martin Moser, Annette Geibel, Andreas Zirlik, Philipp Blanke, Werner Vach, Friedhelm Beyersdorf, Christoph Bode and Manfred Zehender

Chapter 16 **Medium-term outcomes of 78,808 patients after heart valve surgery in a middle-income country** 124
Regina Maria de Aquino Xavier, Vitor Manuel Pereira Azevedo, Paulo Henrique Godoy, Arn Migowski, Antonio Luiz Pinho Ribeiro, Rogério Brant Martins Chaves, Marcelo Goulart Correia, Carolina de Aquino Xavier, Lucas de Aquino Hashimoto, Clara Weksler and Nelson Albuquerque Souza e Silva

Chapter 17 **Role of elevated red cell distribution width on acute kidney injury patients after cardiac surgery** 134
Zhouping Zou, Yamin Zhuang, Lan Liu, Bo Shen, Jiarui Xu, Wuhua Jiang, Zhe Luo, Jie Teng, Chunsheng Wang and Xiaoqiang Ding

Chapter 18 **Implantation of cardiac resynchronization therapypacemaker via the coronary sinus in a patient with triple valve replacement** **141**
Cheng Zheng, Wei-Qian Lin, Yuan-Zheng Lin, Hao Lian, Zhi-Rui Liu, Jia-Hui Chen and Jia-Feng Lin

Chapter 19 **Meta-analysis and systematic review of intravascular ultrasound versus angiography-guided drug eluting stent implantation in left main coronary disease in 4592 patients** **146**
Yue Wang, Gary S. Mintz, Zhichun Gu, Yue Qi, Yue Wang, Mengru Liu and Xiaofan Wu

Chapter 20 **Heart rate in patients with reduced ejection fraction: relationship between single time point measurement and mean heart rate on prolonged implantable cardioverter defibrillator monitoring** **157**
Marlena V. Habal, Kumaraswamy Nanthakumar, Peter C. Austin, Cassandra Freitas, Christopher Labos and Douglas S. Lee

Chapter 21 **Endovascular treatment of transplant renal artery stenosis based on hemodynamic assessment using a pressure wire** **164**
Yoshito Kadoya, Kan Zen and Satoaki Matoba

Chapter 22 **Relationship between high platelet reactivity on clopidogrel and long-term clinical outcomes after drug-eluting stents implantation (PAINT-DES)** **170**
Xiao-Fei Gao, Shu Lu, Zhen Ge, Guang-Feng Zuo, Zhi-Mei Wang, Feng Wang, Xiang-Quan Kong, Da-Yang Chai, Shao-Liang Chen and Jun-Jie Zhang

Chapter 23 **Incomplete intestinal obstruction as the possible main complaint in Behcet's disease after surgery for recurrent abdominal aortic pseudoaneurysms** **180**
Fang Jiang, Hui Xiang and Zhi-Yong Peng

Chapter 24 **Lipoprotein(a) and lipid profiles of patients awaiting coronary artery bypass bypass graft** **186**
E. M. S. Bandara, S. Ekanayake, C. A. Wanigatunge and A. Kapuruge

Chapter 25 **Effects of the cardiac myosin activator Omecamtiv-mecarbil on severe chronic aortic regurgitation in Wistar rats** **192**
Bachar El-Oumeiri, Kathleen Mc Entee, Filippo Annoni, Antoine Herpain, Frédéric Vanden Eynden, Pascal Jespers, Guido Van Nooten and Philippe van de Borne

Permissions

List of Contributors

Index

Preface

This book aims to highlight the current researches and provides a platform to further the scope of innovations in this area. This book is a product of the combined efforts of many researchers and scientists, after going through thorough studies and analysis from different parts of the world. The objective of this book is to provide the readers with the latest information of the field.

The surgery of the heart or the great vessels, performed to correct congenital heart disease or treat valvular disease or complications arising due to ischemic heart disease, is termed as cardiac surgery. The scope of cardiac surgery is wide. The surgery that is performed on the heart after a large incision to the chest to open the rib cage is called an open-heart surgery. Depending on the procedure, it may entail the opening of the heart itself. Such procedures can be better performed in a motionless and bloodless environment. A modern development in cardiology is the procedure of beating-heart surgery, in which the heart continues to beat even during the surgery. Coronary artery bypass grafting is performed with the objective of preventing clot formation, and subsequent heart attack. As opposed to the highly invasive open-heart surgery, minimally invasive surgery requires smaller incisions and can be robot-assisted. Another important area of cardiac surgery is heart transplantation. This book is compiled in such a manner, that it will provide in-depth knowledge about the theory and practice of cardiac surgery. The aim of this book is to present researches that have transformed such surgical techniques and aided their advancement. For someone with an interest and eye for detail, this book covers the most significant topics in this field.

I would like to express my sincere thanks to the authors for their dedicated efforts in the completion of this book. I acknowledge the efforts of the publisher for providing constant support. Lastly, I would like to thank my family for their support in all academic endeavors.

Editor

1

Preoperative serum h-FABP concentration is associated with postoperative incidence of acute kidney injury in patients undergoing cardiac surgery

Mehmet Oezkur[1*], Armin Gorski[1], Jennifer Peltz[1], Martin Wagner[2], Maria Lazariotou[1], Christoph Schimmer[1], Peter U Heuschmann[2,3] and Rainer G Leyh[1]

Abstract

Background: Fatty acid binding protein (FABP) is an intracellular transport protein associated with myocardial damage size in patients undergoing cardiac surgery. Furthermore, elevated FABP serum concentrations are related to a number of common comorbidities, such as heart failure, chronic kidney disease, diabetes mellitus, and metabolic syndrome, which represent important risk factors for postoperative acute kidney injury (AKI). Data are lacking on the association between preoperative FABP serum level and postoperative incidence of AKI.

Methods: This prospective cohort study investigated the association between preoperative h-FABP serum concentrations and postoperative incidence of AKI, hospitalization time and length of ICU treatment. Blood samples were collected according to a predefined schedule. The AKI Network definition of AKI was used as primary endpoint. All associations were analysed using descriptive and univariate analyses.

Results: Between 05/2009 and 09/2009, 70 patients undergoing cardiac surgery were investigated. AKI was observed in 45 patients (64%). Preoperative median (IQR) h-FABP differed between the AKI group (2.9 [1.7–4.1] ng/ml) and patients without AKI (1.7 [1.1–3.3] ng/ml; $p = 0.04$), respectively. Patients with AKI were significantly older. No statistically significant differences were found for gender, type of surgery, operation duration, CPB-, or X-Clamp time, preoperative cardiac enzymes, HbA1c, or CRP between the two groups. Preoperative h-FABP was also correlated with the length of ICU stay ($r_s = 0.32$, $p = 0.007$).

Conclusions: We found a correlation between preoperative serum h-FABP and the postoperative incidence of AKI. Our results suggest a potential role for h-FABP as a biomarker for AKI in cardiac surgery.

Background

Fatty Acid Binding Protein (FABP) is an intracellular transport protein responsible for transporting long chained fatty acids to their destination and has organ specific subtypes (e.g. heart-type, liver-type and brain-type FABP) [1,2]. Heart-type FABP (h-FABP) is a marker for myocardial ischemia and is associated with ECG changes, arrhythmia and mortality after cardiac surgery [3-8]. Furthermore, h-FABP is elevated in patients with heart insufficiency, diabetes mellitus, chronic kidney disease, metabolic syndrome and is positively correlated with age [1,4,9-11]. These entities also represent important risk factors for postoperative acute kidney injury (AKI), which is a common postoperative complication with an incidence of 20 to 40% after cardiac surgery with high impact on postoperative mortality [12-20].

Utilizing h-FABP as a single marker for the described variety of risk factors of AKI seems to be possible. But studies regarding the association of h-FABP's pre-operative serum concentration and post-operative outcomes for patients undergoing operations with cardiopulmonary bypass (CPB) are lacking. Although postoperative l-FABP has been

* Correspondence: Oezkur_m@ukw.de
[1]Department of Cardiovascular Surgery, University Hospital Würzburg, Würzburg, Germany
Full list of author information is available at the end of the article

described as a marker for AKI, pre-operative h-FABP has not been investigated as an AKI marker in a cohort of cardiac surgical patients [14,15,17,21-24].

In the current study, we aimed to explore the association between preoperative h-FABP levels and the occurrence of AKI in patients undergoing cardiac surgery within the setting of a prospective mono-center cohort study.

Methods

The study protocol was approved by the Ethics Committee at the University Hospital of Würzburg. Adult (>18 years) patients scheduled for elective CABG surgery or single valve repair/replacement in the Department of Cardio-Thoracic Surgery at the University Hospital Würzburg, Germany were eligible if they provided written informed consent. Exclusion criteria comprised chronic kidney disease stage 3 or greater (i.e. $eGFR_{CKD\text{-}EPI}$ <30 ml/min/1.73 m^2), off pump surgery, acute inflammation (defined by C-reactive protein (CRP) > 4 mg/dl, and procalcitonin (PCT) > 1.0 µg/l), history of immunological or musculoskeletal disorders, stroke within 30 day prior to admission, preoperative resuscitation, preoperative electrical cardioversion, salvage or urgent operations (defined as preoperative beginning of cardiopulmonary support). All patients were operated with blood cardioplegia at 4°C applied every 20 minutes and in mild hypothermic perfusion (32°C).

Primary endpoint was defined as incidence of AKI according to acute kidney injury network (AKIN) (increase of serum creatinine by ≥0.3 within 48 hours), while baseline was set at admission to hospital, which was usually the day before operation; secondary endpoints were mechanical ventilation time, length of ICU stay, and hospitalization time [16].

Standard demographic data of patients was collected prospectively including sex, age, weight, height and waist circumference at the time of operation. Intraoperative data such as operation time, paracorporal bypass time and aortic cross clamping time were noted. Blood samples were taken at hospital admission, after induction of anaesthesia 30 minutes, 6, 24 and 48 hours after aortic cross clamping. Length of mechanical ventilation, length of ICU stay and hospitalization time was listed.

h-FABP was measured by ELISA (HK402 HUMAN H-FABP ELISE KIT, Hycult biotech, Netherlands) in ng/ml in our own laboratory from blood samples taken after introduction of anaesthesia and 30 minutes after aortic clamping. Creatinine was measured in central laboratory unit of the University of Wurzburg.

Statistical analysis

Continuous variables are presented as mean and standard deviations or as medians and interquartile ranges. Categorical variables are presented in percentages. Normal distribution testing was performed with a Kolmogorov-Smirnov-Test. To test for differences across all groups, χ^2-test, Fisher's exact test, *t*-test, Mann–Whitney-*U*-Test were used. Correlation analyses were performed employing Spearman correlation. In logistic regression analysis modelling we investigated h-FABP, age and eGFR regarding their association with the risk for AKI. To assure normal distribution of h-FABP natural log was used. Two-sided p-values of ≤0.05 were considered as statistically significant. Analyses were performed with SPSS Version 21.

Results

A total of 238 consecutive patients admitted to the department of cardiovascular surgery of the University of Würzburg between 05/2009 and 09/2009 were screened for participation in the study. Of those, 122 patients met the inclusion criteria and 70 were included in the study. Reasons for exclusion were: urgent surgery (32 patients), chronic kidney disease stage 3 or greater (14 patients), off pump surgery (5 patients), acute inflammation (1 patient).

Patient characteristics at baseline are shown in Table 1. Patients were predominantly male (80%) with a mean age of 67(±10) yrs. The mean preoperative eGFR was 88 (±11) ml/min/1.73 m^2, 69% (n = 48) of the cohort received CABG surgery, while 22 (31%) underwent single valve replacement. Preoperative median troponin T was 0.01 [IQR: 0.01–0.01].

A total of 45 patients (64.3%) achieved the primary endpoint of AKI, while only three patients experienced more severe stages of AKI, including the need for dialysis (4.3%).

Postoperative ischemia markers did not differ significantly between the two groups of AKI vs. non-AKI (see Table 2). Patients with AKI had to remain longer on the ICU, however, mechanical ventilation time and overall hospital stay did not differ (Table 3). Preoperative median (IQR) h-FABP differed between the AKI group (2.9 [1.7–4.1] ng/m) and patients without AKI (1.7 [1.1–3.3] ng/ml; p = 0.04), respectively. Preoperative h-FABP was also correlated with the length of ICU stay (r_s = 0.32, p = 0.007) and with hospitalization time (r_s = 0.308; p = 0.009). No relation was found for age with the length of ICU stay (r_s = 0.089, p = 0.47). h-FABP was associated with preoperative creatinine (r_s = 0.404, p = 0.001), eGFR (r_s = −0.603, p < 0.001), and myoglobin levels (r_s = 0.610, p < 0.001).

Although a number of preoperative variables (e.g., age, waist circumference, HbA1c, operation duration, x-clamp time, all p < 0.05) differed between CABG and valve patients, there was no statistically significant difference in the incidence of the primary endpoint AKI (p = 0.29). In logistic regression analysis, the association of elevated h-FABP levels with an increased risk for AKI diminished after adjustment for age and preoperative kidney function (Table 4). However, in the final elimination model only

Table 1 Preoperative characteristics

Variable	All patients (n = 70)	AKI (n = 45)	No AKI (n = 25)	P-value
h-FABP [ng/dl]	2.9 (1.4–3.9)	2.9 (1.7–4.1)	1.7 (1.1–3.3)	0.039
Age (yr)	67 (±10)	69 (±9)	64 (±11)	0.016
Male	56 (80%)	37 (82%)	19 (76%)	0.76
CABG	48 (69%)	33 (73%)	15 (60%)	0.29
Preoperative creatinine [mg/dl]	1.0 (±0.3)	1.0 (±0.2)	0.9 (±0.1)	0.50
eGFR-CKDEPI preoperative [ml/min/1,73 m2]	88 (±11)	87 (±10)	91 (±12)	0.17
Troponin T (mg/dl)	0.01 (0.01–0.01)	0.01 (0.01–0.01)	0.01 (0.01–0.01)	0.28
Waist Circumferrence [cm]	104 (±13)	102 (±13)	104 (±13)	0.86
Operation duration [min]	240 (±60)	244 (±60)	239 (±59)	0.91
CPB duration [min]	113 (±36)	113 (±38)	114 (±34)	0.41
X-Clamp duration [min]	82 (±30)	81 (±29)	85 (±30)	0.90
HbA1c [%]	6.0 (5.6–6.6)	5.9 (5.6–6.4)	6.0 (5.7–7.2)	1.0
CK [mg/dl]	80 (55–116)	80 (60–118)	100 (57–122)	0.97
Myoglobin [mg/dl]	44 (31–54)	46 (32–59)	37 (29–52)	0.15
C-reactive protein [mg/dl]	0.3 (0.1–0.6)	0.3 (0.1–0.6)	0.2 (0.1–0.3)	0.33

Data are mean (±SD), number (%) or median (IQR). CABG: coronary artery bypass grafting, CPB: cardio pulmonary bypass, X-Clamp: Aortic clamping.

h-FABP was associated with the incidence of AKI independent from age and preoperative eGFR.

7 (10%) of the patients had an positive Troponin T (>0.05 mg/dl). Neither in uni- nor in multivariate analyses preoperative troponin T showed a statically significant association with the incidence of AKI ($p > 0.05$).

Discussion

In our study preoperative h-FABP serum concentration was associated with the incidence of postoperative AKI as well as with a longer stay on the ICU.

Previous studies have shown that postoperative h-FABP elevation was a marker for intraoperative myocardial damage with postoperative ECG changings and elevation of established ischemia markers [5,7]. In a similar setting, serum and plasma levels of h-FABP without an ischemic incident were found to be associated with poor outcome in end-stage heart failure patients with circulatory support [25]. The pathophysiology for the poorer outcome was explained by the myocardial damage indicated by h-FABP elevation. None of the studies investigated a possible association between preoperative h-FABP concentrations with postoperative complications, although h-FABP has been linked to preoperative risk factors like heart failure, metabolic syndrome, chronic kidney disease or diabetes mellitus [1,2,9,11,26]. None of the cited studies have approached our hypothesis.

The incidence of AKI is higher in our cohort than in recent literature. This might be due to the rigorous definitions of AKIN with only a slight creatinine increase of 0.3 mg/dl. In particular as our study was performed during the summer months, the preoperative fastening status thus potentially causing hypovolemia might have sensitised the kidney for intraoperative stress and thus the incidence of AKI. It was reassuring though that only few patients experienced more severe stages of AKI including dialysis as we also did not observe any perioperative mortality.

However, postoperative urinary l-FABP has been shown in several recent studies as a promising marker for the

Table 2 Postoperative results

Variable	All patients (n = 70)	AKI (n = 45)	No AKI (n = 25)	P-value
h-FABP [ng/dl]	9.9 (9.5–10.1)	9.9 (9.7–10.4)	9.9 (9.2–10.1)	0.79
Creatinine Peak Within 48 h [mg/dl]	1.4 (±0.6)	1.7 (±0.6)	1.0 (±0.2)	<0.001
C-reactive protein [mg/dl]	0.2 (0.1–0.5)	0.2 (0.1–0.4)	0.1 (0.1–0.2)	0.54
CK [mg/dl]	230 (145–375)	244 (175–438)	254 (138–422)	0.87
Myoglobin [mg/dl]	261 (182–410)	300 (212–424)	210 (137–446)	0.38
Troponin T [μg/l]	0.3 (0.1–0.5)	0.4 (0.2–0.7)	0.2 (0.1–0.5)	0.29

Data are mean (±SD), number (%) or median (IQR). CABG: coronary artery bypass grafting, CPB: cardio pulmonary bypass, X-Clamp: Aortic clamping.

Table 3 Ventilation time, ICU stay and hospitalization time

Variable	All patients (n = 70)	AKI (n = 45)	No AKI (n = 25)	P-value
Hospitalization [d]	12 (11–15)	13 (11–15)	12 (10–15)	0.35
ICU Stay [h]	44 (21–83)	46 (22-92)	22 (18–47)	0.030
Ventilation Time [h]	16 (12–20)	15 (11–20)	15 (12–21)	0.49

Data are mean (±SD), number (%) or median (IQR). CABG: coronary artery bypass grafting, CPB: cardio pulmonary bypass, X-Clamp: Aortic clamping.

extent of AKI [21-24]. Preoperative levels of urinary or serum levels of l-FABP have not been reported to be associated with AKI yet.

h-FABP as a marker for comorbidities

Patients with higher h-FABP values were older, had higher creatinine values and thus lower eGFR in the present study. Age and preoperative h-FABP were related to postoperative AKI. These findings were similar to the results in previous studies. A possible explanation is the association of h-FABP with a wide spectrum of comorbidities evident in patients undergoing cardiac surgery. DM and metabolic syndrome, which have been described as risk factors for AKI after CABG, were known to cause elevated h-FABP levels [11,18,27-31]. We did not screen for all symptoms of metabolic syndrome, but for waist circumference, and HbA1c. Neither waist circumference nor HbA1c were associated with AKI or with elevated preoperative h-FABP. But in CABG patients HbA1c and waist circumference were higher than in patients with valve surgery. In a larger cohort of CABG patients an association between metabolic syndrome, h-FABP and AKI might be detected.

Older age indicates increased risk for AKI after cardiac surgery. Furthermore, elderly patients tend to have higher h-FABP levels [1,2,18-20,30]. Both effects could be observed in our results.

Length of ICU stay

The second finding in the present study was the association between preoperative h-FABP and longer postoperative ICU treatment. A reasonable explanation for this phenomenon was the incidence of AKI, which was associated with a longer ICU stay itself. AKI and renal failure are known factors with an impact on ICU and hospitalization time in cardiac surgical patients [14]. By being associated with the incidence of AKI, h-FABP was also related to the length of ICU stay. Longer ICU stay is associated with higher costs and ICU capacity frequently is a limiting factor for cardiac surgery departments. Predicting possible lengths of stay for risk patients is of crucial importance for the cost-effectiveness and for decent organisation of departments. Therefore predictive markers need to be identified in further studies.

Postoperative h-FABP

Postoperative h-FABP was not associated with AKI in the current study. h-FABP is a proven marker for myocardial damage and is known to be elevated after cardiac surgery. Postoperative h-FABP correlated with the established myocardial damage markers (myoglobin, troponin T and CK/CK-MB) in this study. None of the postoperative markers had an association with AKI, however, we might have missed true associations due to limited sample size and thus limited statistical power.

The presented study with a small number of patients was designed to create hypotheses for future investigations and has several limitations. A larger cohort is needed for multivariate analyses, e.g. to adjust for the effect of age and to investigate the different AKI stages in more detail to also further explore the association with the length of stay on the ICU. The screening for metabolic syndrome was incomplete, as well as was the information on further pathomechanisms for the incidence of AKI, such as red cell count, left ventricular ejection fraction, and hemodynamic instabilities. However, this information is lacking in literature as well. Other subtypes of FABP (liver, brain) might also interfere with h-FABP and should be measured in future studies. If the rather strict definition of AKI by the KDIGO can be transferred unmodified to cardiac surgical patients needs to be discussed as well.

Conclusions

The findings of our study suggest an association between preoperative serum h-FABP levels and postoperative incidence of AKI and the length of ICU stay. The results justify further research of FABP as a possible predictor for adverse events after cardiac surgery within the setting of prospective studies requiring larger sample sizes.

Table 4 Univariate and multivariate models

Variable	Univariate	Model I	Model II	Model III	Model IV	Final model ($p < 0.1$) OR (95% CI)
Ln(h-FABP)	2.29 (1.08–4.88)	2.29 (1.08–4.89)	1.82 (0.78–4.24)	2.24 (1.01–4.94)	1.79 (0.73–4.39)	2.29 (1.08–4.88)
eGFR	0.99 (0.97–1.02)	0.99 (0.97–1.02)	-	-	0.99 (0.96–1.02)	-
Age	1.06 (1.00–1.11)	-	1.04 (0.98–1.10)	-	1.03 (0.97–1.09)	-
Ln(TropT)	1.33 (0.74–2.39)	-	-	1.11 (0.60–2.05)	1.15 (0.62–2.13)	

Determinants of AKI; data is presented as OR (CI95%); ln(h-FABP) to achieve normal distribution ln of FABP was calculated; final model is based on backward elimination.

Abbreviations

AKI: Acute kidney injury; CABG: Coronary artery bypass grafting; CPB: Cardio pulmonary bypass; DM: Diabetes mellitus; ECG: Electrocardiography; FABP: Fatty acid binding protein; h-FABP: Heart-type fatty acid binding protein; ICU: Intensive care unit; l-FABP: Liver-type fatty acid binding protein; IQR: Interquartile range; LV-EF: Left ventricular ejection fraction; SD: Standard deviation.

Competing interests

M Oezkur was supported by a rotational post from the Comprehensive Heart Failure Center Würzburg funded by the German Ministry of Research and Education. PU Heuschmann receives/ received in the recent years research support from the German Ministry of Research and Education (Center for Stroke Research Berlin; Comprehensive Heart Failure Center Würzburg), the European Union (European Implementation Score Collaboration), the German Stroke Foundation, the Charité-Universitätsmedizin Berlin, the Berlin Chamber of Physicians, and the University Hospital of Würzburg.

Authors' contributions

MO concepted, designed, executed the study and had major parts in the statistical analyses. AG substantially contributed to conception and design of the study. JP carried out the patient acquisition, blood sampling and performed the ELISA. ML participated in the laboratory work, especially in the ELISA. PH and MW gave significant input to the statistical analysis and design of the manuscript. CS, RL participated in the design of the study, and gave significant input on the manuscript. All authors read and approved the final manuscript.

Acknowledgements

We thank all patients providing data to the current study as we as we thank the physicians and study personnel for filling in case report forms for study participant and performing study procedures. This publication was funded by the German Research Foundation (DFG) and the University of Wuerzburg in the funding programme Open Access Publishing.
This study was supported by the German Ministry of Education and Research (BMBF) within the setting of the Comprehensive Heart Failure Center Würzburg (BMBF 01EO1004).

Author details

[1]Department of Cardiovascular Surgery, University Hospital Würzburg, Würzburg, Germany. [2]Institute of Clinical Epidemiology and Biometry, Comprehensive Heart Failure Center, University of Würzburg, Würzburg, Germany. [3]Clinical Trial Center Würzburg, University Hospital Würzburg, Würzburg, Germany.

References

1. Azzazy HM, Pelsers MM, Christenson RH: **Unbound free fatty acids and heart-type fatty acid-binding protein: diagnostic assays and clinical applications.** *Clin Chem* 2006, **52**(1):19–29.
2. Glatz JF, van der Vusse GJ: **Cellular fatty acid-binding proteins: their function and physiological significance.** *Prog Lipid Res* 1996, **35**(3):243–282.
3. Fransen EJ, Maessen JG, Hermens WT, Glatz JF, Buurman WA: **Peri-operative myocardial tissue injury and the release of inflammatory mediators in coronary artery bypass graft patients.** *Cardiovasc Res* 2000, **45**(4):853–859.
4. Hayashida N, Chihara S, Akasu K, Oda T, Tayama E, Kai E, Kawara T, Aoyagi S: **Plasma and urinary levels of heart fatty acid-binding protein in patients undergoing cardiac surgery.** *Jpn Circ J* 2000, **64**(1):18–22.
5. Petzold T, Feindt P, Sunderdiek U, Boeken U, Fischer Y, Gams E: **Heart-type fatty acid binding protein (hFABP) in the diagnosis of myocardial damage in coronary artery bypass grafting.** *Eur J Cardiothorac Surg* 2001, **19**(6):859–864.
6. Nakata T, Hashimoto A, Hase M, Tsuchihashi K, Shimamoto K: **Human heart-type fatty acid-binding protein as an early diagnostic and prognostic marker in acute coronary syndrome.** *Cardiology* 2003, **99**(2):96–104.
7. Liu H, Dong GH, Xu B, Shen Y, Jing H: **Heart fatty acid binding protein in the rapid evaluation of myocardial damage following valve replacement surgery.** *Clin Chim Acta* 2005, **356**(1–2):147–153.
8. Colli A, Josa M, Pomar JL, Mestres CA, Gherli T: **Heart fatty acid binding protein in the diagnosis of myocardial infarction: where do we stand today?** *Cardiology* 2007, **108**(1):4–10.
9. Kimura H, Fujii H, Suzuki S, Ono T, Arakawa M, Gejyo F: **Lipid-binding proteins in rat and human kidney.** *Kidney Int Suppl* 1999, **71**:S159–S162.
10. Setsuta K, Seino Y, Kitahara Y, Arau M, Ohbayashi T, Takano T, Mizuno K: **Elevated levels of both cardiomyocyte membrane and myofibril damage markers predict adverse outcomes in patients with chronic heart failure.** *Circ J* 2008, **72**(4):569–574.
11. Akbal E, Ozbek M, Gunes F, Akyurek O, Ureten K, Delibasi T: **Serum heart type fatty acid binding protein levels in metabolic syndrome.** *Endocrine* 2009, **36**(3):433–437.
12. Haase-Fielitz A, Haase M, Bellomo R, Lambert G, Matalanis G, Story D, Doolan L, Buxton B, Gutteridge G, Luft FC, Schnuck W-H, Dragun D: **Decreased catecholamine degradation associates with shock and kidney injury after cardiac surgery.** *J Am Soc Nephrol* 2009, **20**(6):1393–1403.
13. Yan X, Jia S, Meng X, Dong P, Jia M, Wan J, Hou X: **Acute kidney injury in adult postcardiotomy patients with extracorporeal membrane oxygenation: evaluation of the RIFLE classification and the Acute Kidney Injury Network criteria.** *Eur J Cardiothorac Surg* 2010, **37**(2):334–338.
14. Li SY, Chen JY, Yang WC, Chuang CL: **Acute kidney injury network classification predicts in-hospital and long-term mortality in patients undergoing elective coronary artery bypass grafting surgery.** *Eur J Cardiothorac Surg* 2011, **39**(3):323–328.
15. Olsson D, Sartipy U, Braunschweig F, Holzmann MJ: **Acute kidney injury following coronary artery bypass surgery and long-term risk of heart failure.** *Circ Heart Fail* 2013, **6**(1):83–90.
16. Mehta RL, Kellum JA, Shah SV, Molitoris BA, Ronco C, Warnock DG, Levin A, Acute Kidney Injury Network: **Acute Kidney Injury Network: report of an initiative to improve outcomes in acute kidney injury.** *Crit Care* 2007, **11**(2):R31.
17. Haase M, Bellomo R, Devarajan P, Ma Q, Bennett MR, Mockel M, Matalanis G, Dragun D, Haase-Fielitz A: **Novel biomarkers early predict the severity of acute kidney injury after cardiac surgery in adults.** *Ann Thorac Surg* 2009, **88**(1):124–130.
18. Gaudino M, Luciani N, Giungi S, Caradonna E, Nasso G, Schiavello R, Luciani G, Possati G: **Different profiles of patients who require dialysis after cardiac surgery.** *Ann Thorac Surg* 2005, **79**(3):825–829. author reply 829–830.
19. Kuitunen A, Vento A, Suojaranta-Ylinen R, Pettila V: **Acute renal failure after cardiac surgery: evaluation of the RIFLE classification.** *Ann Thorac Surg* 2006, **81**(2):542–546.
20. Haase M, Bellomo R, Matalanis G, Calzavacca P, Dragun D, Haase-Fielitz A: **A comparison of the RIFLE and Acute Kidney Injury Network classifications for cardiac surgery-associated acute kidney injury: a prospective cohort study.** *J Thorac Cardiovasc Surg* 2009, **138**(6):1370–1376.
21. Katagiri D, Doi K, Honda K, Negishi K, Fujita T, Hisagi M, Ono M, Matsubara T, Yahagi N, Iwagami M, Ohtake T, Kobayashi S, Sugaya T, Noiri E: **Combination of two urinary biomarkers predicts acute kidney injury after adult cardiac surgery.** *Ann Thorac Surg* 2012, **93**(2):577–583.
22. Arthur JM, Hill EG, Alge JL, Lewis EC, Neely BA, Janech MG, Tumlin JA, Chawla LS, Shaw AD: **Evaluation of 32 urine biomarkers to predict the progression of acute kidney injury after cardiac surgery.** *Kidney Int* 2014, **85**(2):431–438.
23. Liu S, Che M, Xue S, Xie B, Zhu M, Lu R, Zhang W, Qian J, Yan Y: **Urinary L-FABP and its combination with urinary NGAL in early diagnosis of acute kidney injury after cardiac surgery in adult patients.** *Biomarkers* 2013, **18**(1):95–101.
24. Peco-Antic A, Ivanisevic I, Vulicevic I, Kotur-Stevuljevic J, Ilic S, Ivanisevic J, Miljkovic M, Kocev N: **Biomarkers of acute kidney injury in pediatric cardiac surgery.** *Clin Biochem* 2013, **46**(13 14):1244 1251.
25. Cabiati M, Caselli C, Caruso R, Prescimone T, Verde A, Botta L, Parodi O, Del Ry S, Giannessi D: **High peripheral levels of h-FABP are associated with poor prognosis in end-stage heart failure patients with mechanical circulatory support.** *Biomark Med* 2013, **7**(3):481–492.
26. Pleym H, Tjomsland O, Asberg A, Lydersen S, Wahba A, Bjella L, Dale O, Stenseth R: **Effects of autotransfusion of mediastinal shed blood on biochemical markers of myocardial damage in coronary surgery.** *Acta Anaesthesiol Scand* 2005, **49**(9):1248–1254.
27. The International Expert Committee: **International Expert Committee report on the role of the A1C assay in the diagnosis of diabetes.** *Diabetes Care* 2009, **32**(7):1327–1334.

28. Aronson S, Fontes ML, Miao Y, Mangano DT, Investigators of the Multicenter Study of Perioperative Ischemia Research Group, Ischemia Research and Education Foundation: **Risk index for perioperative renal dysfunction/ failure: critical dependence on pulse pressure hypertension.** *Circulation* 2007, **115**(6):733–742.
29. Nauta FL, Boertien WE, Bakker SJ, van Goor H, van Oeveren W, de Jong PE, Bilo H, Gansevoort RT: **Glomerular and tubular damage markers are elevated in patients with diabetes.** *Diabetes Care* 2011, **34**(4):975–981.
30. Vellinga S, Verbrugghe W, De Paep R, Verpooten GA, Janssen van Doorn K: **Identification of modifiable risk factors for acute kidney injury after cardiac surgery.** *Neth J Med* 2012, **70**(10):450–454.
31. Hong S, Youn Y-N, Yoo K-J: **Metabolic syndrome as a risk factor for postoperative kidney injury after off-pump coronary artery bypass surgery.** *Circ J* 2010, **74**(6):1121–1126.

2

Factors associated with length of stay following trans-catheter aortic valve replacement

Yaron Arbel[1,2,6], Nevena Zivkovic[1,2], Dhruven Mehta[1,2], Sam Radhakrishnan[1,2], Stephen E. Fremes[1,2], Effat Rezaei[2,5], Asim N. Cheema[2,5], Sami Al-Nasser[2,5], Ariel Finkelstein[6] and Harindra C. Wijeysundera[1,2,3,4*]

Abstract

Background: Most patients undergoing Transcatheter aortic valve implantation (TAVR) are elderly with significant co-morbidities and there is limited information available regarding factors that influence length of stay (LOS) post-procedure. The aim of this study was to identify the patient, and procedural factors that affect post-TAVR LOS using a contemporary multinational registry.

Methods: We conducted a retrospective cohort study, with patients recruited from three high volume tertiary institutions. The primary outcome was the LOS post-TAVR procedure. We examined patient and procedural factors in a cause-specific Cox multivariable regression model to elucidate their effect on LOS, accounting for the competing risk of post-procedural death. Hazard ratios (HR) greater than 1 indicate a shorter LOS, while HRs less than 1 indicate a longer LOS.

Results: The cohort consisted of 809 patients. Patient factors associated with longer LOS were older age, prior atrial fibrillation, and greater patient urgency. Patient factors associated with shorter LOS were lower NYHA class, higher ejection fraction and higher mean aortic valve gradients.
Procedural characteristics associated with shorter LOS were conscious sedation (HR = 1.19, 95% CI 1.06–1.35, $p = 0.004$). Transapical access was associated with prolonged LOS (HR = 0.49, 95% CI 0.41–0.58, $p < 0.001$).

Conclusion: This multicenter study identified potentially modifiable patient and procedural factors associated with a prolonged LOS. Future research is needed to determine if interventions focused on these factors will translate to a shorter LOS.

Keywords: Transcatheter aortic valve replacement, Length of stay, Competing risks, Conscious sedation

Background

Aortic stenosis (AS) is the most frequent degenerative valvular heart disease in Western countries with a prevalence that has increased in parallel with the aging demographic of the population [1, 2]. AS patients are typically elderly with multiple co-morbidities, which precludes traditional surgical aortic valve replacement (SAVR) [3, 4]. Transcatheter aortic valve replacement (TAVR) has emerged over the last decade as an innovative procedure to deliver aortic valves percutaneously in a minimally invasive manner; based on landmark studies, guidelines now recommend TAVR as the preferred treatment for severe AS patients who are inoperable, and as a reasonable alternative in patients with high operative risk [5]. Emerging evidence supports the expansion of TAVR indications to intermediate risk patients [6]. As such, there has been an exponential growth in the demand for TAVR which will likely increase in the future.

Given the extensive pre-procedural diagnostic work-up, the complexity of the prosthesis and procedure, and the requirement for close post-procedural follow-up, TAVR is extremely resource intensive [7–9]. Given the current economic environment, there is increasing need

* Correspondence: Harindra.Wijeysundera@sunnybrook.ca
[1]Schulich Heart Centre, Division of Cardiology and Cardiac surgery, Sunnybrook Health Sciences Centre, Toronto, ON, Canada
[2]University of Toronto, Toronto, ON, Canada
Full list of author information is available at the end of the article

to improve the efficiency of health care delivery in complex interventions such as TAVR, in order to improve the overall value of health care and also improve equitable access to this life-saving intervention within strict budgetary constraints. One such area specific to TAVR is improving post-procedural length of stay (LOS). In addition to its economic benefits, optimizing LOS in an elderly population has a number of other potential clinical advantages such as reducing infection rates, increasing rehabilitation rates, avoiding malnutrition, and improving overall psychological status.

Although TAVR has been shown to have shorter hospitalizations compared to SAVR [10], some TAVR patients nonetheless have prolonged post-procedural stay [7, 11]. Moreover, there is a wide variation in reports of TAVR LOS reinforcing the likelihood of inefficient care. For example, some studies report the mean hospital stay following TAVR to be 11–13 days [7, 12], while other contemporary cohorts demonstrate hospitalization duration shorter than three days in approximately 30% of patients [11, 13, 14].

There is a paucity of data on the drivers that impact LOS post-TAVR. Elucidating these factors is important so as to identify potentially modifiable factors that can lead to quality improvement interventions to optimize LOS. To address this gap in knowledge, we sought to identify the major drivers of post-TAVR LOS using a contemporary multinational registry.

Methods

We conducted a retrospective cohort study, with patients recruited from three tertiary institutions, including two in Toronto, Canada (Sites 1 and 3) and one in Tel Aviv, Israel (Site 2). Research ethics board approval was obtained from all centers for the prospective databases. The need for individual patient consent was waived by all the institutional review boards.

Patient selection

Patients were identified from the TAVR registries from each institution. Each registry collects data on all TAVR patients prospectively. Inclusion criteria were all patients that had a TAVR procedure from January 1st, 2012 to December 31st, 2014. This time frame was chosen in order to include only patients receiving a contemporary TAVR valve procedure, and after each site completed at least 100 cases to overcome the learning curve associated with TAVR. We treated in-hospital death as a competing risk and included patients who died during the procedure or during the TAVR hospitalization.

Outcome variable

The primary outcome was the LOS post-TAVR procedure. The day of the TAVR was considered time 0, with each 24-h period after this recorded as 1 day. Additional outcomes of interest included peri-procedural minor and major complications, which were defined according to the Valve Academic Research Consortium (VARC- 2) criteria [15].

Covariates

We also documented the length of time (in days) patients were admitted prior to the TAVR procedure as well as the total LOS, from the date of admission to discharge from the TAVR hospital. For the purpose of analyses, we categorized pre-TAVR admission into 2 groups: a) those admitted electively up to two days prior to the procedure and b) those with a TAVR preadmission of ≥3 days. This categorization was consistent with these hospitals' clinical practice based on the advice of our clinical experts, as patients admitted ≥3 days pre-TAVR have pre-procedural clinical deterioration. We determined if the procedure was done 1 day prior to the weekend and contrasted these from procedures done earlier in the week. Patient characteristics that were abstracted from the registries included age, gender, body-mass index (BMI), co-morbidities, as well as mean gradient across the aortic valve.

Peri-procedural risk of in-hospital/30 day mortality was captured by the Society for Thoracic Surgery (STS) score [16, 17]. This score includes approximately 30 variables, including demographics, risk factors, previous interventions, pre-operative status, hemodynamics, and coronary anatomy, and has been well validated to accurately predict peri-operative mortality and morbidity.

Procedural factors included the access type, transcatheter heart valve type, conscious or general anesthesia, and procedural time. We also included the year of the procedure to account for temporal improvements in care delivery.

Statistical analysis

Data completeness was verified for all covariates and there were <1% missing data in any co-morbidity field with the exception of EuroScore [18]; as such a complete case analysis was conducted. Descriptive statistics were compared across the 3 hospitals for baseline data, procedure characteristics, and complications, with χ^2 tests for categorical variables and one-way analysis of variance (ANOVA) for continuous variables.

In order to identify the drivers of LOS, we developed a cause-specific Cox-proportional hazard model, where the dependent variable was the post-TAVR LOS, measured in days [19, 20]. In our study, this is analogous to modeling the rate (or hazard) of being discharged. Hazard ratios (HR) greater than 1 indicate a shorter LOS, while HRs less than 1 indicate a longer LOS. We built a cause-specific Cox model to account for the competing risk of in-hospital death, which precludes the possibility of the primary outcome (discharge). The models included a sandwich type variance estimator to account for clustering of patients at each of the three institutions. We compared the unadjusted LOS between the 3 hospitals using this model.

Prior to inclusion into the final covariate-adjusted model, we assessed all baseline factors for co-linearity based on the variance inflation factor but found no important multi-colinearities. To build the final covariate adjusted model, we planned to include all variables except for EuroScore due to >5% missing data. The results for creatinine lacked face validity in the adjusted model so it was excluded. All other variables were included as this was an explanatory model. The proportional hazards assumption was tested by computing Martingale residuals for the final model.

A sensitivity analysis was conducted to understand the role of complications in TAVR post-procedural LOS. For each complication, we calculated both an unadjusted HR and one adjusted for all co-variates in the full model. All of the analyses were considered significant at a two-tailed p-value of less than 0.05. All analysis was done with SAS 9.3.

Results

We included a total of 809 patients from three centers over the time period of interest. Mean pre-TAVR LOS differed between the three sites. Site two routinely admitted elective patients one to two days before TAVR, while the other sites generally admitted these patients on the morning of the procedure (Table 1). Figure 1 demonstrates the post-TAVR LOS. Approximately 27.1% of patients had post-procedural LOS between 2 to 3 days. The three sites show no significant differences in terms of post-TAVR or total LOS. The mean post-procedural LOS was 6.6 days, with means of 6.9, 5.8 and 7.7 at the three sites, while mean total LOS was calculated at 8.8 days across sites, with site-specific values of 9.8, 7.9 and 9.4, respectively.

The incidence of complications for the entire cohort is summarized in Additional file 1: Table S1, as is post-procedure aortic regurgitation and post-procedure mitral regurgitation. Thirty patients (3.7%) died in hospital, while 30-day mortality was 4.9%. The rates of complications were comparable to those found in the literature, with 18 (2.2%) having a stroke, 107 (13.2%) requiring a permanent pacemaker, 49 (6.1%) suffering from a major vascular complication, and 37 (4.6%) having major bleeding.

As seen in Table 2, there was a temporal effect on LOS identified in the multivariable models, with patients undergoing TAVR in 2012 having a longer LOS compared to those in 2014. We found the following patient characteristics to be associated with longer length of stay: prior atrial fibrillation (HR = 0.76, 95% CI 0.69–0.84, $p < 0.001$), each one-year increase in patient age (HR = 0.990, 95% CI 0.985–0.995, $p < 0.001$), and patient urgency as indicated by pre-TAVR admission of three or more days (HR = 0.64, 95% CI 0.46–0.90, $p = 0.009$).

Patients were discharged sooner if they were NYHA class 1 or 2 (HR = 1.28, 95% CI 1.10–1.49, $p = 0.001$) or NYHA class 3 (HR =1.16, 95% CI 1.03–1.31, $p = 0.019$) compared to NYHA class 4. Every 10% increase in ejection fraction was associated with shorter length of stay (HR = 1.05, 95% CI 1.03–1.07, $p < 0.001$), as was each one mmHg increase in the pre-procedural mean aortic valve pressure gradient (HR = 1.004, 95% CI 1.002–1.01, $p < 0.001$). Patients who had at least one prior open heart surgery were also discharged sooner (HR = 1.15, 95%CI 1.09–1.21, $p < 0.001$).

Procedure factors had important impact on post-TAVR LOS. Patients receiving conscious sedation, rather than general anesthesia, had a significantly shorter LOS (HR = 1.19, 95% CI 1.06–1.35, $p = 0.004$). Compared to patients receiving TAVR via trans-femoral approach, direct aortic approach was associated with longer LOS (HR = 0.76, 95% CI 0.67–0.85, $p < 0.001$), as was trans-apical approach (HR = 0.49, 95% CI 0.41–0.58, $p < 0.001$). A subclavian or suprasternal approach was associated with earlier discharge compared to transfemoral (HR = 2.42, 95% CI 1.40–4.20, $p = 0.002$); however, there were few patients with these alternative access sites ($n = 3$) in our cohort. Longer TAVR procedure duration was associated with longer LOS (HR = 0.98 for every 10 min increase, 95% CI 0.96–0.99, $p = 0.001$). In terms of valve type, implantation of a Portico trans-catheter heart valve was associated with longer LOS (HR = 0.43, 95% CI 0.25–0.73, $p < 0.001$). A valve in valve procedure was associated with shorter LOS (HR = 1.28, 95% CI 1.15–1.41, $p < 0.001$).

The unadjusted HR suggest that almost all post procedure complications are statistically associated with longer LOS, except for new arrhythmia and myocardial infarction ($p = 0.090$, $p = 0.055$, respectively). When adjusted for baseline characteristics, all post-procedural complications were associated with a statistically significant increase in length of stay (Table 3).

Discussion

In this multi-center study of contemporary TAVR procedures, we found a wide variation in post-TAVR LOS. We identified a number of potentially modifiable factors that influenced LOS, such as access route, type of anesthesia, the timing of the procedure prior to the weekend, procedure time, and valve type. These are potential targets for quality improvement initiatives. Importantly, we found that post-procedural complications were strongly associated with prolonged stay.

Table 1 Baseline Patient and Procedural Characteristics. Cohort baseline and procedural characteristics according to site. All covariates are presented as frequencies and percentages, with the exception of mean values. Mean values include standard deviation

	Total (*N* = 809)	Site 1 (*n* = 164)	Site 2 (*n* = 406)	Site 3 (*n* = 239)	*p* Value
Patient Characteristics					
Age (years)	82.7 ± 6.4	83.7 ± 6.4	82.4 ± 6.2	82.6 ± 6.7	0.095
Female	415 (51.3%)	79 (48.2%)	219 (53.9%)	117 (49.0%)	0.316
BMI	27.1 ± 5.3	27.0 ± 6.1	27.3 ± 5.3	26.6 ± 4.6	0.224
STS	6.0 ± 5.4	4.4 ± 2.8	4.3 ± 2.9	10.0 ± 7.6	<0.001
NYHA					<0.001
1	2 (0.3%)	2 (1.2%)	0	0	
2	99 (12.3%)	15 (9.2%)	55 (13.6%)	29 (12.3%)	
3	505 (62.9%)	120 (73.6%)	227 (56.2%)	158 (67.0%)	
4	197 (24.5%)	26 (16.0%)	122 (30.2%)	49 (20.8%)	
Atrial Fibrillation	280 (34.6%)	68 (41.5%)	135 (33.3%)	77 (32.2%)	0.114
Hypertension	717 (88.6%)	141 (86.0%)	358 (88.2%)	218 (91.2%)	0.245
Diabetes Mellitus	279 (34.5%)	48 (29.3%)	155 (38.2%)	76 (31.8%)	0.075
Dyslipidemia	645 (79.8%)	114 (69.5%)	333 (82.2%)	198 (82.9%)	0.001
COPD	129 (16.0%)	16 (9.8%)	55 (13.6%)	58 (24.3%)	<0.001
Coronary Artery Disease	520 (64.3%)	87 (53.1%)	260 (64.0%)	173 (72.4%)	<0.001
Peripheral Vascular Disease	93 (11.5%)	24 (14.6%)	17 (4.2%)	52 (21.8%)	<0.001
Dialysis	26 (3.2%)	5 (3.1%)	10 (2.5%)	11 (4.6%)	0.328
Permanent Pacemaker	101 (12.5%)	25 (15.2%)	55 (13.6%)	21 (8.8%)	0.103
Prior Stroke	120 (14.8%)	35 (21.3%)	52 (12.8%)	33 (13.8%)	0.030
Prior Cardiac Surgery	203 (25.1%)	46 (28.1%)	89 (21.9%)	68 (28.5%)	0.113
Prior PCI	196 (24.2%)	32 (19.5%)	55 (13.6%)	109 (45.6%)	<0.001
Pre-Procedural Ejection Fraction (%)	54.3 ± 10.7	51.7 ± 9.0	55.1 ± 8.6	54.5 ± 14.3	0.003
Pre-Procedural Mean Pressure Gradient (mmHg)	46.4 ± 15.9	48.8 ± 16.3	46.2 ± 15.0	45.2 ± 16.8	0.071
Pre-Procedural Creatinine (μmol/L)	107.9 ± 64.0	113.6 ± 88.9	104.0 ± 58.9	110.6 ± 50.5	0.203
Procedural Characteristics					
Procedure Year					0.015
2012	224 (27.7%)	42 (25.6%)	129 (31.8%)	53 (22.2%)	
2013	274 (33.9%)	66 (40.2%)	131 (32.3%)	77 (32.2%)	
2014	311 (38.4%)	56 (34.2%)	146 (36.0%)	109 (45.6%)	
Procedure Prior to Weekend[a]	185 (22.9%)	2 (1.2%)	26 (6.4%)	157 (65.7%)	<0.001
Procedure Time (min)	161.1 ± 67.5	87.4 ± 38.8	168.9 ± 50.1	199.6 ± 69.7	<0.001
Access Site					<0.001
Transfemoral	737 (91.1%)	111 (67.7%)	405 (99.8%)	221 (92.5%)	
Subclavian	2 (0.3%)	0	1 (0.3%)	1 (0.4%)	
Suprasternal	1 (0.1%)	1 (0.6%)	0	0	
Direct Aortic	26 (3.2%)	10 (6.1%)	0	16 (6.7%)	
Transapical	43 (5.3%)	42 (25.6%)	0	1 (0.4%)	
Anesthesia Type					<0.001
General Anesthesia	408 (50.4%)	164 (100%)	5 (1.2%)	239 (100%)	
Local/Conscious Sedation	401 (49.6%)	0	401 (98.8%)	0	

Table 1 Baseline Patient and Procedural Characteristics. Cohort baseline and procedural characteristics according to site. All covariates are presented as frequencies and percentages, with the exception of mean values. Mean values include standard deviation *(Continued)*

Valve Used					<0.001
Medtronic CoreValve or Evolut R	458 (56.7%)	1 (0.6%)	253 (62.6%)	204 (85.3%)	
Edwards XT or S3	332 (41.2%)	155 (94.5%)	146 (36.1%)	31 (13%)	
Portico	17 (0.2%)	8 (4.9%)	5 (1.2%)	4 (1.7%)	
Valve in Valve	34 (4.2%)	8 (4.9%)	0	26 (10.9%)	<0.001
Pre-TAVR Admission					<0.001
0 days	305 (37.7%)	115 (70.12%)	1 (0.3%)	189 (79.1%)	
1–2 days	415 (51.3%)	14 (8.54%)	382 (94.1%)	19 (8%)	
≥ 3 days	89 (11%)	35 (21.34%)	23 (5.7%)	31 (13%)	

BMI Body Mass Index, *COPD* Chronic Obstructive Pulmonary Disease, *NYHA* New York Heart Association functional classification, *PCI* percutaneous coronary intervention, *STS* Society of Thoracic Surgeons adult cardiac surgery risk score
[a]Refers to procedures that take place one day prior to the weekend

Improving efficiency of health care delivery is of particular importance in the current era of budgetary constraints such that scarce health care resources are used optimally. One target for improving efficiency is reduction of LOS. Indeed, there is an abundant literature on LOS in different areas of medicine, specifically the drivers of prolonged LOS as well as strategies to improve it. For example, malnutrition measured by recent weight loss or a BMI below 20 has been associated with prolonged LOS [21]. Surgical site infections are a major driver of LOS in the surgical literature with a doubling of the LOS [22]. Early interventions and internal fixations have been associated with reduced LOS in patients with hip fractures [23]. Improving patients' renal function [24] as well as pulmonary function have been associated with shorter LOS in patients undergoing cardiac surgery [25]. Increasing hospital volume has been associated with a reduced LOS [26]. Many of these factors are potentially modifiable and thus targets for quality improvement.

TAVR is an example of a complex intervention, targeted to an elderly patient population, often with multiple comorbidities. Moreover, it is extremely resource intensive, and in many jurisdictions, limited to select tertiary hospitals, each with limited funding. These supply factors,

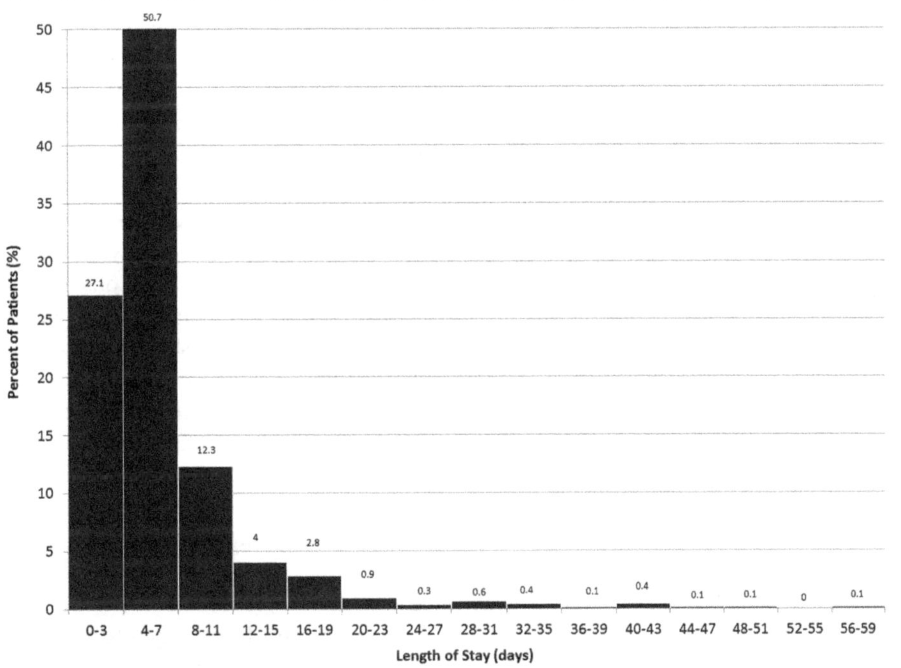

Fig. 1 Distribution of Post-TAVR Length of Stay of Discharged Patients. Figure shows percentage of patients discharged in each time period following TAVR. All patients have a minimum LOS of 2 days

Table 2 Relationship between Baseline and Procedural Characteristics with Post-TAVR Length of Stay, Adjusted by Model Covariates. Multivariable analysis of the variables associated with length of stay

Parameter	Hazard Ratio (95% Confidence Interval)	*p* Value
Year		
2014	Referent	
2012	0.78 (0.68–0.9)	<0.001
2013	0.85 (0.73–0.98)	0.021
Sex		
Female	Referent	
Male	1.12 (0.97–1.3)	0.133
Age	0.99 (0.99–1)	<0.001
Pre-TAVR Admission		
0–2 days	Referent	
≥ 3 days	0.64 (0.46–0.9)	0.009
BMI	1 (0.98–1.02)	0.920
STS Risk Score	0.98 (0.96–1)	0.064
NYHA Class		
4	Referent	
1–2	1.28 (1.1–1.49)	0.001
3	1.16 (1.03–1.31)	0.019
Atrial Fibrillation	0.76 (0.69–0.84)	<0.001
Hypertension	1 (0.83–1.2)	0.960
Diabetes Mellitus	1 (0.89–1.13)	0.986
Dyslipidemia	0.92 (0.68–1.24)	0.577
Coronary Artery Disease	0.98 (0.82–1.16)	0.805
Prior PCI	1.05 (0.84–1.31)	0.670
Prior Open Heart Surgery	1.15 (1.09–1.21)	<0.001
Dialysis	0.95 (0.64–1.41)	0.797
COPD	0.94 (0.75–1.17)	0.558
Peripheral Vascular Disease	1.01 (0.81–1.25)	0.948
Permanent Pacemaker	1.1 (0.74–1.62)	0.644
Stroke	0.81 (0.58–1.13)	0.215
Pre-Procedural Ejection Fraction (1ss0%)	1.05 (1.03–1.07)	<0.001
Pre-Procedural Mean Pressure Gradient	1 (1–1.01)	<0.001
Procedure Time (10 min)	0.98 (0.96–0.99)	0.001
Access Site		
Transfemoral	Referent	
Direct Aortic	0.76 (0.67–0.85)	<0.001
Subclavian or Suprasternal	2.42 (1.4–4.2)	0.002
Transapical	0.49 (0.41–0.58)	<0.001
Anesthesia Type		
General Anesthesia	Referent	
Local/Conscious Sedation	1.19 (1.06–1.35)	0.004

Table 2 Relationship between Baseline and Procedural Characteristics with Post-TAVR Length of Stay, Adjusted by Model Covariates. Multivariable analysis of the variables associated with length of stay *(Continued)*

Valve Used		
Medtronic CoreValve or Evolut-R	Referent	
Edwards XT or S3	0.99 (0.96–1.03)	0.647
Portico	0.43 (0.25–0.73)	0.002
Valve in Valve Procedure	1.28 (1.15–1.41)	<0.001
Procedure prior to Weekend[a]	0.88 (0.77–1.01)	0.061

Hazard ratios above 1 indicate shorter time to discharge and shorter length of stay, whereas the opposite is true for ratios below 1. *STS* Society of Thoracic Surgeons adult cardiac surgery risk score, *NYHA* New York Heart Association functional classification, *COPD* chronic obstructive pulmonary disease, *PCI* percutaneous coronary intervention

[a]Refers to procedures that take place one day prior to the weekend

combined with an exponentially growing demand, in particular as indications expand beyond only inoperable and very high risk patients, make TAVR an especially relevant area to identify potential targets for improving efficiency. The limited data on TAVR LOS currently suggests that there is variation in LOS [13, 27, 28].

In our study, we confirmed this wide variation in LOS, extending from 2 days to 59 days. We were able to identify a number of baseline patient characteristics that were associated with prolonged LOS, including prior atrial fibrillation, age, and lower baseline ejection fraction. Indeed, LOS appears to be a surrogate for the burden of comorbidity. Although these factors are non-modifiable, they nonetheless should alert health care providers of the potential for a longer LOS, and as such, pre-emptive measures could be put into place early to facilitate transitions to the community or in-patient rehabilitation.

We also identified a number of potentially modifiable procedural factors such as procedure done before the weekend, valve type and conscious sedation. Indeed, other groups are evaluating the use of conscious sedation in combination with a care pathway to facilitate next day discharge post TAVR [29–31]. Conscious Sedation and non-surgical access have been associated with less delirium and might explain the shorter LOS. [32] The relationship between length of procedure and higher NYHA with LOS might be explained by the increased incidence of complications in sicker patients. Similarly, in hospital TAVI patients are more frail and await rehabilitation and hence have longer LOS. [33] The relationship between Portico valve and LOS might be attributed to a learning curve since it is a newer valve compared to Corevalve and Sapien valves. Longer LOS when the TAVR procedure is performed prior to the weekend has face validity and may be related to delays in obtaining post-procedural echocardiograms during the weekend, or being able to put into place the necessary transition supports such as homecare. If so,

Table 3 Relationship between Presence of Complication to Post-TAVR Length of Stay, with Unadjusted and Adjusted Analyses. Hazard ratios with 95% confidence intervals for post-TAVR LOS according to presence of different complications. Includes unadjusted analysis as well as multivariable adjustment for baseline and procedural characteristics

	Unadjusted Hazard Ratio	*p* Value	Adjusted Hazard Ratio	*p* Value
Vascular				
Major	0.46 (0.33–0.64)	<0.001	0.42 (0.37–0.49)	<0.001
Minor	0.79 (0.64–0.97)	0.023	0.73 (0.58–0.93)	0.011
Stroke	0.31 (0.19–0.50)	<0.001	0.35 (0.22–0.55)	<0.001
MI	0.33 (0.11–1.02)	0.055	0.6 (0.42–0.84)	0.003
Arrhythmia	0.88 (0.76–1.02)	0.090	0.75 (0.61–0.93)	0.008
Permanent Pacemaker	0.59 (0.48–0.73)	<0.001	0.49 (0.37–0.64)	<0.001
Bleeding				
Life Threatening	0.30 (0.17–0.55)	<0.001	0.28 (0.17–0.46)	<0.001
Major	0.54 (0.38–0.76)	<0.001	0.56 (0.46–0.68)	<0.001
Minor	0.69 (0.49–0.98)	0.036	0.82 (0.7–0.95)	0.009
Transfusion	0.56 (0.46–0.68)	<0.001	0.59 (0.54–0.65)	<0.001
Cardio-pulmonary bypass	0.32 (0.12–0.87)	0.025	0.27 (0.18–0.41)	<0.001
Emergency operation	0.31 (0.15–0.65)	0.002	0.31 (0.11–0.91)	0.033
Open heart surgery	0.29 (0.09–0.89)	0.030	0.27 (0.18–0.41)	<0.001
Any Major Complication[a]	0.44 (0.37–0.52)	<0.001	0.38 (0.28–0.5)	<0.001

Hazard ratios >1 indicate shorter time to discharge, while hazard ratios <1 indicate prolonged time to discharge. *MI* myocardial infarction
[a]Patient with any of the following complications: major vascular, stroke, MI, new permanent pacemaker, life-threatening bleeding, major bleeding, cardio-pulmonary bypass, emergency operation, or open heart surgery

this suggests that development of strategies to mitigate these delays; one such strategy could be performing echocardiography immediately post procedure. These are all potential areas for future study.

It is important to note the complex relationship between pre-procedural LOS and post-procedural hospitalization duration. We grouped patients admitted to hospital 0–2 days pre-TAVR as they likely received an elective TAVR. It is clear that elective pre-admission did not impact post-TAVR LOS. In contrast, patients who were admitted for longer periods prior to their TAVR likely represent patients who had decompensated heart failure. This group has a substantially longer LOS; this illustrates that once TAVR patients deteriorate while waiting for their procedure, this translates into a slower recovery post-procedure. This reinforces the importance of diligent wait-time management for TAVR patients.

In addition, there are some general measures that have been shown to help reduce LOS which might also be relevant to TAVR patients. Patients with expected long LOS might benefit from preemptive interventions [34, 35] including geriatric care and pre-procedural rehab [36, 37], nutrition supplementation [38], reducing bleeding risk [39], optimize periprocedural practice [29, 40, 41], and post procedural rehabilitation [42].

Our study provides a number of new insights to the literature. First, we used competing risk models to include all TAVR patients in our analyses, not only those who survived to discharge. This eliminates the potential biases introduced by only studying patients selected for survival. In addition, we have shown that in TAVR the occurrence of a post-procedural complication has a remarkable influence on LOS and one can hypothesize that the occurrence of complications may be one of the causal pathways by which the factors identified in our models impact LOS. The extended LOS likely explains in part the increased costs associated with complications [8, 39].

Our study must be interpreted in the context of several limitations that merit discussion. Although we had a relatively larger sample size across two countries, and used a clustered model to account for potential site related factors, our cohort was limited to three tertiary care hospitals that had wide variability in clinical practice (access site, sedation type, etc.), which impacts the generalizability of our findings. Second, although we identified factors associated with LOS, it does not follow necessarily that changing those factors will translate to shorter LOS. Instead, potential strategies impacting those factors must be empirically tested. Third, we did not have data on frailty or social status. The number of portico cases was small as were subclavian and direct aortic access routes and therefore, any conclusions regarding these variables may be explained by the learning curve. Finally, our study was an observational study, and there may have residual confounders that we did not account for. As such, our results should be considered hypothesis generating and not conclusive.

Conclusions

In conclusion, this multicenter study identified a number of important modifiable patient and procedural factors associated with LOS. Future studies should evaluate if interventions focused on these potentially modifiable factors will translate to shorter LOS.

Abbreviations

AS: Aortic Stenosis; CI: Confidence Interval; HR: Hazard ratio; LOS: Length of stay; NYHA: New York Heart association; STS: Society of Thoracic surgeons; TAVR: Transcatheter aortic valve replacement

Acknowledgements

NA.

Funding

This study was funded in part by Schulich Heart Center and the Sunnybrook Research Institute. Dr. H. Wijeysundera is supported by a Distinguished Clinical Scientist Award from the Heart and Stroke Foundation of Canada. Dr. S. Fremes is supported in part by the Bernard S. Goldman Chair in Cardiovascular Surgery. None of the funding bodies had any role in the design of the study and collection, analysis, and interpretation of data and in writing the manuscript. The authors take full responsibility for the manuscript.

Authors' contributions

YA, NZ, DM, SR, SEF, ER, AC, SALN, AF, HCW were involved in the writing and/or review process. YA, NZ and HW were involved in the data acquisition and analysis. All authors have read and approved the final version of the manuscript.

Competing interests

Dr. Wijeysundera receives research support from Edwards Lifesciences and Medtronic Inc. Dr. Radhakrishnan is a proctor for Medtronic Inc. Dr. Finkelstein is a proctor for Medronic and Edwards Inc.

Author details

[1]Schulich Heart Centre, Division of Cardiology and Cardiac surgery, Sunnybrook Health Sciences Centre, Toronto, ON, Canada. [2]University of Toronto, Toronto, ON, Canada. [3]Institute for Clinical Evaluative Sciences (ICES), 2075 Bayview Avenue, Suite A202, Toronto, ON M4N 3M5, Canada. [4]Sunnybrook Research Institute (SRI), Dept. of Medicine & Institute of Health Policy, Management and Evaluation, University of Toronto, Toronto, ON, Canada. [5]St. Michael's Hospital, Toronto, ON, Canada. [6]Department of Cardiology, Tel Aviv Medical Center, Tel Aviv, affiliated to the Sackler School of Medicine, Tel Aviv University, Tel Aviv, Israel.

References

1. Kamperidis V, Delgado V, van Mieghem NM, Kappetein AP, Leon MB, Bax JJ. Diagnosis and management of aortic valve stenosis in patients with heart failure. Eur J Heart Fail. 2016;18(5):469-81.
2. Nkomo VT, Gardin JM, Skelton TN, Gottdiener JS, Scott CG, Enriquez-Sarano M. Burden of valvular heart diseases: a population-based study. Lancet. 2006;368:1005–11.
3. Reinohl J, Kaier K, Reinecke H, Schmoor C, Frankenstein L, Vach W, et al. Effect of Availability of Transcatheter Aortic-Valve Replacement on Clinical Practice. N Engl J Med. 2015;373:2438–47.
4. Leon MB, Smith CR, Mack M, Miller DC, Moses JW, Svensson LG, et al. Transcatheter aortic-valve implantation for aortic stenosis in patients who cannot undergo surgery. N Engl J Med. 2010;363:1597–607.
5. Smith CR, Leon MB, Mack MJ, Miller DC, Moses JW, Svensson LG, et al. Transcatheter versus surgical aortic-valve replacement in high-risk patients. N Engl J Med. 2011;364:2187–98.
6. Leon MB, Smith CR, Mack MJ, Makkar RR, Svensson LG, Kodali SK, et al. Transcatheter or Surgical Aortic-Valve Replacement in Intermediate-Risk Patients. N Engl J Med. 2016;28:1609–20.
7. Reinohl J, Kaier K, Gutmann A, Sorg S, von Zur MC, Siepe M, et al. In-hospital resource utilization in surgical and transcatheter aortic valve replacement. BMC Cardiovasc Disord. 2015;15:132.
8. Gutmann A, Kaier K, Sorg S, von Zur MC, Siepe M, Moser M, et al. Analysis of the additional costs of clinical complications in patients undergoing transcatheter aortic valve replacement in the German Health Care System. Int J Cardiol. 2015;179:231–7.
9. Barbanti M, Petronio AS, Ettori F, Latib A, Bedogni F, De Marco F, et al. 5-Year Outcomes After Transcatheter Aortic Valve Implantation With CoreValve Prosthesis. JACC Cardiovasc Interv. 2015;8:1084–91.
10. Minutello RM, Wong SC, Swaminathan RV, Feldman DN, Kaple RK, Horn EM, et al. Costs and in-hospital outcomes of transcatheter aortic valve implantation versus surgical aortic valve replacement in commercial cases using a propensity score matched model. Am J Cardiol. 2015;115(10):1443-7.
11. Noad RL, Johnston N, McKinley A, Dougherty M, Nzewi OC, Jeganathan R, et al. A pathway to earlier discharge following TAVI: Assessment of safety and resource utilization. Catheter Cardiovasc Interv. 2015. doi:10.1002/ccd.26005.
12. Gilard M, Eltchaninoff H, Iung B, Donzeau-Gouge P, Chevreul K, Fajadet J, et al. Registry of transcatheter aortic-valve implantation in high-risk patients. N Engl J Med. 2012;366:1705–15.
13. Durand E, Eltchaninoff H, Canville A, Bouhzam N, Godin M, Tron C, et al. Feasibility and safety of early discharge after transfemoral transcatheter aortic valve implantation with the Edwards SAPIEN-XT prosthesis. Am J Cardiol. 2015;115:1116–22.
14. Barbanti M, Capranzano P, Ohno Y, Attizzani GF, Gulino S, Imme S, et al. Early discharge after transfemoral transcatheter aortic valve implantation. Heart. 2015;101:1485–90.
15. Kappetein AP, Head SJ, Genereux P, Piazza N, van Mieghem NM, Blackstone EH, et al. Updated standardized endpoint definitions for transcatheter aortic valve implantation: the Valve Academic Research Consortium-2 consensus document. J Thorac Cardiovasc Surg. 2013;145:6–23.
16. Shahian DM, He X, Jacobs JP, Rankin JS, Welke KF, Filardo G, et al. The Society of Thoracic Surgeons Isolated Aortic Valve Replacement (AVR) Composite Score: a report of the STS Quality Measurement Task Force. Ann Thorac Surg. 2012;94:2166–71.
17. Shahian DM, He X, Jacobs JP, Rankin JS, Welke KF, Edwards FH, et al. The STS AVR+CABG composite score: a report of the STS Quality Measurement Task Force. Ann Thorac Surg. 2014;97:1604–9.
18. Nashef SA, Roques F, Michel P, Gauducheau E, Lemeshow S, Salamon R. European system for cardiac operative risk evaluation (EuroSCORE). Eur J Cardiothorac Surg. 1999;16:9–13.
19. Konigstein M, Ben-Assa E, Banai S, Shacham Y, Ziv-Baran T, Abramowitz Y, et al. Periprocedural bleeding, acute kidney injury, and long-term mortality after transcatheter aortic valve implantation. Can J Cardiol. 2015;31:56–62.
20. Fine JP, Gray RJ. A Proportional Hazards Model for the Subdistribution of a Competing Risk. J Am Stat Assoc. 1999;94:496–509.
21. van Venrooij LM, de Vos R, Borgmeijer-Hoelen MM, Haaring C, de Mol BA. Preoperative unintended weight loss and low body mass index in relation to complications and length of stay after cardiac surgery. Am J Clin Nutr. 2008;87:1656–61.
22. Kusachi S, Kashimura N, Konishi T, Shimizu J, Kusunoki M, Oka M, et al. Length of stay and cost for surgical site infection after abdominal and cardiac surgery in Japanese hospitals: multi-center surveillance. Surg Infect. 2012;13:257–65.
23. Buller LT, Best MJ, Quinnan SM. A Nationwide Analysis of Pelvic Ring Fractures: Incidence and Trends in Treatment, Length of Stay, and Mortality. Geriatr Orthop Surg Rehabil. 2016;7:9–17.
24. LaPar DJ, Rich JB, Isbell JM, Brooks CH, Crosby IK, Yarboro LT, et al. Preoperative Renal Function Predicts Hospital Costs and Length of Stay in Coronary Artery Bypass Grafting. Ann Thorac Surg. 2016;101:606–12.
25. Sasaki J, Dykes JC, Sosa LJ, Salvaggio JL, Tablante MD, Ojito J, et al. Risk Factors for Longer Hospital Stay Following the Fontan Operation. Pediatr Crit Care Med. 2016;17(5):411-9.

26. Shinjo D, Fushimi K. Preoperative factors affecting cost and length of stay for isolated off-pump coronary artery bypass grafting: hierarchical linear model analysis. BMJ Open. 2015;5:e008750.
27. Babaliaros V, Devireddy C, Lerakis S, Leonardi R, Iturra SA, Mavromatis K, et al. Comparison of transfemoral transcatheter aortic valve replacement performed in the catheterization laboratory (minimalist approach) versus hybrid operating room (standard approach): outcomes and cost analysis. JACC Cardiovasc Interv. 2014;7:898–904.
28. Serletis-Bizios A, Durand E, Cellier G, Tron C, Bauer F, Glinel B, Dacher JN, Cribier A, Eltchaninoff H. A Prospective Analysis of Early Discharge After Transfemoral Transcatheter Aortic Valve Implantation. Am J Cardiol. 2016; 118(6):866-72. doi: 10.1016/j.amjcard.2016.06.035. Epub 2016 Jun 27.
29. Lauck SB, Wood DA, Achtem L, Baumbusch J, Boone RH, Cheung A, et al. Risk stratification and clinical pathways to optimize length of stay after transcatheter aortic valve replacement. Can J Cardiol. 2014;30:1583–7.
30. Wood DA, Poulter R, Cook R, Stub D, Leipsic JA, Ye J, et al. TCT-701 A Multidisciplinary, Multimodality, but Minimalist (3M) approach to transfemoral transcatheter aortic valve replacement facilitates safe next day discharge home in high risk patients: 1 year follow up. J Am Coll Cardiol. 2014;64
31. Lauck SB, Wood DA, Baumbusch J, Kwon JY, Stub D, Achtem L, et al. Vancouver Transcatheter Aortic Valve Replacement Clinical Pathway: Minimalist Approach, Standardized Care, and Discharge Criteria to Reduce Length of Stay. Circ Cardiov Qual Outcomes. 2016;9:312–21.
32. Abawi M, Nijhoff F, Agostoni P, Emmelot-Vonk MH, de Vries R, Doevendans PA, et al. Incidence, Predictive Factors, and Effect of Delirium After Transcatheter Aortic Valve Replacement. JACC Cardiovasc Interv. 2016;9:160–8.
33. Huded CP, Huded JM, Friedman JL, Benck LR, Lindquist LA, Holly TA, et al. Frailty Status and Outcomes After Transcatheter Aortic Valve Implantation. Am J Cardiol. 2016;117:1966–71.
34. Goodman H, Parsons A, Davison J, Preedy M, Peters E, Shuldham C, et al. A randomised controlled trial to evaluate a nurse-led programme of support and lifestyle management for patients awaiting cardiac surgery 'Fit for surgery: Fit for life' study. Eur J Cardiovasc Nurs. 2008;7:189–95.
35. Arthur HM, Daniels C, McKelvie R, Hirsh J, Rush B. Effect of a preoperative intervention on preoperative and postoperative outcomes in low-risk patients awaiting elective coronary artery bypass graft surgery. A randomized, controlled trial. Ann Intern Med. 2000;133:253–62.
36. Opasich C, Patrignani A, Mazza A, Gualco A, Cobelli F, Pinna GD. An elderly-centered, personalized, physiotherapy program early after cardiac surgery. Eur J Cardiovasc Prev Rehabil. 2010;17:582–7.
37. Furze G, Dumville JC, Miles JN, Irvine K, Thompson DR, Lewin RJ. "Prehabilitation" prior to CABG surgery improves physical functioning and depression. Int J Cardiol. 2009;132:51–8.
38. van Venrooij LM, de Vos R, Zijlstra E, Borgmeijer-Hoelen MM, van Leeuwen PA, de Mol BA. The impact of low preoperative fat-free body mass on infections and length of stay after cardiac surgery: a prospective cohort study. J Thorac Cardiovasc Surg. 2011;142:1263–9.
39. Reinohl J, Gutmann A, Kollum M, von Zur MC, Baumbach H, Avlar M, et al. Transfemoral aortic valve implantation: bleeding events, related costs and outcomes. J Thromb Thrombolysis. 2013;35:469–75.
40. Shuvy M, Mewa J, Wolff R, Hutson J, Austin PC, Bentley D, et al. Preprocedure Anemia Management Decreases Transfusion Rates in Patients Undergoing Transcatheter Aortic Valve Implantation. Can J Cardiol. 2015. Doi: 10.1016/j.cjca.2015.08.018.
41. Arbel Y, Ben-Assa E, Halkin A, Keren G, Schwartz AL, Havakuk O, et al. Forced diuresis with matched hydration in reducing acute kidney injury during transcatheter aortic valve implantation (Reduce-AKI): study protocol for a randomized sham-controlled trial. Trials. 2014;15:262.
42. Russo N, Compostella L, Tarantini G, Setzu T, Napodano M, Bottio T, et al. Cardiac rehabilitation after transcatheter versus surgical prosthetic valve implantation for aortic stenosis in the elderly. Eur J Prev Cardiol. 2014;21:1341–8.

3

IgG4-positive cell infiltration in various cardiovascular disorders - results from histopathological analysis of surgical samples

Ryoto Hourai[1†], Satomi Kasashima[2†], Koichi Sohmiya[1], Yohei Yamauchi[1], Hideki Ozawa[3], Yoshinobu Hirose[4], Yasuhiro Ogino[4], Takahiro Katsumata[3], Masahiro Daimon[3], Shu-ichi Fujita[1], Masaaki Hoshiga[1] and Nobukazu Ishizaka[1*]

Abstract

Background: The diagnosis of Immunoglobulin G4 (IgG4)-related disease (IgG4-RD), in general, depends on serum IgG4 concentrations and histopathological findings; therefore, diagnosis of IgG4-RD in cardiovascular organs/tissues is often difficult owing to the risk of tissue sampling.

Methods: Prevalence of IgG4-positive lymphoplasmacytic infiltration in 103 consecutive cardiovascular surgical samples from 98 patients with various cardiovascular diseases was analyzed immunohistochemically.

Results: The diagnoses of the enrolled patients included aortic aneurysm (abdominal, $n = 8$; thoracic, $n = 9$); aortic dissection ($n = 20$); aortic stenosis ($n = 24$), aortic regurgitation ($n = 10$), and mitral stenosis/regurgitation ($n = 17$). In total, 10 (9.7%) of the 103 specimens showed IgG4-positive cell infiltration with various intensities; five of these were aortic valve specimens from aortic stenosis, and IgG4-positive cell infiltration was present at >10 /HPF in three of them. In one aortic wall sample from an abdominal aortic aneurysm, various histopathological features of IgG4-RD, such as IgG4-positive cell infiltration, obliterating phlebitis, and storiform fibrosis, were observed.

Conclusions: IgG4-positive cell infiltration was observed in 9.7% of the surgical cardiovascular specimens, mainly in the aortic valve from aortic stenosis and in the aortic wall from aortic aneurysm. Whether IgG4-positive cell infiltration has pathophysiological importance in the development or progression of cardiovascular diseases should be investigated in future studies.

Keywords: IgG4-related disease, Aortic valve, Aortic stenosis, Aortic wall, Aortic aneurysm

Background

Immunoglobulin G4 (IgG4)-related disease (IgG4-RD), first documented by Hamano et al. in 2001 [1], is characterized by clinical (organ enlargement or nodular/hyperplastic lesions; serum IgG4 concentration ≥135 mg/dL) and histopathological (IgG4-positive cells infiltration, >10/HPF; IgG4 /IgG ratio, >40%) findings. IgG4-RD may affect a wide variety of organs concurrently or metachronously, [2, 3]. At present, IgG4-RD can be diagnosed either by comprehensive diagnostic criteria [4] or by organ specific diagnostic criteria [5–7], although there are no heart/artery-specific diagnostic criteria for IgG4-RD.

Several previous reports have demonstrated IgG4-RD in various-size arteries and pericardium [8–13]. Most, but not all, cases of IgG4-RD in cardiovascular organs have diagnosed on the basis of histopathological findings in samples obtained either at the time of surgery or by autopsy. Biopsy of these vital organs in other situations is generally associated with considerable risk; therefore, IgG4-RD in cardiovascular organs may be underdiagnosed. In the current study, we have investigated the

* Correspondence: ishizaka@osaka-med.ac.jp
†Equal contributors
[1]Department of Cardiology, Osaka Medical College, Daigaku-machi 2-7, Takatsuki, Osaka 569-8686, Japan
Full list of author information is available at the end of the article

prevalence and the extent of IgG4-positive lymphoplasmacytic infiltration observed in tissue samples of various cardiovascular diseases obtained at the time of surgery.

Methods

Histology specimens and patients

In this study, histological analysis was carried out on 103 consecutive histologic specimens obtained from 98 patients who underwent cardiovascular surgery at Department of Thoracic and Cardiovascular Surgery, Osaka Medical College between January 2014 and December 2014. None of the enrolled patients had been diagnosed with or was suspected to have IgG4-RD at the time of surgery. Due to the retrospective design of the current study, serum IgG4 concentrations of the enrolled patients at the time of surgery were not available. Histological evaluation was carried out on formalin-fixed and paraffin embedded specimens. Immunostaining was performed with mouse monoclonal antibody against IgG4 (MC011, Biding Site, Birmingham, UK). IgG staining was performed with anti-IgG antibody (DAKO, Glostrup, Denmark). For some specimens, owing to the high background of IgG staining, anti-human CD138 antibody (AbD, Serotec, Oxford, UK) was used to stain plasma cells. In specimens where IgG4-positive cell infiltration was observed, we counted three ×40 fields with the highest number of IgG4-positive plasma cells, and then calculated the average number of IgG4-positive plasma cells within these fields. For the purpose of calculating the IgG4-to-IgG, or IgG4-CD138, ratio, the same three fields were counted [14].

Table 1 Baseline characteristics of the study patients

No. of subjects	98
Male gender, n (%)	58 (59.2)
Age, years	68.9 ± 11.7
BMI, kg/m^2	22.4 ± 3.6
Chronic hemodialysis, n (%)	9 (9.2)
Co-morbidities	
Hypertension, n (%)	62 (63.3)
Diabetes, n (%)	25 (25.5)
Collagen vascular diseases, n (%)	5 (5.1)
Malignant disorders, n (%)	20 (20.4)
Smoking status	
Never (%)	48 (49.0)
Former (%)	41 (41.8)
Current (%)	9 (9.2)
Laboratory data	
White blood cell count, ×10^3/μL	6.5 ± 3.4
Eosinophil count, /μL	188 ± 154
Hemoglobin, g/dL	12.6 ± 2.0
Platelet count, ×10^4/μL	19.8 ± 5.9
Total protein, g/dL	6.8 ± 0.6
Albumin, g/dL	3.8 ± 0.5
Creatinine[a], mg/dL	1.0 ± 0.4
eGFR[a], mL/min/1.73 m^2	59.2 ± 20.0
C-reactive protein, median (IQR) mg/dL	0.14 (0.04–1.65)
Amylase, U/L	90.9 ± 42.7

[a]Excluding those undergoing chronic hemodialysis. IQR indicates interquartile range. Data indicate mean ± standard deviation unless otherwise described

Results

Patients and histology samples

In total, 103 histological samples from 98 patients were analyzed. About one fifth of the patients had a history of malignancy, and nine patients were undergoing chronic hemodialysis (Table 1). The most common diagnosis among the cardiovascular conditions was aortic stenosis (24 patients), followed by aortic dissection (20 patients) (Table 2). Aortic aneurysm, either abdominal ($n = 8$) or thoracic ($n = 9$), was diagnosed for 17 patients. There were no patients who were diagnosed with inflammatory aortic aneurysm. From patients with either mitral stenosis ($n = 4$) or mitral regurgitation ($n = 7$), 11 mitral valve samples and 6 myocyte samples were obtained. Five tumors were analyzed, comprising atrial myxoma ($n = 3$), thymoma ($n = 1$), and pulmonary artery sarcoma ($n = 1$).

Prevalence of IgG4-positive cell infiltration in cardiovascular samples

Of the 103 histological samples, IgG4-positive cell infiltration was demonstrated immunohistochemically in 10 samples (10 patients): five in aortic valve samples, and five in aortic wall specimens (Table 3). Of note, all five aortic valve specimens that showed positive IgG4-cell infiltration were from patients with aortic stenosis; therefore the prevalence of of IgG4-positive cell infiltration positivity in aortic valve samples from aortic stenosis was as calculated to be 21% (5/24). The prevalence of IgG4-positivity in the cardiovascular specimen tended to be higher among patients with aortic stenosis (21%) than among patients without aortic stenosis (5/74, 7%, $P = 0.062$ by Fisher's exact test).th=tlb=

Three of the 10 patients with a histological sample showing IgG4-positive cell infiltration were undergoing chronic hemodialysis; this prevalence of hemodialysis (30%) was significantly higher than that among patients without IgG4-positive cell infiltration (6/88, 7%; $P = 0.047$ by Fisher's exact test). IgG4-positive cell infiltration was not observed in any of the mitral valve samples ($n = 11$), myocardium samples ($n = 6$), cardiac tumors ($n = 3$), pericardium samples ($n = 3$), mediastinal thymoma ($n = 1$), or pulmonary artery sarcoma ($n = 1$).

Table 2 Number and type of sampled cardiovascular tissues by clinical diagnosis

		Sampled tissues							
Clinical diagnosis	Pt. no.	Aortic wall	Arterial wall	Aortic valve	Mitral valve	Myocardium	Pericardium	Tumor	Thrombus
Abdominal aortic aneurysm	8	8							
Thoracic aortic aneurysm	9	9							
Aortic dissection (type A)	15	15							
Aortic dissection (type B)	5	5							
Annuloaortic ectasia	1	1							
Annuloaortic ectasia + aortic regurgitation	3	3		3					
Iliac arterial aneurysm	1		1						
Aortic stenosis	22			22					
Aortic regurgitation	4			4					
Aortic stenosis + regurgitation	2			2					
Aortic regurgitation + mitral stenosis	1			1	1				
Mitral stenosis	2				2				
Mitral regurgitation	11				5	6			
Mitral stenosis + regurgitation	2				2				
Mitral stenosis + mediastinal tumor	1				1			1	
Pericarditis	3						3		
Atrial myxoma	3							3	
Intra-pulmonary arterial tumor	1							1	
Pulmonary thrombosis	1								1
Arteriosclerosis obliterans	2	2							
Right aortic arch	1	1							
	Total	Total of tissues sampled (103 sampled regions)							
	98 pts.	44	1	32	11	6	3	5	1

IgG4-positive cell infiltration in aortic valve specimens

Five of 24 aortic valve specimens showed IgG4-positive cell infiltration; therefore, the ratio of IgG4-positive infiltration among patients with aortic stenosis was calculated to be 21% (Table 3). The stenosed aortic valves associated with IgG4-positive cell infiltration were tricuspid in four patients and bicuspid in one patient (case 10), and all these stenosed aortic valves were atherosclerotic (i.e., non-rheumatic) in nature.

The histopathological findings in two cases (case 6 and case 8) are demonstrated in Fig. 1. In case 6, an 84-year female patient, the IgG4/CD138 ratio was greater than 40% (Figs. 1a-d). In case 8, a 67-year male patient, the sample showed abundant infiltration of CD138-positive (CD138+) plasma cells; however, only a minor proportion of them were IgG4-positive (IgG4-positive/CD138+, <20%) (Figs. 1e-h). Based on the low IgG4-positive/CD138+ ratio and absence of characteristic histologic features, such as obliterating phlebitis and storiform fibrosis, none of the five aortic valve specimens with IgG4-positive cell infiltration (cases 6–10) was considered to indicate IgG4-RD.

According to clinical records, during the median follow-up period of 464 days (range, 316–636 days), neither occurrence of IgG4-RD nor dysfunction of the prosthetic valve (one bioprosthetic and four mechanical) was noted in any of the five patients with positive IgG4-positive cell infiltration in their aortic valve sample.

IgG4-positive cell infiltration in aortic wall specimens

The remaining five samples with IgG4-positive cell infiltration were from patients with abdominal aortic aneurysm (AAA, $n = 2$), aortic dissection ($n = 2$), and thoracic aortic aneurysm (TAA, $n = 1$) (Table 3). The prevalence of IgG4-positive cell infiltration among patients with aortic aneurysm and aortic dissection was thus calculated to be 20% (3/15) and 10% (2/20), respectively. In case 4, the specimen showed IgG4-positive plasmacytic infiltration with an IgG4-positive/IgG-positive ratio above 40% but obliterating phlebitis was not observed; therefore, the suspected diagnosis was reactive infiltration of lymphoid cells with IgG4-positive cell infiltration (Fig. 2).

Table 3 Clinical and histopathological findings of the 10 cases with IgG4-positive cell infiltration

Case no.	Case 1	case 2	Case 3	case 4	Case 5	Case 6	Case 7	Case 8	Case 9	Case 10
Sex	male	female	female	male	female	female	female	male	female	male
Age	67	93	72	66	56	84	74	67	64	63
Cardiovascular disorder	Abdominal aortic aneurysm	Aortic dissection (type A)	Aortic dissection (type A)	Thoracic aortic aneurysm	Abdominal aortic aneurysm	Aortic stenosis	Aortic stenosis + regurgitation	Aortic stenosis + regurgitation	Aortic stenosis	Aortic stenosis
Tissue sampled	aortic wall	aortic wall	aortic wall	aortic wall	aortic wall	aortic valve	aortic valve	aortic valve	aortic valve	aortic valve
IgG4 (/HPF)	101	18.7	35	37.5	5.2	73	3	20	3	23.5
IgG4/IgG (CD138) ratio (%)	75	41.3	46.7	51.3	12.4	44.8[a]	8[a]	17.4[a]	30[a]	31.5[a]
Obliterating phlebitis	+	-	-	-	-	-	-	-	-	-
Storiform fibrosis	+	-	-	+	-	-	-	-	-	-
Lymphoid follicle	+	-	-	+	+	-	-	-	-	-
Eosinophil infiltration	+	-	-	-	-	-	-	-	-	-
Neutrophil infiltration	-	+	-	-	-	-	-	-	-	-
Perineural inflammation	+	-	-	-	-	-	-	-	-	-
Granuloma	-	-	-	-	-	-	-	-	-	-
Thickness of adventitial fibrosis, mm	2.4	1	2	1.2	0.1	N/A	N/A	N/A	N/A	N/A
Hemosiderin deposition	-	+	+	-	+	+	+	-	-	+

N/A Not assessable
[a]CD138 staining was performed in the place of IgG staining

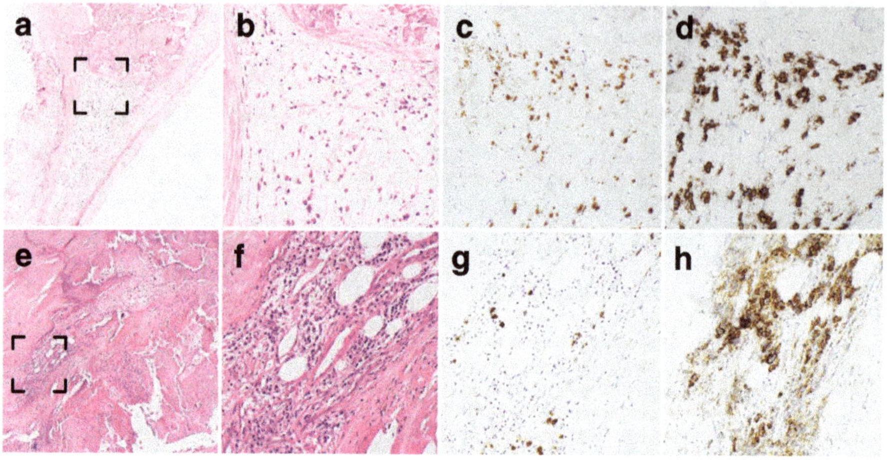

Fig. 1 Histopathological findings of tissue samples obtained from two patients with aortic stenosis (case 6 and case 8). **a-d** Case 6. **e-h** Case 8. **a**, **b**, **e**, **f** Hematoxylin and eosin (HE) staining. **c**, **g** IgG4 staining. **d**, **h** CD138 staining. **b** Higher magnification image of the bracketed area in **a**. The number of IgG4-positive cells was 73/HPF and the IgG4/CD138 ratio was 45%. **f** Higher magnification image of the bracketed area in **e**. Original magnification, ×40 (**a**, **e**), and × 200 (**b-d**, **f-h**). The number of IgG4-positive cells was 20/HPF and IgG4/CD138 ratio was 17%

The sample of case 1, who was diagnosed with AAA, showed not only IgG4-positive cell infiltration, but also other pathological features that are characteristic of IgG4-RD, such as adventitial thickening, lymphoid follicle formation, eosinophil infiltration, perineural infiltration, storiform fibrosis, and obliterating phlebitis (Fig. 3). Based on these observations, IgG4-RD was strongly suggested histopathologically in this patient. The patient also had TAA (Fig. 4) and underwent thoracic endovascular aortic repair 8 months after surgery for the AAA.

According to clinical records, during the median follow-up of 367 days (range, 50–795 days), occurrence of IgG4-RD in tissues other than cardiovascular tissues was not noted in any of the five patients with positive IgG4-positive cell infiltration in the aortic wall samples. In addition, in case 1, neither clinically significant systemic inflammation nor graft problems occurred during the follow up period.

Discussion

In the current study, whether, and if so to what extent, IgG4-positive cell infiltration was present in 103 consecutive surgical samples from 98 patients undergoing cardiovascular surgery. In total, IgG4-positive cell infiltration was observed in 10 histological samples. IgG4-positive cell infiltration was most frequently observed in aortic wall of the AAA (3/8, 38%) followed by the aortic valve of aortic stenosis (5/24, 21%), and the aortic wall of dissecting aneurysm (2/20, 10%). On the other hand, IgG4-positive cell infiltration was not observed among the remaining 93 histological specimens. These findings indicate that IgG4-positive cell infiltration may occur in certain limited cardiovascular disease. In one patient with AAA (case 1), in addition to IgG4-positive cell infiltration, other histopathologic features characteristic of IgG4-RD listed in the International Consensus Diagnostic Criteria (ICDC) [15] were observed, such as storiform fibrosis and obliterating phlebitis (Fig. 3), leading to the increased possibility of an IgG4-related aortic lesion.

There are several previous studies examining the prevalence of IgG4-RD or IgG4-positive lymphoplasmacytic infiltration in cardiovascular histological specimens. Kasashima et al. reported that 13 (5.2%) of 252 surgically-treated AAA cases [8] and 5 (7.0%) of 71 surgically-treated

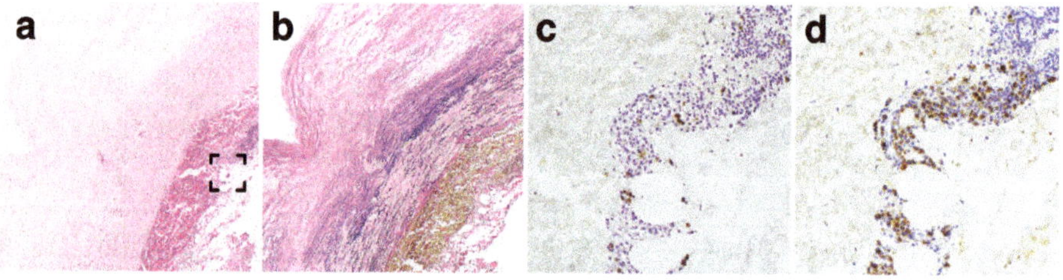

Fig. 2 Histopathological findings of tissue samples obtained from patients with thoracic aortic aneurysm and suspected reactive inflammatory cell infiltration (case 4). **a** HE staining. **b** Elastica van Gieson staining. **c** IgG4 staining. **d** IgG staining. **c** and **d** show higher magnification images of the bracketed area in A. Original magnification, ×40 (**a**, **b**), and × 200 (**c**, **d**)

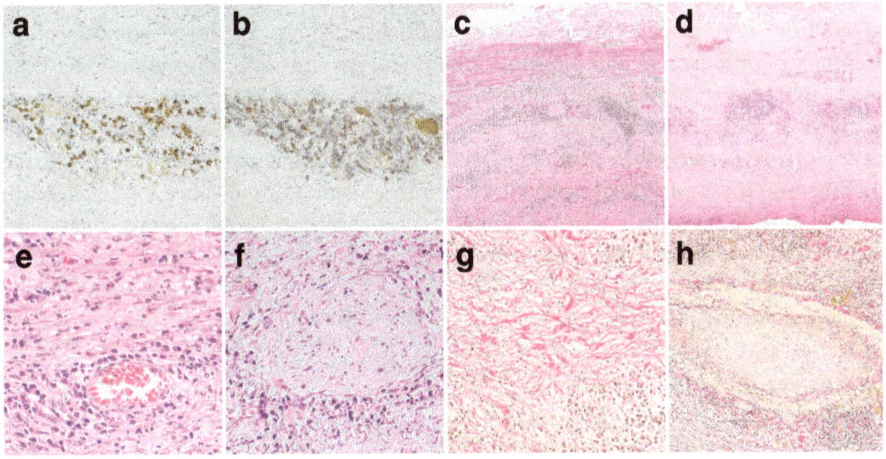

Fig. 3 Histopathological findings of tissue samples from case 1. **a** IgG4 staining. **b** IgG staining. **c**, **g**, **h** Elastica van Gieson staining. **d-f**, HE staining. **a**, **b** The IgG4-positive/IgG-positive ratio was >70%. **c**, **d** Prominent adventitial thickening (**c**) with formation of lymphoid follicles (**d**) were observed. **e** Infiltration of eosinophils. **f** Perineural inflammatory cell infiltration. **g** Storiform fibrosis. **h** Obliterative phlebitis. Original magnification, ×200 (**a**, **b**, **g**), ×40 (**c**, **d**), ×400 (**e**, **f**), and × 100 (**h**)

TAA cases [16] may have belonged to IgG4-RD. In the current study, if case 1 were diagnosed with IgG4-RD, the prevalence of undiagnosed IgG4-RD among AAA might be calculated as 1/8 (13%). It should be noted, however, that elevation of serum IgG4 levels-information that was not available for this patient-is indispensable for the definitive diagnosis of IgG4-RD [4, 8, 17]. Regarding other organ-specific diagnostic criteria, such as those targeting IgG4-related sialodacryoadenitis and autoimmune pancreatitis, it may be possible to diagnose IgG4-RD without serum IgG4 levels; however, there are currently no organ-specific diagnostic criteria for IgG4-related cardiovascular lesions in Japan, Thus, what we showed in the current study was not the prevalence of IgG4-related disease, but the prevalence of IgG-positive cell infiltration in cardiovascular surgical samples.

Lymphocytic infiltration in calcified aortic stenosis has been reported in several previous studies. Wallby et al. showed that infiltration of T lymphocytes and plasma cells has been frequently observed in non-rheumatic stenosed tricuspid or bicuspid aortic valves [18]. In addition, Wu et al. proposed that lymphocytic infiltration may not represent a secondary response to inflammation, but may provide components of the valvular injury responsible for aortic stenosis [19]. There are also a few reports regarding IgG4-positive cell infiltration in aortic stenosis. Steiner et al. reported that 13 (87%) of 15 stenosed aortic valve samples showed IgG4-positive cell

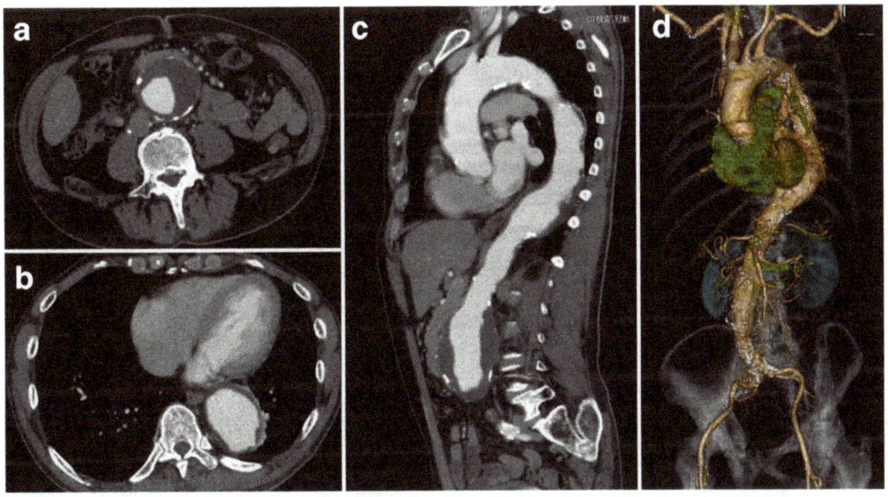

Fig. 4 Contrast enhanced computed tomography of case 1 before the operation for abdominal and thoracic aortic aneurysm. **a**, **b** Axial view. **a** Aneurysmal dilatation with intraluminal thrombus was observed in the abdominal aorta. **b** The thoracic aorta was also enlarged. **c**, **d** Sagittal reconstruction (**c**) and 3-dimensional reconstruction (**d**), demonstrating the morphology of the thoracic and abdominal aorta and branches

infiltration [20]. In their study, 15 stenosed aortic valve samples were selected from a total of 178 aortic valve samples by the presence of intense cellular infiltration (≥100 cells/HPF); therefore, the true percentage of samples with IgG4-positive cell infiltration among the overall (i.e., 178) cases of aortic stenosis could not be determined. It should be noted that in the current study, we did not select aortic specimens with intense cellular infiltration (≥100 cells/HPF) before IgG4-staining; therefore, we cannot simply compare the prevalence of IgG4-cell infiltration in stenosed aortic valve samples between Steiner et al.'s study and ours.

Chronic hemodialysis was more prevalent among patients with histological samples showing IgG4-positive cell infiltration. Krediet et al. reported that serum IgG4 subclass was decreased among those undergoing ambulatory peritoneal dialysis and was not significantly different among those undergoing hemodialysis as compared with healthy volunteers [21]. Although the possibility exists that IgG4-related kidney disease might have preceded the introduction of hemodialysis [22] for some patients in whom IgG4-positive cell infiltration was shown, whether there is a causal or resultant relationship between these conditions awaits further large-scale studies.

There are some limitations in the current study. First, due to the study design, data on serum IgG4 concentrations at the time of surgery were not available. Second, owing to the cross-sectional nature of the study, the pathophysiological importance of IgG4-positive cell infiltration in cardiovascular tissues cannot be addressed. Whether cardiovascular patients with IgG4-positive cell infiltration have a different clinical course [23] and an altered responsiveness to drug therapy as compared with those without IgG4-positive cell infiltration should be analyzed in future longitudinal studies. Third, IgG4-positive lymphoplasmacytic infiltration is not a feature exclusive to IgG4-RD; it may be observed in several immune and/or inflammatory disorders such as Castleman disease [24], Rosai-Dorfman disease [25], Wegener granulomatosis [26], and sialadenitis caused by sialolithiasis [27]. Lastly, we examined the presence or absence of IgG4-positive cell infiltration in one slide for each of the 103 samples; therefore, the true prevalence of IgG4-positive cell infiltration among these surgical samples might have been greater than what we have observed. The strength of the current study, on the other hand, was that by means of a comprehensive histopathological analysis, we have been able to estimate the prevalence and extent of IgG4-positive cell infiltration in various cardiovascular diseases.

Conclusion

In conclusion, by analyzing 103 consecutive surgical samples obtained from 98 patients undergoing cardiovascular surgery, IgG4-positive cell infiltration was noted in 5 (21%) cases of 24 aortic stenosis and 5 cases of aortic aneurysm or aortic dissection. These findings collectively indicate that IgG4-positive cell infiltration is not a rare finding in cardiovascular diseases, especially in aortic stenosis, aortic aneurysm, and aortic dissection. The pathophysiological importance of IgG4-positive infiltration in these disorders should be investigated in further studies.

Abbreviations

AAA: Abdominal aortic aneurysm; IgG4: Immunoglobulin G4; IgG4-RD: IgG4-related disease; TAA: Thoracic aortic aneurysm

Acknowledgements

We are highly appreciative of Megumi Hashimoto for her excellent technical assistance.

Funding

This work was supported in part by Grants in Aid for Scientific Research from the Ministry of Education, Science, and Culture of Japan (No. 15 K09106). There are no relationships with the company relating to employment, consultancy, patents, products in development or marketed products.

Authors' contributions

KS, RH: creating database. MH: performed statistical analysis. SK: performed histological analysis and interpretation of the results. YY, HO, TK, MD: obtained informed consent, performed surgery, checked manuscript. YH, YO: performed histological assessment. NI: designing the study, statistical assessment. All authors read and approved the final manuscript.

Competing interests

Authors do not have a financial relationship with the organization that sponsored the research.

This work was supported in part by Grants in Aid for Scientific Research from the Ministry of Education, Science, and Culture of Japan (No. 15 K09106).

Author details

[1]Department of Cardiology, Osaka Medical College, Daigaku-machi 2-7, Takatsuki, Osaka 569-8686, Japan. [2]Department of Pathology, National Hospital Organization, Kanazawa Medical Center, Kanazawa, Japan. [3]Department of Thoracic and Cardiovascular Surgery, Osaka Medical College, Osaka, Japan. [4]Department of Pathology Osaka Medical College, Osaka, Japan.

References

1. Hamano H, Kawa S, Horiuchi A, Unno H, Furuya N, Akamatsu T, Fukushima M, Nikaido T, Nakayama K, Usuda N, Kiyosawa K. High serum IgG4 concentrations in patients with sclerosing pancreatitis. N Engl J Med. 2001;344(10):732–8.
2. Stone JH, Zen Y, Deshpande V. IgG4-related disease. N Engl J Med. 2012;366(6):539–51.
3. Kamisawa T, Zen Y, Pillai S, Stone JH. IgG4-related disease. Lancet. 2015;385(9976):1460–71.

4. Okazaki K, Umehara H. Are Classification Criteria for IgG4-RD Now Possible? The Concept of IgG4-Related Disease and Proposal of Comprehensive Diagnostic Criteria in Japan. Int J Rheumatol. 2012;2012:357071.
5. Okazaki K, Uchida K, Matsushita M, Takaoka M. How to diagnose autoimmune pancreatitis by the revised Japanese clinical criteria. J Gastroenterol. 2007;42 Suppl 18:32–8.
6. Masaki Y, Sugai S, Umehara H. IgG4-related diseases including Mikulicz's disease and sclerosing pancreatitis: diagnostic insights. J Rheumatol. 2010;37(7):1380–5.
7. Kawano M, Saeki T, Nakashima H, Nishi S, Yamaguchi Y, Hisano S, Yamanaka N, Inoue D, Yamamoto M, Takahashi H, Nomura H, Taguchi T, Umehara H, Makino H, Saito T. Proposal for diagnostic criteria for IgG4-related kidney disease. Clin Exp Nephrol. 2011;15(5):615–26.
8. Kasashima S, Zen Y, Kawashima A, Endo M, Matsumoto Y, Kasashima F. A new clinicopathological entity of IgG4-related inflammatory abdominal aortic aneurysm. J Vasc Surg. 2009;49(5):1264–71. discussion 1271.
9. Tanigawa J, Daimon M, Murai M, Katsumata T, Tsuji M, Ishizaka N. Immunoglobulin G4-related coronary periarteritis in a patient presenting with myocardial ischemia. Hum Pathol. 2012;43(7):1131–4.
10. Ishizaka N. IgG4-related disease underlying the pathogenesis of coronary artery disease. Clin Chim Acta. 2013;415:220–5.
11. Hourai R, Miyamura M, Tasaki R, Iwata A, Takeda Y, Morita H, Hanaoka N, Tanigawa J, Shibata K, Takeshita A, Kawano M, Sato Y, Hirose Y, Ishizaka N. A case of IgG4-related lymphadenopathy, pericarditis, coronary artery periarteritis and luminal stenosis. Heart Vessels. 2016;31(10):1709–13.
12. Tanigawa J, Daimon M, Takeda Y, Katsumata T, Ishizaka N. Temporal changes in serum IgG4 levels after coronary artery bypass graft surgery. Hum Pathol. 2012;43(11):2093–5.
13. Sakamoto A, Nagai R, Saito K, Imai Y, Takahashi M, Hosoya Y, Takeda N, Hirano K, Koike K, Enomoto Y, Kume H, Homma Y, Maeda D, Yamada H, Fukayama M, Hirata Y, Ishizaka N. Idiopathic retroperitoneal fibrosis, inflammatory aortic aneurysm, and inflammatory pericarditis-retrospective analysis of 11 case histories. J Cardiol. 2012;59(2):139–46.
14. Deshpande V, Zen Y, Chan JK, Yi EE, Sato Y, Yoshino T, Kloppel G, Heathcote JG, Khosroshahi A, Ferry JA, Aalberse RC, Bloch DB, Brugge WR, Bateman AC, Carruthers MN, Chari ST, Cheuk W, Cornell LD, Fernandez-Del Castillo C, Forcione DG, Hamilos DL, Kamisawa T, Kasashima S, Kawa S, Kawano M, Lauwers GY, Masaki Y, Nakanuma Y, Notohara K, Okazaki K, et al. Consensus statement on the pathology of IgG4-related disease. Mod Pathol. 2012;25(9):1181–92.
15. Shimosegawa T, Chari ST, Frulloni L, Kamisawa T, Kawa S, Mino-Kenudson M, Kim MH, Kloppel G, Lerch MM, Lohr M, Notohara K, Okazaki K, Schneider A, Zhang L. International consensus diagnostic criteria for autoimmune pancreatitis: guidelines of the International Association of Pancreatology. Pancreas. 2011;40(3):352–8.
16. Kasashima S, Zen Y, Kawashima A, Endo M, Matsumoto Y, Kasashima F, Ohtake H, Nakanuma Y. A clinicopathologic study of immunoglobulin G4-related sclerosing disease of the thoracic aorta. J Vasc Surg. 2010;52(6):1587–95.
17. Kasashima S, Zen Y. IgG4-related inflammatory abdominal aortic aneurysm. Curr Opin Rheumatol. 2011;23(1):18–23.
18. Wallby L, Janerot-Sjoberg B, Steffensen T, Broqvist M. T lymphocyte infiltration in non-rheumatic aortic stenosis: a comparative descriptive study between tricuspid and bicuspid aortic valves. Heart. 2002;88(4):348–51.
19. Wu HD, Maurer MS, Friedman RA, Marboe CC, Ruiz-Vazquez EM, Ramakrishnan R, Schwartz A, Tilson MD, Stewart AS, Winchester R. The lymphocytic infiltration in calcific aortic stenosis predominantly consists of clonally expanded T cells. J Immunol. 2007;178(8):5329–39.
20. Steiner I, Krbal L, Rozkos T, Harrer J, Laco J. Calcific aortic valve stenosis: Immunohistochemical analysis of inflammatory infiltrate. Pathol Res Pract. 2012;208(4):231–4.
21. Krediet RT, Koomen GC, Vlug A, Struijk DG, Buis B, van Olden RW, Imholz AL. IgG subclasses in CAPD patients. Perit Dial Int. 1996;16(3):288–94.
22. Saeki T, Kawano M, Mizushima I, Yamamoto M, Wada Y, Nakashima H, Homma N, Tsubata Y, Takahashi H, Ito T, Yamazaki H, Saito T, Narita I. The clinical course of patients with IgG4-related kidney disease. Kidney Int. 2013;84(4):826–33.
23. Maleszewski JJ, Tazelaar HD, Horcher HM, Hinkamp TJ, Conte JV, Porterfield JK, Halushka MK. IgG4-related disease of the aortic valve: a report of two cases and review of the literature. Cardiovasc Pathol. 2015;24(1):56–9.
24. Izumi Y, Takeshita H, Moriwaki Y, Hisatomi K, Matsuda M, Yamashita N, Kawahara C, Shigemitsu Y, Iwanaga N, Kawakami A, Kurohama H, Niino D, Ito M, Migita K. Multicentric Castleman disease mimicking IgG4-related disease: A case report. Mod Rheumatol. 2014;22:1–4.
25. Apperley ST, Hyjek EM, Musani R, Thenganatt J. Intrathoracic Rosai Dorfman Disease with Focal Aggregates of IgG4-bearing Plasma Cells. Case Report and Literature Review. Ann Am Thorac Soc. 2016;13(5):666–70.
26. Chang SY, Keogh KA, Lewis JE, Ryu JH, Cornell LD, Garrity JA, Yi ES. IgG4-positive plasma cells in granulomatosis with polyangiitis (Wegener's): a clinicopathologic and immunohistochemical study on 43 granulomatosis with polyangiitis and 20 control cases. Hum Pathol. 2013;44(11):2432–7.
27. Strehl JD, Hartmann A, Agaimy A. Numerous IgG4-positive plasma cells are ubiquitous in diverse localised non-specific chronic inflammatory conditions and need to be distinguished from IgG4-related systemic disorders. J Clin Pathol. 2011;64(3):237–43.

4

Pre- and post-surgical evaluation of the inflammatory response in patients with aortic stenosis treated with different types of prosthesis

Maria Elena Soto[1*], Jose Luis Salas[2], Jesus Vargas-Barron[3], Ricardo Marquez[1], Alejandra Rodriguez-Hernandez[4], Rafael Bojalil-Parra[1], Israel Pérez-Torres[5] and Veronica Guarner-Lans[6]

Abstract

Background: The inflammatory process in aortic valvular stenosis persists after surgery to replace the valve in almost half of the patients. No association has been found to its persistence. The main objective of this study was to evaluate the inflammatory response in patients with aortic stenosis through the determination of several biomarkers in plasma measured before and after the valvular replacement and to seek an association with the type of prosthesis used.

Methods: This is an observational study with a follow up of 6 months in subjects with severe aortic stenosis. Seric concentrations of TNFa, IL-1, IL-6 and ICAM and echocardiographic variables were quantified previous to the surgery and a week and 6 months after it. A group of control subjects paired by age and gender was included.

Results: Seventy-nine subjects were studied of which 57% were male; the average age was of 59 (± 11.4) years. Previous to surgery, the concentration of cytokines was higher in patients than in control subjects. A biological prosthesis was implanted in 48 patients and a mechanical prosthesis in 31. Both, types of prosthesis have components made of titanium. The echocardiograms 1 week and 6 months after the surgery showed a decrease in the mean aortic gradient and an increase in the valvular area ($p = 0.001$). Half of the patients still showed high proinflammatory cytokine levels. There were no differences according to the type of prosthesis implanted after adjustments for demographic variables, comorbidities and echocardiographic data.

Conclusions: The inflammatory response caused by both types of valvular prothesis at 6 months after implantation were similar. Both types of prosthesis are recommended, they had similarities in hemodynamic profiles registered with Doppler echocardiography. Age of the patient or the suitability use of anticoagulants determines the type of prosthesis to be used.

Keywords: Aortic valve, Aortic stenosis, Inflammatory response, Heart surgery

Background

Aortic stenosis (AS) is a disease that develops with a high local inflammatory response. Its physiopathogeny resembles that of the atherosclerotic process. It is characterized by an initial lesion in the valvular endothelium followed by an active inflammatory infiltrate that leads to progressive calcification, reduction of the valvular area and an increase in the left ventricular (LV) afterload [1–3].

Accordingly, dramatically increased levels of intracellular adhesion molecule 1 (ICAM1) and proinflammatory cytokines such as tumoral necrosis factor-α (TNF-α), interleukin 6 (IL-6) and interleukin 1 (IL-1) are found in patients with AS [4–6]. The only effective treatment in severe AS is the surgical replacement of the aortic valve. However, even after the surgical procedure, the inflammatory state persists in almost half of the patients [7].

* Correspondence: mesoto50@hotmail.com
[1]Immunology Department, Instituto Nacional de Cardiología "Ignacio Chávez", Juan Badiano número 1, Colonia Sección XVI, Delegación Tlalpan, Mexico CP 14080, Mexico
Full list of author information is available at the end of the article

However, recently, it has been proposed that the technical approach determines the inflammatory response after surgical and transcatheter aortic valve replacement [8].

Previous studies have not found a correlation between age, gender, smoking habit, ventricular geometry, transvalvular aortic gradient, atherosclerosis risk factors or infection by *Chlamydia pneumoniae* and the persistence of the inflammatory state after the replacement of the aortic valve [9, 10].

The factors triggering or perpetuating the chronic inflammatory process after the valvular replacement are multiple and some of them might even coexist [11]. Therefore, it might be likely that some of the materials with which the different kinds of prosthesis are manufactured could induce the inflammatory mechanisms. [12].

It is well known that mechanical and biological prosthesis are manufactured with different types of materials. In the biological prosthesis, the incomplete process of removing cells from the original animal tissue could lead the presence of protein residues in the valves that might act as immunogens. [13] The metallic components present in mechanical prosthesis such as titanium could also trigger an inflammatory response [14, 15]. It is still unknown if the hemodynamic profile of the patients correlates with the type of inflammatory response or if this response is in correlation with the type of prosthesis implanted.

The main objective of this study was to evaluate the inflammatory response in patients with aortic stenosis through the determination of several biomarkers in plasma measured before and after the valvular replacement and to seek an association with the type of prosthesis used.

Methods

This is an observational, longitudinal, prospective follow-up study of 6 months. A cohort of patients with aortic stenosis recruited consecutively from September 2013 to January 2015 was studied.

Inclusion criteria

Subjects of any gender, aged 40 years or more and hospitalized with the diagnosis of severe aortic stenosis determined by nonrheumatic clinical criteria and by echocardiography criteria were included [16]. They agreed to participate by signing an informed consent form.

Exclusion criteria

Patients with moderate or severe aortic insufficiency, patients having other moderate or severe valvular disease, patients with coronary artery disease, subjects that required other cardiac surgery in addition to aortic valve replacement, patients with autoimmune or oncologic diseases and patients using immunosuppressant were excluded. The use of Non-steroidal anti-inflammatory drugs (NSAIDs) and/or caffeinated foods was suspended 1 day before the blood sampling and 1 week in the case of statins. An elimination criteria was the development of any intra-hospital infection.

Control group

Forty healthy subjects were matched by age and gender and the age of some controls could be matched with more than one case. Control subjects underwent physical examination, complete transthoracic echocardiography to rule out structural cardiac abnormalities and collection of peripheral blood samples by venopunction for the quantification of inflammatory mediators.

Sample size

With a confidence of 95% and a power of 90%, a sample of 35 patients per group was estimated by difference in proportions based on the concentration of TNF α obtained in previous studies [10].

Study design

The study was divided into three phases: preoperative (7 days before surgery), early postoperative (7 days after surgery) and late postoperative (6 months after surgery). In each of the phases an interrogation and physical examination directed to discard active infectious foci was conducted. In the pre-surgical protocol of patients in which cardiac surgery is performed a multidisciplinary team mis involved where the ginecology, odontology and infectology departments intervene. An exhaustive physical examination aimed to determine the clinical diagnosis of active infections is practiced including the performance of an uroculture and nasal and vaginal cultures. In the event of a positive culture, patients are excluded from the surgical programming until they have received antibiotic treatment and a negative culture is obtained. The results from the cultures of every patient previous to surgery were negative and the results from the leucocyte measurement had a mean value of 5600 ± 800. A transthoracic echocardiography study was done and peripheral blood samples for quantification of inflammatory mediators were obtained.

Determination of cytokines

10 ml of peripheral blood were centrifuged at 2500 rpm/10 min at 4 °C; then 500 ml aliquots of serum were made and stored at −75 °C until cytokine determination. Subsequently, TNF, IL-1, IL-6 and ICAM-1 were determined by enzyme-linked immunosorbent assay (ELISA) sandwich using commercial systems DuoSet (R & D Systems, Minneapolis, MN) according to the instructions provided by the manufacturer [17].

Echocardiographic study

The echocardiographic study was conducted by two experts' echocardiographists as is actually recommended [18]. An ultrasound system Philips iE33 xMATRIX (Philips, AndoverMassachusetts) with a transducer ×5 was employed. The LV dimensions were measured using the long parasternal axis; the volumes of the left atrium and LV were calculated with the method of Simpson. The aortic valve area was estimated with the equation of continuity. LV mass was estimated with the method of Devereaux. The mean and maximum aortic transvalvular gradient were obtained from the apical projection of three or five chambers, where an appropriate continuous spectrum from the Doppler was found and where the most transaortic velocity was observed. Systolic pulmonary artery pressure was estimated by the addition of the right atrial pressure to the gradient of tricuspid regurgitation.

Type of prosthesis implanted

The decision on the type of prosthesis to be implanted was made by the medical team. After aortic valve replacement, the surgery population was divided into two groups according to the type of prosthesis used; biological or mechanical. Biological prostheses manufactured in the National Institute of Cardiology "Ignacio Chavez" from bovine pericardium and titanium metal support were implanted. Mechanical prostheses were bileaflet which are made of pyrolytic carbon and mounted on a support of pyrocarbon covered with Dacron St. Jude Medical™ Masters HP series. A follow up of 6 months from the date of surgery was done.

Ethical aspects

The study included the signature of an informed consent form that is in accordance with the Declaration of Helsinki and the protocol was approved by the scientific and institutional bioethics committee.

Statistical analysis

The categorical variables were expressed in proportions, when there was a continuity in mean ± standard deviation or median interquartile range according to distribution. The comparisons were done using Chi Square or Fisher's exact test for categorical variables; for dimensional variables, Student's t or Mann-Whitney's U tests were applied. The correlations were done with Pearson's r for quantitative variables or with Spearman's rho for qualitative variables. Related samples, where repeated measurements were done, were analyzed with ANOVA and Friedman's test or with a distribution with a post hoc test to identify differences between groups. The differences were considered as statistically significant when the p value was <0.05.

The statistical analysis was done with the SPSS program version 22 (SPSS Inc. Chicago, Illinois).

Results

We studied 150 consecutive patients with aortic stenosis, of which 90 met inclusion criteria; Patients were eliminated due to the development of serious intrahospital infection (n = 2) and to the concomitant finding of arterial coronary disease (n = 9), leaving a final population of 79 cases (Fig. 1).

Of the total cases, 45 (57%) were men with an average age of 59 (± 11.4) years, the average age in men with AS was lower (57 ± 12) than in women with AS (62 ± 8.6), p = 0.025. Table 1 shows percentage of demograhic characteristics between cases and controls. 10 (12.5%), cases with diabetes, 29(36%) Hypertension and 7 (8.8%) smoking habits. The total prosthesis, biologic and mechanical, implanted were 48(61%) and 31 (39%) by each type of co morbidity were implanted: in patients with diabetes 4(8%) and 6(19%), with hypertension 18 (38%) and 11(35%), and with smooking habits 4(8%) and 3 (10%) respectively.

In the initial echocardiogram all patients had severe aortic stenosis with a valve area of 0.67 (± 0.2) cm2, mean aortic gradient of 59 (± 16) mmHg and maximum velocity of flow of 4.8 (± 0.6) m/s. The mean LVEF was 53% (± 17). In 30 patients TNFa concentrations were higher than in controls (38%). In 26 patients (33%) the IL-1 concentrations were elevated and in 30 (38%) there was an elevation of IL-6. All patients had elevated levels of ICAM-1. When comparing the group of patients who had elevated levels of cytokines with those who had normal values no significant differences in age, gender or echocardiographic parameters of aortic stenosis were found. When the comparison between the groups was made for values of inflammatory mediators, there was a tendency to an increase in TNF-α, IL-1, IL-6 and ICAM-1concentrations in AS patients versus controls, with p values of 0.08, 0.09, 0.10 and 0.07 respectively (Table 2).

There were no significant differences in the concentration of cytokines in relation to gender (TNFa: p = 0.071, IL-1: p = 0.31, IL-6: 0.76 and ICAM-1: p = 0.5). As well as no differences in the concentrations of cytokines between the older and younger than 60 years of age subjects (p = 0.15, IL-1: p = 0.3, IL-6 and ICAM-1 0.2: p = 0.9 TNFa).

Early post surgical stage

In 61% (n = 48) of the patients a biological prosthesis was implanted, and in 39% (n = 31) a mechanical valve was used. Women are more frequently implanted with a biological prosthesis than men (73% vs 51%), p = 0.043. An overall significant improvement in echocardiographic parameters was found with an increase in aortic valve area, a decreased mean aortic transvalvular gradient and a decreased in flow velocity. When

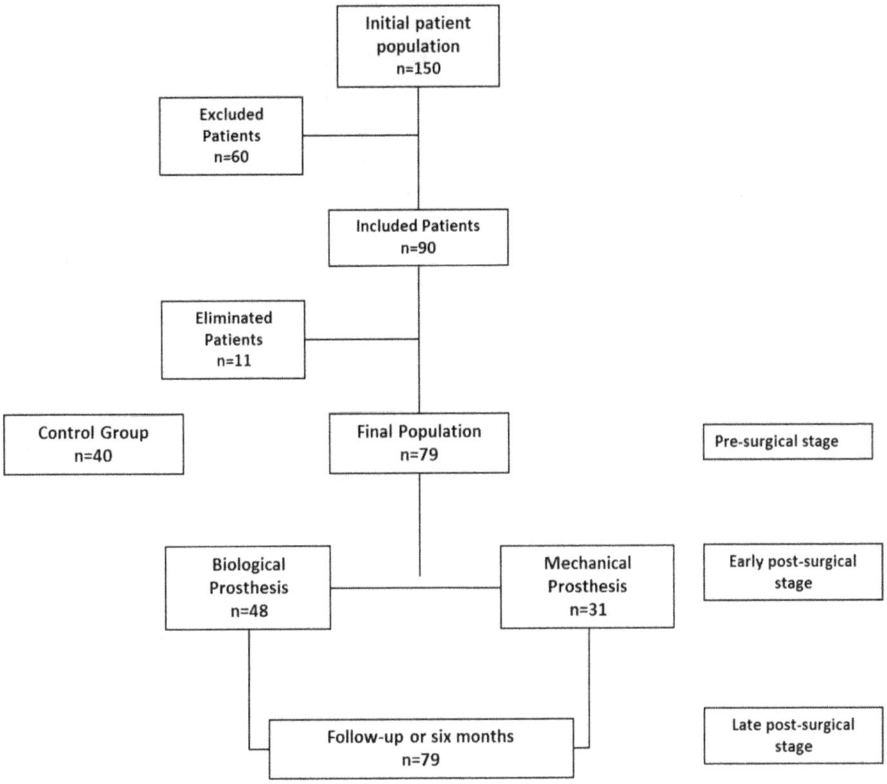

Fig. 1 The design of study and flow of patients

the ventricular geometry was analyzed, there was a decrease in LV mass (p = 0.001). A significant increase in the concentration of cytokines was found when compared to the preoperative values (Table 3).

Late post surgical stage

At a follow-up period of 6 months an additional decrease in mean aortic gradient and maximum velocity, and an increase in aortic valve area were observed. There was also a decrease in left ventricular mass (Table 3). About half of the patients still had elevated levels of cytokines at this stage, TNFa: 60% (n = 47), IL-1: 42% (n = 33) and IL-6: 53% (n = 42) and all of the patients maintained high levels of ICAM-1. There was a greater concentration of

Table 1 Demographic characteristics of the AS patient and the control groups

Variables Mean (±) SD *n* (%)	AS *n* = 79	CONTROL *n* = 40	*p*
Age (yr)	59 (11)	58 (11)	0.25
Men	45 (57)	23 (57)	0.68
Women	34 (43)	17 (43)	0.72
Weight (Kg)	69 (11.2)	65 (10)	0.36
Height (cm)	161 (8.8)	165 (9)	0.58
BSA (m^2)	1.71 (0.17)	1.74 (0.2)	0.87
Diabetes	8 (10)	0	
Hypertension	22 (27.8)	0	

AS aortic stenosis, *BSA* body surface area

Table 2 Echocardiographic variables and interleukin levels of AS patients and control groups

Variables mean(±SD)	AS *n* = 79	CONTROL *n* = 40	*p*
LV mass (gr/m^{2}BSA)	144 (45)	73 (8)	0.001
AoV area (cm^2)	0.67 (0.2)	2.9 (0.4)	0.001
Ao Mean Gr (mmHg)	59 (16)	2 (0.4)	0.001
Ao Max Vel (m/s)	4.8 (0.6)	0.9 (0.2)	0.001
Ao annulus (mm)	21 (2.6)	22 (3)	NS
LVEF (%)	52 (13)	67 (4.2)	0.001
PASP (mmHg)	36 (13)	22 (2.5)	0.001
TNFα (pg/cc)	0 (0-65)[a]	0 (0-30)[a]	0.08
IL-1 (pg/cc)	0 (0-36)[a]	0 (0-15.7)[a]	0.09
IL-6 (pg/cc)	0 (0-30)[a]	0 (0-10.7)[a]	0.1
ICAM-1 (pg/cc)	3610 (3060-6854)[a]	3555 (3199-3849)[a]	0.07

[a]median (IQR 25-75)
AS Aortic stenosis, *LV* left ventricle, *Ao* aortic, *V* valve, *Gr* gradient, *Max* maximum, *Vel* velocity, *Vol* volume, *LVEF* LV expulsion fraction, *PASP* pulmonary artery systolic pressure, *IQR* interquartile range

Table 3 Comparison between surgical stages in all type of prosthesis

Variable mean(±SD)	Preoperative	Early PostCx	LatePostCx	p
LV mass (gr/m^2 BSA)	144 (45)	131 (38)	115 (28)	0.001
AoV area (cm^2)	0.67 (0.2)	1.5 (0.25)	1.7 (0.15)	0.001
Ao Mean Gr (mmHg)	59 (16)	18 (8)	15 (5.5)	0.001
Ao Max Vel (m/s)	4.8 (0.6)	2.6 (0.6)	2.3 (0.4)	0.01
LVEF (%)	52 (13)	52 (12)	56 (9)	0.01
PASP (mmHg)	36 (13)	34 (9)	28 (5.4)	0.001
TNFα (pg/cc)	0 (0-65)[a]	0 (0-269)[a]	60 (0-204)[a]	0.001
IL-1 (pg/cc)	0 (0-36)[a]	0 (0-90)[a]	0 (0-65)[a]	0.01
IL-6 (pg/cc)	0 (0-30)[a]	18 (0-98)[a]	16 (0-80)[a]	0.048
ICAM-1 (pg/cc)	3610 (3060-6854)[a]	6306 (4984-7058)[a]	3782 (3138-6460)[a]	0.001

[a]median (IQR 25-75)
BSA body surface area, *LV* left ventricle, *Ao* aortic, *V* valve, *Vol* volume, *Gr* gradient, *Max* maximum, *Vel* velocity, *LVEF* LV expulsion fraction, *PASP* pulmonary artery systolic pressure, *IQR* interquartile range

inflammatory cytokines (TNFa: p = 0.001, IL-1: p = 0.05, IL-6 and ICAM-1 0003: p = 0.039) when compared with the control group. The post-hoc analysis of Friedman test showed that at the late postoperative stage, the cytokine concentrations were higher than before the surgery (TNF: p = 0.001, IL-1: p = 0.001, IL-6 and ICAM 0.034 1: p = 0.001). Comparing the late postoperative stage with the early postoperative stage, there were no significant decreases in the concentrations of TNF (p = 0.62) and IL-6 (p = 0.24), but a downward tendency in IL-1 (p = 0.08) and a significant decrease in ICAM-1 (0016). An inverse correlation was found between ICAM-1 and the maximum aortic velocity (r = −0.22, p = 0.05) and the mean aortic gradient (r = 0.25, p = 0.02).

When the population was divided according to the type of prosthesis implanted (biological or mechanical) no significant differences in the parameters of echocardiography were found in the early and late postsurgical stages, nor in the concentration of inflammatory mediators (Table 4).

Discussion

After surgery for aortic valve replacement, approximately 50% of the patients continued to have an active systemic inflammatory state that was even higher than the one present in the preoperative stage. Our data is consistent with that of previous studies where a significant proportion of subjects remained with high levels of inflammatory mediators [7]. We did not find significant differences in the concentration of cytokines in our population according to the type of valve implanted even when the valve prostheses are manufactured with different materials. Biological valvular prostheses are made from animal tissue that is subjected to a decellularization process and glutaraldehyde fixation in order to reduce their immunogenicity [19, 20]. The artificial valves are manufactured from various synthetic materials, including carbon graphite, pyrolytic carbon and titanium [21]. It has been reported that the residual phospholipids in biological tissue prosthesis could trigger an inflammatory response that might explain the high concentration of cytokines in the subjects who received this type of prosthesis [22]. It is also known that some types of implanted prostheses manufactured with titanium may trigger a chronic inflammatory response, which is not necessarily acute, and where the mechanism might be mediated by Toll receptors [23].

Titanium has high resistance to corrosion in biological environments and it is for this reason that it is the biomaterial of choice for manufacturing implant devices used in various sites in the body. The contact between the biological tissue and the metal promotes the formation of a stable layer of titanium oxide on the surface of the implant [24]. In tissues surrounding the biomaterial and in regional lymph nodes, titanium ions can be found. Despite its biocompatibility there are excellent studies that show that titanium is an allergen capable of triggering an immune response [25].

In experimental mouse models spread of titanium nanoparticles from the intra-articular injection site to the rest of the body has been found [26]. Similarly, neuroinflammation induced by titanium has been found in mice [27]. The results shown here agree with the previously published medical literature. There are studies on inflammation in patients that received mechanical and biological aortic prosthesis where no significant differences between the types of materials were found after an implantation time of 6 months to 2 years similar to those studied here. After some time of the implantation of the biological or mechanical valves, a deposit of extracellular matrix and calcification in the bioprosthetic tissue or the appearance of pannus in the mechanical valves begins, which correlates with prosthetic dysfunction [28].

Oxidative damage and lipid peroxidation was also observed in the synovium of patients with implanted devices which induced the expression of proinflammatory cytokines such as TNFa and IL-1 [29]. Other studies have found toxicity in cells of the heart tissue after exposure to titanium dioxide. There are also well known hiperesensibility reactions to titanium after implantation of this material in dentistry and orthopedics. There are also reports of systemic inflammation caused by titanium nanoparticles [15] and of

Table 4 Comparison of echocardiographic characteristics and biomarkers among the type of implanted prosthetic aortic valve

	Early Postsurgical			Late Postsurgical		
VARIABLES	Biologic	Mechanic	*p*	Biologic	Mechanic	*p*
mean (±SD)	*n* = 48	*n* = 31		*n* = 48	*n* = 31	
LV mass (gr/m^2 BSA)	132 (39)	129 (37)	0.75	117 (30)	112 (27)	0.45
AoV area (cm^2)	1.5 (0.24)	1.5 (0.26)	0.41	1.7 (0.14)	1.7 (0.16)	0.2
Ao Mean Gr (mmHg)	17 (7.9)	19 (8.2)	0.33	15 (5)	17 (6)	0.09
Ao Max Vel (m/s)	2.5 (0.62)	2.7 (0.59)	0.32	2.2 (0.46)	2.4 (0.44)	0.17
LVEF (%)	53 (11)	51 (14)	0.57	56 (8)	56 (11)	0.8
PASP (mmHg)	35 (8)	33 (9)	0.37	29 (5)	28 (6)	0.6
TNFα (pg/cc)	16 (0-264)[a]	0 (0-387)[a]	0.61	0 (60-252)[a]	0 (62-150)[a]	0.41
IL-1 (pg/cm^3)	9 (0-84)[a]	0 (0-146)[a]	0.7	0 (0-66)[a]	0 (0-65)[a]	0.64
IL-6 (pg/cc)	17 (0-106)[a]	44 (0-92)[a]	0.91	18 (0-78)[a]	0 (0-82)[a]	0.41
ICAM-1 (pg/cc)	6336 (5041-41,060)[a]	6066 (4534-6822)[a]	0.46	4287 (3161-43,985)[a]	3632 (3052-5986)[a]	0.24

[a]median (IQR 25-75)
BSA body surface area, *LV* left ventricle, *Ao* aortic, *V* valve, *Gr* gradient, *Max* maximum, *Vel* velocity, *Vol* volume, *LVEF* LV expulsion fraction, *PASP:* pulmonary artery systolic pressure, *IQR:* interquartile range

activation of the immune system with retarded hypersensitivity reactions.

This suggests that the sustained inflammatory response after replacement of the aortic valve may be due to an immune response to components of implanted prostheses such as titanium which is present in both biological and mechanical prosthesis. A striking finding of this study is that the increase in interleukins was similar in patients that had been implanted with any kind of valvular prosthesis. Therefore, we consider that it would be convenient to study the inflammatory response in other types of valvular prosthesis containing titanium and other metallic alloys such as nickel chromium.

The results of this study are consistent with previously published experience. There are studies of inflammation in biological and mechanical aortic prostheses in which no significant differences were found between both manufacturing materials with implantation time from 6 months to 2 years. Problems associated to the durability of the prosthesis and the appearance of dysfunction occurs in a similar rate in mechanical and biological valves. A requirement of another intervention is necessary in up to 60% of the implants for both types of prosthesis [30, 31].

The deposition of extracellular matrix and the formation of pannus leads to the dysfunction of mechanical prostheses. On the other hand, in the dysfunction of biological prostheses calcification and inflammation play an important role [32]. Recent studies have shown that the pathologic calcification in these prosthesis, might be regulated by inductor and inhibitor factors similar to those regulating bone mineralization. The pathophysiology of calcification of biological valves has been evaluated in-vitro and in animal models [33, 34]. For a better comprehension, several aspects should be analyzed such as the determinants of mineralization and their regulating mechanisms. Among these determinants, the metabolism of the host plays an important role. Other mechanical factors include the structure and the chemistry of the implant. Regarding regulation, the pre-treatment of these valves with high doses of glutaraldehide should be considered [35, 36].

Without taking into account the type of prosthesis, inflammation biomarkers have not shown a direct correlation with alterations in the echocardiographic parameters since high levels of cytokines can be found in normal valvular prosthesis and low levels have been found in subjects with dysfunctional ones [37]. This finding was also observed in the present series of patients.

The diversity of the damage mechanisms in each type of prosthesis has been widely discussed and is important when deciding the better therapeutic approach. The decision should take into account the inflammatory, degenerative or calcifying activity of each type of prosthesis. The determination of which type of valve should be used for each patient should include the medical and non-medical conditions, the knowledge of the mechanisms associated to the material to be implanted, and the risk/benefit ratio.

Since the durability of both types of prosthesis is similar, we believe factors such as the cost/effectivity, risk/benefit ratios and quality of life of the patient should be more deeply investigated to decide which type of valve should be implanted.

Conclusion

The inflammatory response caused by biological valvular prosthesis after 6 months of having been installed is similar to that produced mechanical prostheses. In addition, the similarity in the hemodynamic profiles registered with Doppler echocardiography in patients that had received any of the prosthesis allows us to conclude that both types of valve prostheses are recommended. The decision of the type of valve prosthesis implanted is related more to factors such as age of the patient or the suitability of the use of anticoagulant agents.

Abbreviations

AS: Aortic stenosis; ICAM: Intercellular adhesion molecules; IL-1: Interleukin 1; IL-6: Interleukin-6; LV: Left ventriculum; NSAIDs: Non-steroidal anti-inflammatory drugs; TNFa: Tumor necrosis factor alfa

Acknowledgments

We gratefully acknowledge the contribution of all patients.

Funding

This work was supported by a doctoral grant from the Instituto Nacional de Cardiología "Ignacio Chavez".

Authors' contribution

Each author made substantial contributions to the submitted work. Conception and design of study: MES, JVB, JS. Determination of cytokines were carried out by: RM RB. Optimization and initiation of echocardiography study JS, JVB. Performing acquisition of data: JS AR, Revision language VG and Analysis and interpretation of data: MES and JS Drafting the article and/or revising it critically for important intellectual and content: MES JS, JVB, RM, RB, VG and MES edited the revised version. All authors approved the final manuscript.

Competing interests

The authors declare that they have no competing interests.

Author details

[1]Immunology Department, Instituto Nacional de Cardiología "Ignacio Chávez", Juan Badiano número 1, Colonia Sección XVI, Delegación Tlalpan, Mexico CP 14080, Mexico. [2]Echocardiography Department, Instituto Nacional de Cardiología "Ignacio Chávez", Mexico, Mexico. [3]Investigation Department, Instituto Nacional de Cardiología "Ignacio Chávez", Mexico, Mexico. [4]Intensive care Department, Instituto Nacional de Cardiología "Ignacio Chavez", Mexico, Mexico. [5]Department of Pathology, Instituto Nacional de Cardiología "Ignacio Chavez", Mexico, Mexico. [6]Department of Physiology, Instituto Nacional de Cardiología "Ignacio Chávez", Mexico, Mexico.

References

1. Otto CM, Kuusisto J, Reichenback DD, Gown AM, O'Brien KD. Characterization of the early lesion of "degenerative" valvular aortic stenosis. Histological and immunohistochemical studies. Circulation. 1994;90:844–53.
2. Olsson M, Dalsgaard CJ, Haegerstrand A, Rosenqvist M, Ryden L, Nilsson J. Accumulation of T lymphocytes and expression of interleukin-2 receptors in nonrheumatic stenotic aortic valves. J Am Coll Cardiol. 1994;23:1162–70.
3. Mohler ERI, Gannon F, Reynolds C, Zimmerman R, Keane MG, Kaplan FS. Bone formation and inflammation in cardiac valves. Circulation. 2001;103:1522–8.
4. Shavelle DM, Katz R, Takasu J, et al. Soluble intercellular adhesion molecule-1 (sICAM-1) and aortic valve calcification in the multi-ethnic study of atherosclerosis (MESA)J Heart Valve Dis. 2008;17:388–95.
5. Galeone A, Brunetti G, Oranger A, et al. Aortic valvular interstitial cells apoptosis and calcification are mediated by TNF-related apoptosis-inducing ligand. Int J Cardiol. 2013;169:296–30.
6. Kaden JJ, Dempfle CE, Grobholz R, et al. Interleukin-1 beta promotes matrix metalloproteinase expression and cell proliferation in calcific aortic valve stenosis. Atherosclerosis. 2003;170:205–11.
7. Gerber I, Stewart R, Hammett C, et al. Effect of aortic valve replacement on C - reactive protein in nonrheumatic aortic stenosis. Am J Cardiol. 2003;92:1129–32.
8. Erdoes G, Lippuner C, Kocsis I, et al. Technical approach determines inflammatory response after surgical and trans catheter aortic valve replacement. PLoS ONE. 2015;10:e0143089. doi:10.1371/journal.pone.0143089.
9. Agmon Y, Khandheria BK, Jamil Tajik A, et al. Inflammation, infection, and aortic valve sclerosis; insights from the Olmsted County (Minnesota) population. Atherosclerosis. 2004;174:337–42.
10. Kastellanos SS, Toumpoulis IK, Aggeli C, et al. The role of sex and biochemical markers of inflammation in left ventricular remodeling, before and after surgery, in elderly patients with aortic valve stenosis. Hell J Cardiol. 2009;50:26–36.
11. Ramamurthi A, Pandian NG, Gangadharamurthy D, et al. The syndrome of degenerative calcific aortic stenosis: prevalence of multiple pathophysiologic disorders in association with valvular stenosis and their implications. Echocardiography. 2013;30:1–7.
12. Anderson JM, Rodriguez A, Chang DT. Foreign body reaction to biomaterials. Semin Immunol. 2008;20:86–100.
13. Barone A, Benktander J, Teneberg S, Breimer ME. Characterization of acid and non-acid glycosphingolipids of porcine heart valve cusps as potential immune targets in biological heart valve grafts. Xenotransplantation. 2014;21:510–22.
14. Vesely I. Heart valve tissue engineering. Circ Res. 2005;97:743–55.
15. Schanen B, Karakoti A, Drake D, et al. Exposure to titanium dioxide Nanomaterials provokes inflammation of an in vitro human immune construct. ACS Nano. 2009;3:2523–32.
16. Nishimura RA, Otto CM, Bonow RO, et al. Cardiology/American Heart Association task force on practice guidelines. 2014 AHA/ACC guideline for the management of patients with valvular heart disease: a report of the American College of Cardiology/American Heart Association task force on practice guidelines. J Am Coll Cardiol. 2014;63:e57–185.
17. Crowther JR. ELISA. Theory and practice. Methods Mol. Biol. 1995;42:1–218.
18. Lang RM, Badano LP, Mor-Avi V, et al. Recommendations for cardiac chamber quantification by echocardiography in adults: an update from the American Society of Echocardiography and the European Association of Cardiovascular Imaging. Am Soc Echocardiogr. 2015;28:1–39.
19. Lim HG, Kim SH, Choi SY, Kim YJ. Anticalcification effects of decellularization, solvent, and detoxification treatment for genipin and glutaraldehyde fixation of bovine pericardium. Eur J Cardiothorac Surg. 2012;41:383–90.
20. Lim HG, Kim GB, Jeong S, Kim YJ. Development of a next-generation tissue valve using a glutaraldehyde-fixed porcine aortic valve treated with decellularization, α-galactosidase, space filler, organic solvent and detoxification. Eur J Cardiothorac Surg. 2015;48:104–13.
21. Elizondo DR, Boland ED, Ambrus JR, Kurk JL. Mechanical cardiac valve prostheses: wear characteristics and magnitudes in three bileaflet valves. J Heart Valve Dis. 1996;1:S115–23.
22. Pathak CP, Adams AK, Simpson T, Phillips Jr RE, Moore MA. Treatment of bioprosthetic heart valve tissue with long chain alcohol solution to lower calcification potential. J Biomed Mater Res A. 2004;69:140–4.
23. Takagi M, Tamaki Y, Hasegawa H, et al. Toll-like receptors in the interface membrane around loosening total hip replacement implants. J Biomed Mater Res A. 2007;81:1017–26.
24. Kim YS, Shin SY, Moon SK, Yang SM. Surface properties correlated with the human gingival fibroblasts attachment on various materials for implantabutments: a multiple regression analysis. Acta Odontol Scand. 2015;73:38–47.
25. Weingart D, Steinemann S, Schilli W, et al. Titanium deposition in regional lymph nodes after insertion of titanium screw implants in maxillofacial region. Int J Oral Maxillofac Surg. 1994;23:450–2.
26. Wang JX, Fan YB, Gao Y, Hu QH, Wang TC. TiO2 nanoparticles translocation and potential toxicological effect in rats after intraarticular injection. Biomaterials. 2009;30:4590–600.

27. Ze Y, Sheng L, Zhao X, et al. TiO2 nanoparticles induced hippocampal neuroinflammation in mice. PLoS One. 2014;9:e92230.
28. Rodriguez Bacci M, Murad N, Breda JR, et al. Inflammatory biomarker kinetic after mechanical and biopsothetic valve replacement. Rev Assoc Med Bras. 2015;61:58–60.
29. Wang J, Ma J, Dong L, Hou Y, Jia X, Niu X, Fan Y. Effect of anatase TiO2 nanoparticles on the growth of RSC-364 rat synovial cell. J Nanosci Nanotechnol. 2013;13:3874–9.
30. Bloomfield P, Wheatley DJ, Prescott RJ, et al. Twelve yeaqr comparison of a Bjork-Shiley mechanical heart valve with porcine bioprostheses. N Engl J Med. 1991;324:573–9.
31. Hammermeister KE, Sethi GK, Henderson WG, et al. Outcomes 15 years after valve replacement with a mechanical versus a bioprosthetic valve: final report of the veterans affairs. Randomized Trial J Am Coll Cardiol. 2000;36:1152–8.
32. Schoen FJ, Hobson CE. Anatomic analysis of removed prosthetic heart valves: causes of failure of 33 mechanical valves and 58 bioprostheses. 1980 to 1983. Hum Pathol. 1985;16:549.
33. Schoen FJ, Golomb Levy RJ. Calcification of bio prosthetic heart valves: a perspective on models. J Heart Valve Dis. 1992;1:110–4.
34. Bernacca GM, Tobsanick G, Wheatley DJ, et al. Dynamic in-vitro calcification of porcine valve casps. J Heart Valve Dis. 1994;3:684–7.
35. Walley VM, Keon WJ, et al. Patterns of failure in Ionescu-Shiley bovine pericardial bioprosthetic valves. J Thorac Cardiovasc Surg. 1987;93:925–33.
36. Zilla P, Weissenstein C, Human P, Dower T, et al. High glutaraldehyde concentrations mitigate bioprosthetic root calcification in the sheep model. Ann Thorac Sur. 2000;70:2091–5.
37. Kastellanos SS, Toumpoulis IK, Aggeli C, et al. Time course of C reactive protein, tumor necrosis factor-alpha and Monocyte chemoattractant protein-1.Following the surgical treatment of patients with aoirtic valve stenosis. Hellenie J Cardiol. 2007;48:5–14.

5

Mapping strategy for multiple atrial tachyarrhythmias in a transplant heart

Qi Jin[1,2], Steen Pehrson[1], Peter Karl Jacobsen[1] and Xu Chen[1*]

Abstract

Background: Different atrial arrhythmias can coexist in the recipient and donor atria after heart transplantation.

Case presentation: We report an unusual case of a patient with three different types of atrial arrhythmia after heart transplantation: an atrial fibrillation in the recipient atria, and a cavotricuspid isthmus dependent atrial flutter and a focal atrial tachycardia in the donor atria. 3D electroanatomical mapping and ablation were guided by remote magnetic navigation (RMN). Atrial fibrillation continued in the recipient atria even after the donor heart was converted to sinus rhythm by ablation.

Conclusions: It is critical to understand the surgical anatomy of a bi-atrial anastomosis and its relevant electrical activation pattern before ablation. Appropriate electroanatomical mapping strategy with RMN can facilitate the successful ablation of post-transplant atrial arrhythmias.

Keywords: Atrial arrhythmias, Heart transplantation, Remote magnetic navigation

Background

Although the incidence of atrial arrhythmias after heart transplantation has been decreasing in the past decades, it has still ranged from 10 to 20 % in recent studies [1, 2]. Different supraventricular rhythms can coexist in the recipient atria and donor atria [3–5]. Better understanding of the surgical anatomy of a bi-atrial anastomosis and the electrical activation patterns by 3D electroanatomical mapping allowed us to identify the mechanisms of different atrial arrhythmias, and thus, approach their successful ablation [5]. Here, we reported an unusual case of a patient with three different types of atrial arrhythmia after heart transplantation: an atrial fibrillation (Af) in the recipient atria, and a cavotricuspid isthmus (CTI) dependent atrial flutter (AFL) and a focal atrial tachycardia (AT) in the donor atria.

Case presentation

A 65-year-old man underwent orthotopic heart transplantation with bi-atrial anastomosis due to dilated cardiomyopathy in 1995. The patient developed symptomatic persistent AFL that was refractory to anti-arrhythmic drugs for 6 months before the procedure. The surface ECG showed a positive P wave in lead V1 with P-P interval of 230 ms, and 2:1 relation of P/QRS. After the patient signed an informed consent, an electrophysiological study was performed to elucidate the mechanism of the AFL. A 6F steerable catheter (Inquiry, St Jude Medical, Inc., Irvine, CA, USA) and a 5F quadripolar catheter (Medtronic, Inc., Minneapolis, MN, USA) were positioned within the coronary sinus (CS) and at the apex of right ventricle via the left femoral vein, respectively. CS activation pattern and entrainment mapping from CS indicated the clinical AFL originating from right atria (RA) (Fig. 1C). An open irrigated magnetic ablation catheter (Navistar Thermocool-RMT, Biosense Webster Inc., Diamond Bar, CA, USA) was used to perform 3D RA electroanatomic mapping and ablation by the CARTO RMT system and the remote magnetic navigation system (RMN, Stereotaxis Inc., St. Louis, MO, USA). During the initial activation mapping, four different activation patterns coexisted in the donor and recipient atria: 1) AFL with a cycle length of 230 ms at the anterior and septal wall of the donor atria; 2) Af in the recipient atria; 3) scar tissue between the donor and recipient atria; 4) 2:1 conduction from AFL at the

* Correspondence: Xu.Chen@regionh.dk
[1]Department of Cardiology, The Heart Centre, Rigshospitalet, University of Copenhagen, Copenhagen, Denmark
Full list of author information is available at the end of the article

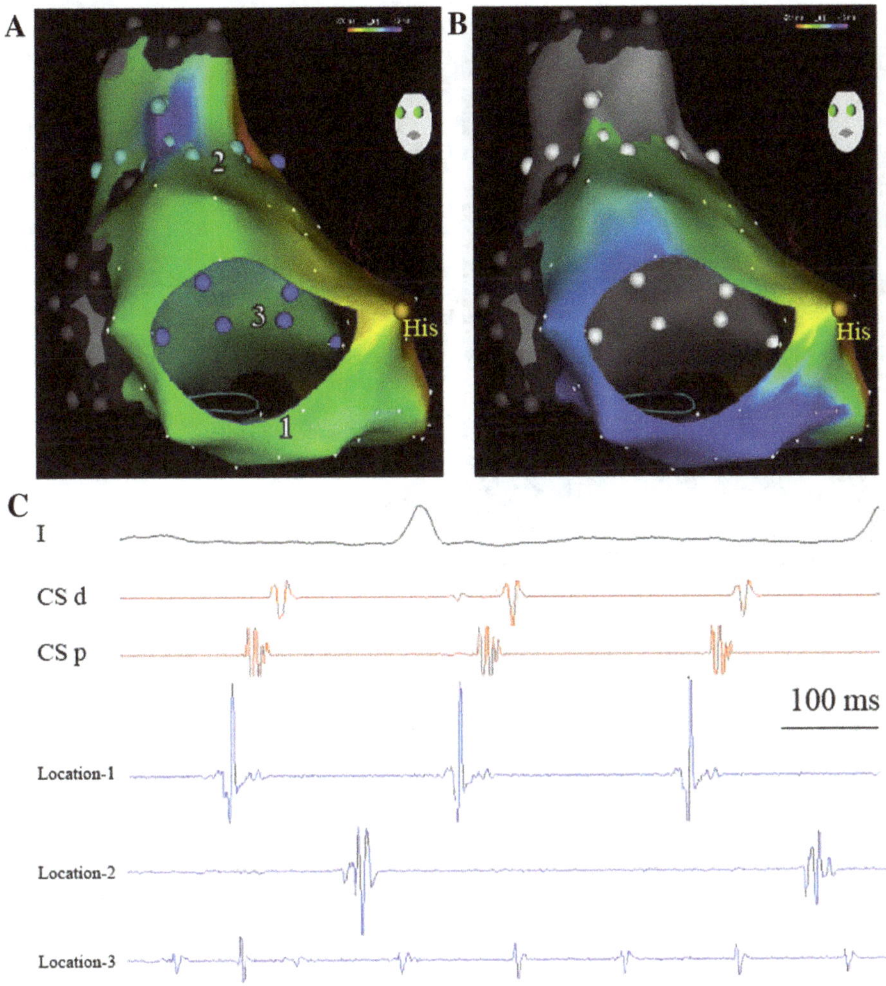

Fig. 1 Panel **A** shows a left anterior oblique (*LAO*) view on a CARTO activation map in the recipient and donor atria. The *red color* represents the earliest activation. The *light blue points* represent the sites of 2:1 conduction block at the border zone. The *blue points* represent the sites with Af activation in the recipient atria. The *grey points* represent scar areas. In Panel **B**, only activation mapping of the clinical AFL in the recipient RA is performed. The activations of Af and 2:1 conduction are both tagged only by location (*white points*). A counterclockwise CTI-dependent AFL is present in this modified activation map. Panel **C** shows the different activation electrograms of the ablation catheter at the different sites. Location *1* is at six clock relative to the TA. Location *2* and *3* are at the anterior-superior wall and posterior-inferior wall respectively

zone between AFL area and scar area (Fig. 1). An activation map containing of the donor and recipient atria led to the complexity of understanding the mechanism of the clinical AFL (Fig. 1A). Thus, we performed the activation mapping only focusing on the AFL in the recipient RA by defining all other areas as scar or location only. A counterclockwise CTI-dependent AFL in the donor atria appeared in the modified activation map (Fig. 1B). Linear ablation guided by RMN was performed at the inferior wall between the atrial suture and the tricuspid annulus (TA). After termination of AFL, an AT with the cycle length of 310 ms was induced in the donor atria by atrial stimulation. A re-map showed a focal AT, which was converted to sinus rhythm by ablation at the focal existence at the border zone between recipient and donor atria (Fig. 2). Af in the recipient atria still continued, indicating that the two atria were electrically dissociated (Fig. 2). The fluoroscopy time was 3 min. No complications occurred during the procedure.

Discussion

Post-transplant atrial arrhythmias were most commonly due to atrial macro-reentry including CTI-dependent and scar-related circuits [1, 6, 7]. Focal AT originating in low-voltage or border zones adjacent to the bi-atrial anastomosis was another possible mechanism [8]. In this case, these two different mechanisms of atrial arrhythmias were detected in the donor atria. Similar to typical AFL in non-transplanted patients, the reentrant circuit of the clinical AFL in this case was around the TA (Fig. 1B). Differently, the ablation line was designed to be relatively narrow for the active component of the

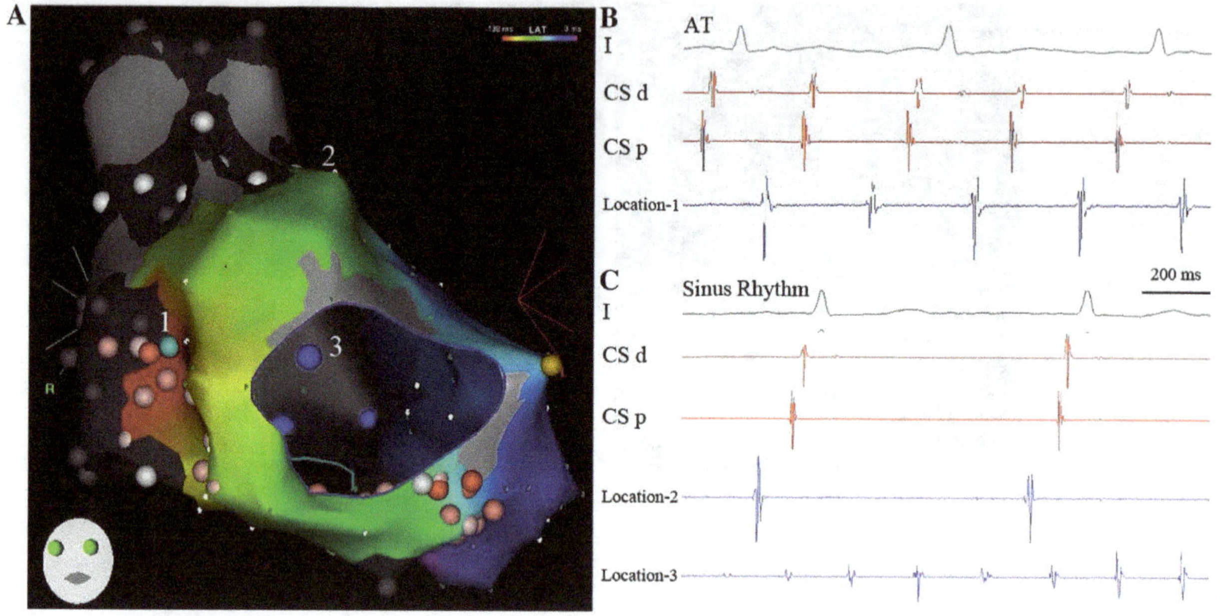

Fig. 2 In Panels **A** and **B**, activation mapping from the donor atria indicates an origin of a focal *AT* at the suture line (border zone, location *1*). The *red color* represents the earliest activation. At this site, radiofrequency current is applied and terminates *AT*. *Red* and *pink points* indicate the ablation areas. The color's strength represents the duration of ablation delivery. Panel **C** shows the patient's sinus rhythm with a cycle length of 800 ms. The ablation catheter at location *2* (anterior-superior wall of the donor atrium) indicates *sinus rhythm*. Af at the ablation catheter in the recipient atria (*blue point*, location *3*) is not changed, but the two atria are electrically dissociated

isthmus from the TA to the atrial suture line rather than to the inferior vena cava (Fig. 2). Radiofrequency energy can achieve isthmus block. An ectopic focus at the border zone induced a non-clinical AT in the donor atria, which was also successfully ablated. This case indicated the importance for the operator to realize that multiple electrical mechanisms can coexist in a transplant heart with bi-atrial anastomosis.

Mapping strategy in the evaluation of atrial arrhythmias in a transplant heart is a key factor to achieve successful ablation [3]. Activation mapping requires generation of complete and dense maps and correct annotation of electrograms may be challenging, especially when activation of the entire atria continued more than the cycle length of the tachycardia [9]. As described above in this case, coexisting donor AFL, recipient Af and the zone with 2:1 AFL conduction made the initial activation mapping strategy of the entire atria impossible to explore the mechanism of the clinical AFL (Fig. 1A). Better understanding the surgical anatomy of bi-atrial anastomosis and its possible electrical correlates helped us to adjust the activation mapping strategy, and thus, elucidate the real mechanism.

Of note, this case was performed by RMN. Mapping and ablation using RMN may offer advantages during some complex procedures compared to manual techniques [10]. RMN systems can help the operator to manipulate the catheter to map the critical regions with high density and complete the designed ablation line in a transplant heart with relatively shorter fluoroscopy time (3 min in this case).

Many factors could be related to atrial tachyarrhythmias after heart transplantation. One of limitations in this study is that we cannot rule out the role of previous transplant rejection or chronic vasculopathy because we did not perform the biological test before or after the ablation procedure.

Conclusions

To our knowledge, it's the first report for a heart transplant patient in whom these two different mechanisms of atrial arrhythmias were observed in the donor atria. Appropriate electroanatomical mapping strategy with RMN may facilitate successful catheter ablation for the multiple atrial tachyarrhythmias in a transplant heart.

Consent

Written informed consent was obtained from the patient for publication of this case report and any accompanying images. A copy of the written consent is available for review by the Editor of this journal.

Abbreviations

Af: Atrial fibrillation; AFL: Atrial flutter; AT: Atrial tachycardia; CTI: Cavotricuspid isthmus; TA: Tricuspid annulus; RMN: Remote magnetic navigation.

Competing interests

The authors declare that they have no competing interests.

Authors' contributions

QJ drafted the manuscript and acquired the images. PS and JP interpreted the electrical mechanism by surface ECG and intra-cardiac electrical correlates. XC performed the procedure and revised the manuscript. All authors read and approved the final manuscript.

Author details

[1]Department of Cardiology, The Heart Centre, Rigshospitalet, University of Copenhagen, Copenhagen, Denmark. [2]Department of Cardiology, Shanghai Ruijin Hospital, Shanghai Jiao Tong University School of Medicine, Shanghai, China.

References

1. Vaseghi M, Boyle NG, Kedia R, Patel JK, Cesario DA, Wiener I, et al. Supraventricular tachycardia after orthotopic cardiac transplantation. J Am Coll Cardiol. 2008;51:2241–9.
2. Dasari TW, Pavlovic-Surjancev B, Patel N, Williams AA, Ezidinma P, Rupani A, et al. Incidence, risk factors, and clinical outcomes of atrial fibrillation and atrial flutter after heart transplantation. Am J Cardiol. 2010;106:737–41.
3. Frogner F, Arya A, Piorkowski C, Hindricks G. Two concomitant arrhythmias in atransplanted heart. Clin Res Cardiol. 2009;98:571–2.
4. D'Alto M, Lord S, Bourke J, Santarpia G, Sarubbi B, Russo MG, et al. Orthotopic heart transplantation: two parts of the heart with two different arrhythmias. J Cardiovasc Med. 2011;12:193–6.
5. Laksman ZW, Skanes AC, Klein GJ, Manlucu J. Dual atrial tachycardia in a transplant heart: when is "in" really "out"? J Cardiovasc Electrophysiol. 2013;24:1428–31.
6. Nof E, Stevenson WG, Epstein LM, Tedrow UB, Koplan BA. Catheter ablation of atrial arrhythmias after cardiac transplantation: findings at ep study utility of 3-d mapping and outcomes. J Cardiovasc Electrophysiol. 2013;24:498–502.
7. Rodriguez-Entem F, Exposito V, Gonzalez-Enriquez S, Garcia-Camarero T, Olalla J. Atrial flutter after heart transplantation: mechanism and catheter ablation. Transplant Proc. 2010;42:2697–701.
8. Elsik M, Teh A, Ling LH, Virdee M, Parameshwar J, Fynn SP, et al. Supraventricular arrhythmias late after orthotopic cardiac transplantation: electrocardiographic and electrophysiological characterization and radiofrequency ablation. Europace. 2012;14:1498–505.
9. Roten L, Tanner H, Goy JJ, Delacretaz E. Three-dimensional electroanatomic entrainment map in atypical atrial flutter late after heart transplantation. Europace. 2010;12:290–2.
10. Akca F, Onsesveren I, Jordaens L, Szili-Torok T. Safety and efficacy of the remote magnetic navigation for ablation of ventricular tachycardias–a systematic review. J Interv Card Electrophysiol. 2012;34:65–71.

Efficacy and safety of transcatheter aortic valve replacement in aortic stenosis patients at low to moderate surgical risk

Ahmed Elmaraezy[1,2], Ammar Ismail[1,2], Abdelrahman Ibrahim Abushouk[2,3], Moutaz Eltoomy[4], Soha Saad[5], Ahmed Negida[6], Osama Mahmoud Abdelaty[7], Ahmed Ramadan Abdallah[8], Ahmed Magdy Aboelfotoh[8], Hossam Mahmoud Hassan[9], Aya Gamal Elmaraezy[10], Mahmoud Morsi[10], Farah Althaher[11], Moath Althaher[11] and Ammar M. AlSafadi[12*]

Abstract

Background: Recently, transcatheter aortic valve replacement (TAVR) has become the procedure of choice in high surgical risk patients with aortic stenosis (AS). However, its value is still debated in operable AS cases. We performed this meta-analysis to compare the safety and efficacy of TAVR to surgical aortic valve replacement (SAVR) in low-to-moderate surgical risk patients with AS.

Methods: A systematic search of five authentic databases retrieved 11 eligible studies (20,056 patients). Relevant Data were pooled as risk ratios (RRs) or standardized mean differences (SMD), with their 95% confidence interval, using Comprehensive Meta-Analysis and RevMan software for windows.

Results: At one-year of follow-up, the pooled effect-estimates showed no significant difference between TAVR and SAVR groups in terms of all-cause mortality (RR 1.02, 95% CI [0.83, 1.26], stroke (RR 0.83, 95%CI [0.56, 1.21]), myocardial infarction (RR 0.82, 95% CI [0.57, 1.19]), and length of hospital stay (SMD -0.04, 95% CI [−0.34, 0.26]). The incidence of major bleeding (RR 0.45, 95% CI [0.24, 0.86]) and acute kidney injury (RR 0.52, 95% CI [0.30, 0.88]) was significantly lower in the TAVR group, compared to the SAVR group. However, TAVR was associated with a higher risk of permanent pacemaker implantation (RR 2.57, 95% CI [1.36, 4.86]), vascular-access complications at 1 year (RR 1.99, 95%CI [1.04, 3. 80]), and paravalvular aortic regurgitation at 30 days (RR 3.90, 95% CI [1.25, 12.12]), compared to SAVR.

Conclusions: Due to the comparable mortality rates in SAVR and TAVR groups and the lower risk of life-threatening complications in the TAVR group, TAVR can be an acceptable alternative to SAVR in low-to-moderate risk patients with AS. However, larger trials with longer follow-up periods are required to compare the long-term outcomes of both techniques.

Keywords: Aortic stenosis, Aortic valve replacement, Meta-analysis, Surgical, Transcatheter

* Correspondence: Ammar.m.alsafadi@gmail.com
[12]Faculty of Medicine, Damascus University, Damascus, Syria
Full list of author information is available at the end of the article

Background

Aortic stenosis (AS) is the most prevalent valvular heart disease in the elderly [1]. An epidemiological study estimated that more than one in eight individuals over the age of 75 years has a moderate to severe AS [2]. Another meta-analysis revealed that the pooled prevalence of the disease among the elderly is 12.4% and estimated that there are more than 291,000 candidates for aortic valve replacement in North America and Europe [3].

Although surgery is still considered the intervention of choice in operable cases of severe AS, transcatheter aortic valve replacement (TAVR) is continuously gaining ground in these lower risk groups [4]. This growing trend is justified by multiple reasons including the remarkable technical advances in the valve replacement procedure which now allows for easy repositioning and removal, the minimally invasive approach that permits performing under local anesthesia [5], as well as the fact that TAVR is a common patient preference among surgically fit cases due to its shorter hospital stay, lower risk of bleeding and mild post-interventional symptoms [6].

Nevertheless, the increasing TAVR drift towards lower surgical risk strata lacks a solid ground of evidence and does not adhere to the well-established guidelines [7]. In fact, only four randomized controlled trials (RCTs) addressed this issue including the PARTNER-II, US pivotal, NOTION, and the prematurely-terminated STACATTO trial [8–11]. Given this paucity of RCTs, observational studies are rendered a legitimate strategy to assess the comparative effectiveness of both procedures in operable patients [12].

We aimed to synthesize level I evidence from published randomized trials and observational studies as to whether or not TAVR could be compared to surgery in terms of efficacy and safety outcomes in low-to-moderate surgical risk patients with AS.

Methods

We performed this meta-analysis in accordance to the guidelines of the Cochrane handbook for systematic reviews of interventions [13] and the Preferred Reporting Items for Systematic Reviews and Meta-analyses (PRISMA statement guidelines) [14].

Literature search strategy

We performed a comprehensive search of five authentic databases (PubMed, Scopus, Web of science, Embase, and Cochrane Central Register of Controlled Trials (CENTRAL)) using the following strategy: [Aortic Stenosis OR Aortic Valve Stenosis OR Aortic Valve Replacement OR Aortic Valve Implantation OR Heart Valve Replacement AND Transcatheter OR TAVR OR Transfemoral OR Transapical AND Surgical Aortic Valve Replacement OR SAVR OR Surgical AVR AND Low Risk OR Moderate Risk OR Intermediate Risk]. There was no restriction by the language of the study or year of publication. We screened the bibliography of eligible articles for any relevant studies and the clinical trial registry (Clinicaltrials.gov) for any ongoing or unpublished studies.

Eligibility criteria and study selection

We included both RCTs and non-randomized studies (prospective and retrospective observational studies) if they matched the following criteria: (1) Population: Patients with severe AS and a low-to-moderate surgical risk [defined as a logistic Euroscore for cardiac operative risk evaluation (≤ 20%) or a Society of Thoracic Surgeons (STS) score below 8%], (2) Intervention: Transcatheter Aortic Valve Replacement (TAVR: through all routes including transfemoral, transapical, and transaxillary routes), (3) Comparator: Surgical Aortic Valve Replacement (SAVR), and (4) Outcomes: Studies that at least included one efficacy (mortality) or safety outcome.

We excluded case reports, case series, and studies that exclusively enrolled patients with high surgical risk. Eligibility screening was conducted in a two step-wise manner (title/abstract screening and full-text screening). Each step was conducted by three reviewers and consensus was obtained upon consulting a fourth reviewer (Abushouk AI).

Data extraction

Three independent authors extracted the relevant data and another reviewer (Elmaraezy A) resolved disagreements. The extracted data included (1) Study year and design, (2) Baseline characteristics of enrolled patients, and (3) Outcomes including the length of hospital stay and the incidence of all-Cause mortality (efficacy outcome), major adverse cardiovascular and cerebrovascular events (MAACE), stroke, myocardial infarction (MI), major life-threatening bleeding, acute kidney injury (AKI), vascular access complications (VAC), paravalvular aortic regurgitation (AR), and permanent pacemaker implantation (PPI).

Risk of bias assessment

Three independent reviewers used the Cochrane risk of bias tool, clearly described in (chapter 8.5) of the Cochrane handbook for systematic reviews of interventions 5.1.0 [13], to assess the risk of bias within included RCTs. For cohort and case-control studies, we used the Newcastle Ottawa scale (NOS) for detection of bias in non-randomized studies [15]. This tool assesses the risk of bias in observational studies based on reporting of three important domains: selection of the study subjects, comparability of groups regarding demographic characteristics and important potential confounders, and ascertainment of the prespecified outcome. Whenever an outcome included 10 or more studies, we assessed for publication bias, using the Egger's test [16].

Data synthesis

Dichotomous data for efficacy and safety outcomes were pooled as risk ratios (RRs), using the Mantel-Haenszel method. Data for hospital stay duration were pooled as a standardized mean difference (SMD), using the Inverse Variance (I-V) method. All statistical analyses in this study were performed using the Comprehensive Meta-Analysis (Biostat Inc) and RevMan (version 5.3) software for windows. Heterogeneity was assessed using the Chi-Square test and its extent was measured using the I-Square test. When a significant heterogeneity was found, the analysis was conducted under the random-effects model. In each included outcome, we performed a subgroup analysis by the endpoint of assessment (30 days, 1, 2, or 3 years after the procedure).

Results

Literature search results

Our literature search retrieved 4587 studies. Of them, 27 full text articles were assessed for eligibility. Finally, 11 studies (reported in 15 published articles) [7–12, 17–25] were included in this meta-analysis [20,056 Patients]. The flow of study selection is shown in our PRISMA flow diagram (Fig. 1). Four eligible studies were RCTs, while the remaining seven studies included five prospective cohort and two retrospective studies. The summary of included studies and baseline characteristics of enrolled patients are shown in Table 1 and Table 2, respectively.

Risk of bias in included studies

The risk of bias in included RCTs ranged from low to moderate as assessed by the Cochrane Risk of Bias tool. Authors' judgements on the risk of bias in included RCTs are illustrated in Additional file 1. The risk of bias in included observational studies was low as assessed by the Newcastle Ottawa scale (mean = 8 out of 9 asterisks).

Safety and efficacy outcomes

All-cause mortality

The overall RR did not favor either of the two groups in terms of in-hospital mortality (RR 1.11, 95% CI [0.63 to 1.95]), 30-day morality (RR 0.95, 95% CI [0.74 to 1.21]), 1-year mortality (RR 1.02, 95% CI [0.83 to 1.26]), or 2-year mortality (RR 0.91, 95% CI [0.76 to 1.08]). These findings were consistent with another scenario in which we considered pooling of data from RCTs only. The RR of 3-year mortality was reported only by the OBSERVENT study, which showed a significantly higher risk of mortality in the TAVR group than the SAVR group (RR 1.63, 95% CI [1.21 to 2.19]) (Fig. 2).

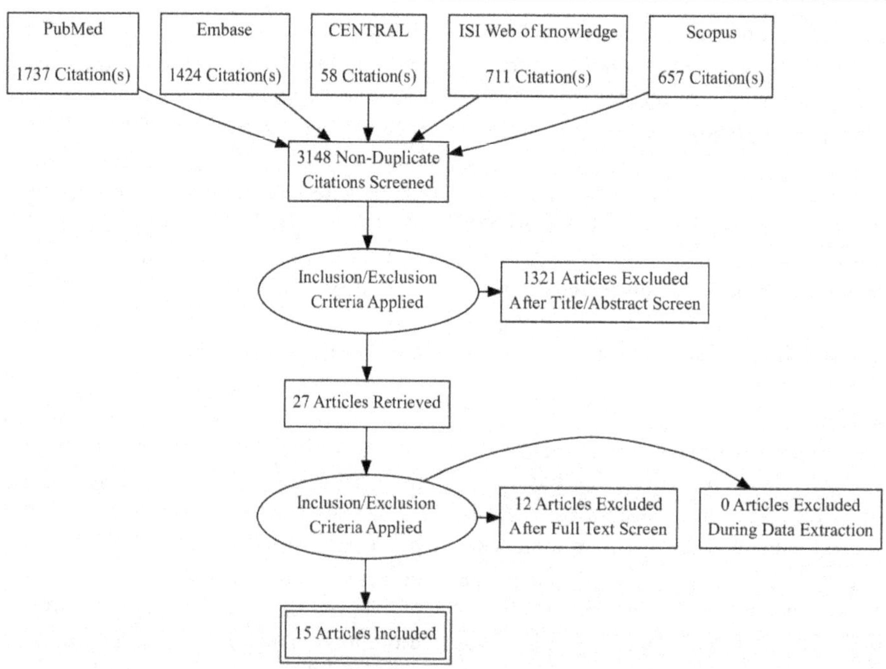

Fig. 1 PRISMA Flow Diagram of literature search and study selection process

Table 1 shows a summary of the design and main findings of included studies

Study ID	Study Design	Population	Valve for TAVR	Follow up	Main Finding
I. Randomized Controlled Trials					
PARTNER II Trial [8]	Prospective, multicenter, randomized trials	Intermediate surgical risk patients who had senile degenerative aortic valve stenosis with Echo-derived criteria: mean gradient >40 mmHg or jet velocity greater than 4.0 m/s and an initial aortic valve area of <0.8 cm2.	Edwards SAPIEN XT	2 years	SAVR and TAVR procedures were similar in the rate of mortality and disabling stroke. However, TAVR was associated with lower rates of bleeding, AKI, and new-onset AF, while SAVR was associated with lower rates of VAC and paravalvular AR.
STACATTO Trial [11]	Prospective, randomized trial	Operable patients, older than 75 years old with sever aortic stenosis (valve area < 1 cm^2)	Edwards SAPIEN	3 months	Despite the premature termination, the authors concluded that transapical TAVR has more complications and lower success rates than SAVR in low risk patients.
NOTION Trial [9]	Multicenter, randomized, superiority trial	Patients > 70 years old with severe aortic valve stenosis and no significant coronary artery disease	CoreValve	2 years	After 2 years of follow up, the rates of mortality, stroke, and myocardial infarction were similar in both SAVR and TAVR groups.
US PIVOTAL Trial [10]	Multicenter, randomized, non-inferiority trial	Intermediate surgical risk patients with severe aortic stenosis and an aortic valve Area ≤ 0.8 cm^2 or an AVA index ≤0.5 cm2/m^2	CoreValve	2 years	The rates of 2-year death or stroke were lower in the TAVR group, compared to the SAVR group.
II. Observational (Prospective and Retrospective Studies)					
OBSERVENT Study [12]	Observational, prospective, multicenter cohort study	Adult patients with a diagnosis of severe AS and low surgical risk	Edwards SAPIEN XT, CoreValve	3 years	SAVR patients are at a higher risk of blood transfusion, while TAVR patients have a higher risk of VAC, paravalvular AR, and atrioventricular block.
Osnabrugge et al. 2012 [21]	Prospective, Cohort study	Patient with severe aortic stenosis and an intermediate surgical risk	CoreValve	1 year	At 1 year follow up, the costs of TAVR were significantly higher than SAVR in intermediate risk patients owing to the higher cost of the transcatheter valve.
Piazza et al. 2013 [22]	Prospective, cohort study	Intermediate surgical risk patients with severe aortic stenosis and an aortic valvular orifice area of <1.0 cm^2	CoreValve	1 year	In intermediate risk patients, TAVR and SAVR had comparable rates of in-hospital and 30-day mortality, with more benefit of TAVR in women
Schymik et al. 2015 [24]	Prospective, cohort study	Patients ≥75 years old with sever aortic stenosis and less than high surgical risk	Edwards SAPIEN XT, CoreValve	3 years	Both groups had comparable mortality rates. However, the rates of VAC, PPI, and AR were higher in the TAVR group and the risk of major bleeding was higher in the SAVR group.
Castrodeza et al. 2016 [18]	Prospective cohort study	Patients with severe aortic stenosis and low to intermediate surgical risk	Edwards SAPIEN XT, CoreValve	1 year	In intermediate risk patients, TAVR is feasible and has comparable mortality and stroke rates to SAVR.
Latib et al. 2012 [19]	Case control study	Intermediate surgical risk patients with severe symptomatic aortic stenosis.	Edwards SAPIEN XT, CoreValve	1 year	The rates of mortality and stroke were comparable in both groups; however, transfemoral TAVR group had a higher incidence of VAC and SAVR group had a higher incidence of AKI.
Möllmann et al. 2016 [20]	Retrospective cohort study	Patients with severe aortic stenosis at low, intermediate, and high surgical risk.	–	1 year	Compared to SAVR, transfemoral TAVR has similar in-hospital mortality in low risk patients and lower in-hospital mortality in intermediate-to-high risk patients.

Abbreviations: ***AF*** **Atrial fibrillation,** ***AKI*** **Acute kidney injury,** ***AR*** **Aortic regurgitation,** ***AVA*** **Aortic valve area,** ***PPI*** **Permanent pacemaker implantation,** ***SAVR*** **Surgical aortic valve replacement,** ***TAVR*** **Transcatheter aortic valve replacement,** ***VAC*** **Vascular access complications**

Table 2 shows baseline characteristics of enrolled patients in included studies

Study ID	Arm	Demographics			Surgical Risk		Comorbidities					
		Sample Size	Age	Male sex (%)	EURO score	STS score	CAD	Previous PCI	HTN	Cerebral Vascular Disease	Peripheral Vascular Disease	Diabetes Mellitus
I. Randomized Controlled Trials												
PARTNER II trial [8]	SAVR	1021	81.7 ± 6.7	560 (54.8)	NA	5.8 ± 1.9	679 (66.5)	282 (27.6)	NA	317 (31)	336 (32.9)	349 (34.2)
	TAVR	1011	81.5 ± 6.7	548 (54.2)	NA	5.8 ± 2.1	700 (69.2)	274 (27.1)	NA	325 (32.1)	282 (27.9)	381 (37.7)
STACATTO trial [11]	SAVR	36	82 ± 4.4	12 (33.3)	10.3 ± 5.8	3.4 ± 1.2	NA	NA	NA	1 (2.8)	3 (8.3)	3 (8.3)
	TAVR-TA	34	80 ± 3.6	9 (26.5)	9.4 ± 3.9	3.1 ± 1.5	NA	NA	NA	1 (2.9)	2 (5.9)	1 (2.9)
NOTION trial [9]	SAVR	135	79 ± 4.7	71 (52.6)	8.9 ± 5.5	3.1 ± 1.7	6 (4.4)	12 (8.9)	103 (76.3)	22 (16.3)	9 (6.7)	28 (20.7)
	TAVR	145	79.2 ± 4.9	78 (53.8)	8.4 ± 4	2.9 ± 1.6	8 (5.5)	11 (7.6)	103 (71)	24 (16.6)	6 (4.1)	26 (17.9)
US PIVOTAL trial [10]	SAVR	359	83.3 ± 6.3	188 (52.4)	18.8 ± 13.2	7.5 ± 3.3	273 (76)	135 (37.6)	345 (96.1)	NA	150 (42)	162 (45.1)
	TAVR	391	83.2 ± 7.1	207 (52.9)	17.7 ± 13	7.3 ± 3.0	295 (75.4)	134 (34.3)	372 (95.1)	NA	159 (41)	136 (34.8)
II. Observational (Prospective and Retrospective Studies)												
OBSERVENT Study [12]	SAVR	1383	72 ± 9	768 (55.5)	6.1 ± 7.1	NA	NA	95 (6.8)	NA	NA	176 (12.7)	346 (25)
	TAVR-TA	602	82 ± 6	243 (40.4)	15.2 ± 14.3	NA	NA	151 (25.1)	NA	NA	114 (18.9)	145 (24.1)
	TAVR-TF	123	82 ± 7	54 (43.9)	14.7 ± 11.3	NA	NA	31 (25.2)	NA	NA	47 (38.2)	34 (27.6)
Osnabrugge et al. 2012 [21]	SAVR	42[a]	79.3 ± 5.5	22 (52.4)	12.5 ± 6.4	NA	20 (47.6)	NA	NA	2 (4.8)	4 (9.5)	8 (19)
	TAVR	42[a]	78.8 ± 6.6	21 (50)	12.9 ± 6.8	NA	20 (47.6)	NA	NA	2 (4.8)	3 (7.1)	11 (26.2)
Piazza et al. 2013 [22]	SAVR	405	79.4 ± 4.8	179 (44.1)	17.5 ± 12.1	NA	96 (57.8)	NA	286 (81.7)	30 (7.4)	41 (10.1)	98 (25.7)
	TAVR	405	79.9 ± 6	175 (43.2)	17.1 ± 10.7	NA	94 (56.6)	NA	301 (86)	40 (9.9)	33 (8.2)	111 (27.4)
Schymik et al. 2015 [24]	SAVR	216	78.2 ± 4.6	51.4%	8.8 ± 2.8	NA	48.1%	NA	NA	NA	6.9%	NA
	TAVR	216	78.3 ± 5.2	46.3%	8.7 ± 2.7	NA	48.1%	NA	NA	NA	5.1%	NA
Castrodeza et al. 2016 [18]	SAVR	70	78 ± 5.6	34 (48.6)	9.3 ± 3.9	4.3 ± 2.4	NA	NA	51 (72.9)	NA	NA	18 (25.7%)
	TAVR	70	79 ± 7.7	36 (51.4)	9.4 ± 3.8	4.6 ± 2.1	NA	NA	45 (64.3)	NA	NA	26 (37.1%)
Latib et al. 2012 [19]	SAVR	111	79.4 ± 3	49 (44.1)	24.4 ± 13.4	4.6 ± 2.6	51 (45.9)	NA	77 (69.4)	20 (18)	38 (34.2)	24 (21.6)
	TAVR	111	80.5 ± 6.9	49 (44.1)	23.2 ± 15.1	4.6 ± 2.3	44 (39.6)	NA	78 (70.3)	16 (14.4)	29 (26.1)	21 (18.9)
Möllmann et al. 2016 [20]	SAVR	9899	68.1 ± 11	60.4%	NA	NA	21.1%	8.9%	NA	5%	4.5%	24.1%
	TAVR-TF	7620	81.2 ± 6.1	44.5%	NA	NA	55%	29.6%	NA	7.8%	14.4%	33.6%
	TAVR-TA	2821	80.3 ± 6.6	52.4%	NA	NA	60.8%	30.4%	NA	9.2%	32%	33.4%

[a]Following propensity score matching. The presented data are either frequency (%) or mean ± standard deviation, unless stated otherwise

Abbreviations: *CAD* Coronary artery disease, *HTN* Hypertension, *NA* Not Available, *PCI* Percutaneous coronary intervention, *SAVR* Surgical aortic valve replacement, *STS* Society of Thoracic Surgeons, *TAVR* Transcatheter aortic valve replacement, *TA* Trans-Apical, *TF* Trans-Femoral

MACCE

The pooled analysis of two RCTs, reporting 1- and 2-year MACCE, favored the TAVR group over the SAVR group (1-year MACCE: RR 0.77, 95% CI [0.61 to 0.98]; and 2-year MACCE: RR 0.79, 95% CI [0.65 to 0.95]). The 30-day MACCE was reported by the US pivotal study only, which showed comparable rates of MACCE between the two groups (RR 0.74, 95% CI [0.47 to 1.18]). Similarly, the 3-year MACCE was reported only by the OBSERVENT study, which favored the SAVR over TAVR (RR 1.70, 95% CI [1.31 to 2.21]) in this regard (Fig. 3).

Stroke

The overall RR did not favor either of the two groups in terms of stroke incidence within 30 days (RR 0.99, 95% CI [0.73 to 1.35]), 1 year (RR 0.83, 95% CI [0.56 to 1.21]), or 2 years (RR 0.88, 95% CI [0.63 to 1.23]) after the procedure. The OBSERVENT study reported a higher 3-year

Study or Subgroup	TAVR Events	TAVR Total	SAVR Events	SAVR Total	Weight	Risk Ratio M-H, Random, 95% CI
1.1.1 In-hospital mortality						
Castrodeza et al. 2016 - Full cohort - 30 days	7	103	9	259	20.2%	1.96 [0.75, 5.11]
Mollman et al. 2016	198	5204	204	7513	46.1%	1.40 [1.16, 1.70]
NOTION - 30 days	1	142	2	134	5.0%	0.47 [0.04, 5.14]
Observant - 30 days	13	650	22	650	28.7%	0.59 [0.30, 1.16]
Subtotal (95% CI)		**6099**		**8556**	**100.0%**	**1.11 [0.63, 1.95]**
Total events	219		237			
Heterogeneity: Tau² = 0.17; Chi² = 7.15, df = 3 (P = 0.07); I² = 58%						
Test for overall effect: Z = 0.35 (P = 0.72)						
1.1.2 30-day mortality						
Latib et al. 2012 - propenity matched - 30 days	2	111	2	111	1.6%	1.00 [0.14, 6.97]
NOTION - 30 days	3	142	5	134	3.0%	0.57 [0.14, 2.32]
Observant - 30 days	20	650	24	650	17.5%	0.83 [0.47, 1.49]
Osnabrugge et al. 2012 - 30 days	2	42	3	42	2.0%	0.67 [0.12, 3.79]
PARTNER II - 30 days	39	1011	41	1021	32.2%	0.96 [0.63, 1.48]
Piazza et al. 2013 - 30 days	33	405	25	405	23.7%	1.32 [0.80, 2.18]
Schymik 2015 - Full cohort - 30 days	7	419	17	722	7.8%	0.71 [0.30, 1.70]
STACATTO	2	34	0	36	0.7%	5.29 [0.26, 106.27]
US Pivotal - 30 days	13	390	16	357	11.6%	0.74 [0.36, 1.52]
Subtotal (95% CI)		**3204**		**3478**	**100.0%**	**0.95 [0.74, 1.21]**
Total events	121		133			
Heterogeneity: Tau² = 0.00; Chi² = 4.66, df = 8 (P = 0.79); I² = 0%						
Test for overall effect: Z = 0.43 (P = 0.66)						
1.1.3 1 year mortality						
Castrodeza et al. 2016 - Full cohort - 1 year	13	103	12	259	6.2%	2.72 [1.29, 5.77]
Latib et al. 2012 - propenity matched - 1 year	7	111	9	111	4.2%	0.78 [0.30, 2.02]
NOTION - 1 year	7	142	10	134	4.3%	0.66 [0.26, 1.69]
Observant - 1 year	83	650	82	650	20.4%	1.01 [0.76, 1.35]
Osnabrugge et al. 2012 - 30 days	7	42	5	42	3.4%	1.40 [0.48, 4.06]
PARTNER II - 1 year	123	1011	124	1021	23.3%	1.00 [0.79, 1.27]
Piazza et al. 2013 - 1 year	71	405	67	405	19.4%	1.06 [0.78, 1.44]
STACATTO	4	34	0	36	0.5%	9.51 [0.53, 170.33]
US Pivotal - 1 year	55	390	67	357	18.2%	0.75 [0.54, 1.04]
Subtotal (95% CI)		**2888**		**3015**	**100.0%**	**1.02 [0.83, 1.26]**
Total events	370		376			
Heterogeneity: Tau² = 0.03; Chi² = 13.69, df = 8 (P = 0.09); I² = 42%						
Test for overall effect: Z = 0.18 (P = 0.86)						
1.1.4 2-year mortality						
NOTION - 2 years	11	142	13	134	5.0%	0.80 [0.37, 1.72]
PARTNER II - 2 years	166	1011	170	1021	68.5%	0.99 [0.81, 1.20]
US Pivotal - 2 years	55	390	67	357	26.5%	0.75 [0.54, 1.04]
Subtotal (95% CI)		**1543**		**1512**	**100.0%**	**0.91 [0.76, 1.08]**
Total events	232		250			
Heterogeneity: Tau² = 0.00; Chi² = 2.08, df = 2 (P = 0.35); I² = 4%						
Test for overall effect: Z = 1.10 (P = 0.27)						
1.1.5 3-year mortality						
Observant - 3 years	91	355	56	355	100.0%	1.63 [1.21, 2.19]
Subtotal (95% CI)		**355**		**355**	**100.0%**	**1.63 [1.21, 2.19]**
Total events	91		56			
Heterogeneity: Not applicable						
Test for overall effect: Z = 3.19 (P = 0.001)						

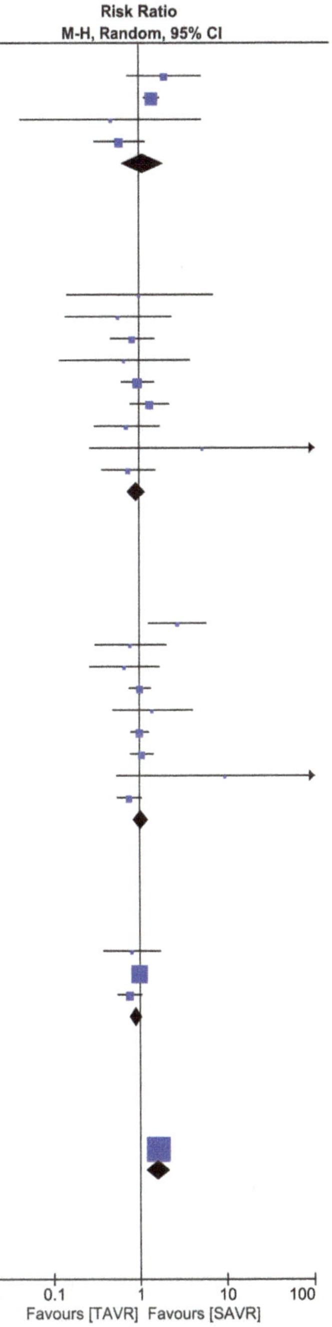

Test for subgroup differences: Chi² = 11.53, df = 4 (P = 0.02), I² = 65.3%

Fig. 2 Forest plot of risk ratio of all-cause mortality

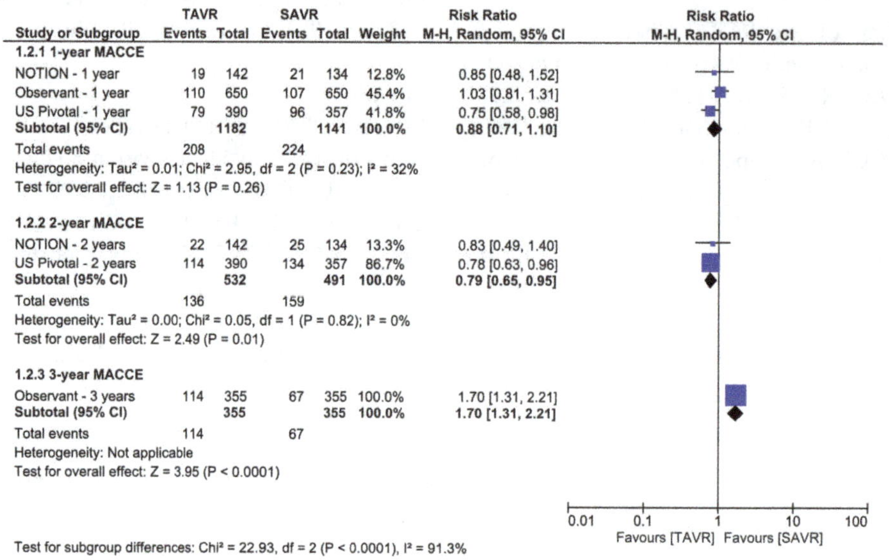

Fig. 3 Forest plot of risk ratio of major adverse cardiovascular and cerebrovascular events

risk of stroke in the TAVR group (RR 2.54, 95% CI [1.36 to 4.74]), compared to SAVR group. For the risk of stroke at 30 days, there was no evidence of publication bias (p = 0.66) (Fig. 4).

Myocardial infarction

The overall RR did not favor either of the two groups in terms of myocardial infarction rate within 30 days (RR 0.64, 95% CI [0.39 to 1.04]), 1 year (RR 0.82, 95% CI [0.57 to 1.19]), 2 years (RR 0.96, 95% CI [0.52 to 1.76]), or 3 years (RR 1.20, 95% CI [0.37 to 3.90]). These findings were consistent when we considered pooling data from RCTs only.

Major life threatening bleeding

The RR of major bleeding was heterogeneous across studies for 30-day and 1- and 2-year endpoints (I^2 = 96%, I^2 = 97%, and I^2 = 97%, respectively). Out of the 9 studies reporting the risk of major bleeding, seven studies (n = 4864 patients) reported a lower incidence of major bleeding in the TAVR group compared with the SAVR group. The STACCATO study showed comparable risk of bleeding between the two groups (1/34 vs. 1/36, respectively), while the ninth study (OBSERVENT) showed a relatively higher incidence of major bleeding in the TAVR group than the SAVR group. When considering data from RCTs only, the pooled RR supported that TAVR has a significantly lower risk of major bleeding than SAVR after 30 days (RR 0.44, 95% CI [0.22 to 0.92]), 1 year (RR 0.45, 95% CI [0.24 to 0.86]), and 2 years (RR 0.48, 95% CI [0.27 to 0.88]).

Acute kidney injury

The overall RR of AKI was lower in the TAVR group than the SAVR group at the endpoints of 30 days (RR 0.45, 95% CI [0.34 to 0.59]), 1 year (RR 0.52, 95% CI [0.30 to 0.88]), and 2 years (RR 0.52, 95% CI [0.33 to 0.80]). These findings were consistent with the other scenario in which we considered pooling of data from RCTs only.

Vascular access complications

The overall RR showed a higher risk of VAC in the TAVR group compared to the SAVR group at the endpoints of 30 days (RR 12.38, 95% CI [2.46 to 62.28]), 1 year (RR 1.99, 95% CI [1.04 to 3.80]), and 2 years (RR 2.16, 95% CI [1.00 to 4.67]). These findings were consistent when we considered pooling data from RCTs only.

Paravalvular aortic regurgitation

The RR of paravalvular AR at 30 days showed a higher incidence of AR in the TAVR group than the SAVR group (RR 3.90, 95% CI [1.25 to 12.12]). Similar results were obtained when pooling data of RCTs only with stratification of AR into mild vs. moderate/severe. The subtotal effect estimates were as follows: (Mild AR: RR 10.21, 95% CI [5.76 to 18.09]; and Moderate/Severe AR: RR 9.30, 95% CI [3.14 to 27.58]).

Permanent pacemaker implantation

Compared to SAVR, the risk of PPI was higher in the TAVR group at 30 days (RR 3.31, 95% CI [2.05 to 5.35]), 1 year (RR 2.57, 95% CI [1.36 to 4.86]), but

Study or Subgroup	TAVR Events	TAVR Total	SAVR Events	SAVR Total	Weight	Risk Ratio M-H, Random, 95% CI
1.3.1 30-day						
Castrodeza et al. 2016 - Full cohort - 30 days	2	103	14	259	4.0%	0.36 [0.08, 1.55]
Latib et al. 2012 - propenity matched - 30 days	1	111	2	111	1.6%	0.50 [0.05, 5.43]
Mollman et al. 2016	131	5233	130	6712	31.2%	1.29 [1.02, 1.64]
NOTION - 30 days	2	142	4	134	3.1%	0.47 [0.09, 2.53]
Observant - 30 days	8	650	14	650	9.6%	0.57 [0.24, 1.35]
Osnabrugge et al. 2012 - 30 days	4	42	1	42	2.0%	4.00 [0.47, 34.31]
PARTNER II - 30 days	55	1011	61	1021	25.6%	0.91 [0.64, 1.30]
Schymik 2015 - Full cohort - 30 days	6	419	4	722	5.2%	2.58 [0.73, 9.11]
STACATTO	3	34	1	36	1.9%	3.18 [0.35, 29.07]
US Pivotal - 30 days	19	390	22	357	15.8%	0.79 [0.44, 1.44]
Subtotal (95% CI)		**8135**		**10044**	**100.0%**	**0.99 [0.73, 1.35]**
Total events	231		253			
Heterogeneity: Tau² = 0.06; Chi² = 13.88, df = 9 (P = 0.13); I² = 35%						
Test for overall effect: Z = 0.08 (P = 0.94)						
1.3.2 1-year						
Castrodeza et al. 2016 - Full cohort - 1 year	3	103	37	259	8.7%	0.20 [0.06, 0.65]
Latib et al. 2012 - propenity matched - 1 year	1	111	3	111	2.7%	0.33 [0.04, 3.16]
NOTION - 1 year	4	142	6	134	7.7%	0.63 [0.18, 2.18]
Observant - 1 year	37	650	29	650	24.8%	1.28 [0.79, 2.05]
PARTNER II - 1 year	78	1011	79	1021	31.9%	1.00 [0.74, 1.35]
Piazza et al. 2013 - 1 year	0	0	0	0		Not estimable
US Pivotal - 1 year	28	390	31	357	24.1%	0.83 [0.51, 1.35]
Subtotal (95% CI)		**2407**		**2532**	**100.0%**	**0.83 [0.56, 1.21]**
Total events	151		185			
Heterogeneity: Tau² = 0.10; Chi² = 10.16, df = 5 (P = 0.07); I² = 51%						
Test for overall effect: Z = 0.97 (P = 0.33)						
1.3.3 2-year						
NOTION - 2 years	5	142	7	134	8.2%	0.67 [0.22, 2.07]
PARTNER II - 2 years	91	1011	85	1021	52.2%	1.08 [0.82, 1.43]
US Pivotal - 2 years	40	390	52	357	39.6%	0.70 [0.48, 1.04]
Subtotal (95% CI)		**1543**		**1512**	**100.0%**	**0.88 [0.63, 1.23]**
Total events	136		144			
Heterogeneity: Tau² = 0.04; Chi² = 3.39, df = 2 (P = 0.18); I² = 41%						
Test for overall effect: Z = 0.76 (P = 0.45)						
1.3.4 3-year						
Observant - 3 years	33	355	13	355	100.0%	2.54 [1.36, 4.74]
Subtotal (95% CI)		**355**		**355**	**100.0%**	**2.54 [1.36, 4.74]**
Total events	33		13			
Heterogeneity: Not applicable						
Test for overall effect: Z = 2.92 (P = 0.003)						

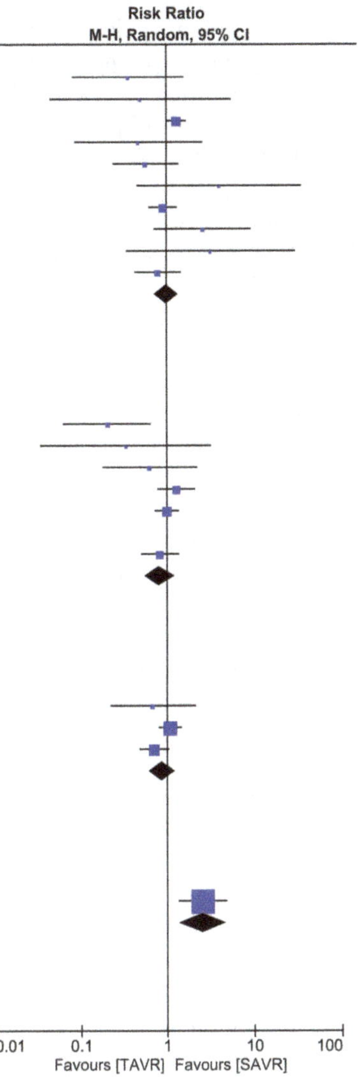

Test for subgroup differences: Chi² = 10.06, df = 3 (P = 0.02), I² = 70.2%

Fig. 4 Forest plot of risk ratio of stroke

not after 2 years (RR 1.57, 95% CI [0.91 to 2.70]), probably due to the small number of included studies at the 2-year endpoint. When analyzing data from RCTs only, the effect estimate favored the SAVR group over the TAVR group at all endpoints (30-day and one- and two-years).

Hospital stay

Six studies reported the duration of hospital stay. Of them, 4 studies showed significantly less hospital stay after TAVR, compared to SAVR. However, the fifth study showed the reverse and the sixth study did not favor either of the two groups. The pooled effect size of hospital stay did not favor either of the two groups (SMD -0.04, 95% CI [−0.34 to 0.26]). However, as we mentioned, this effect size was heterogeneous (I^2 = 95%).

Discussion

Since its introduction in 2002, TAVR has attracted the interest of interventional cardiologists as a possible alternative to SAVR [26]. Recently, the clinical practice guidelines of the European Society of Cardiology (ESC) and American College of Cardiology /American Heart Association (ACC/AHA) recommended TAVR as the procedure of choice in high surgical risk patients [27, 28]. However, its value is still debated in AS patients with a low-to-moderate surgical risk. Recently, the ACC added TAVR as a grade IIa recommendation in AS patients with an intermediate surgical risk [29].

Our analysis of data from over 20,000 low-to-moderate risk patients showed no significant difference between SAVR and TAVR in terms of the incidence of all-cause mortality, myocardial infarction, stroke, and

MACCE, as well as the length of hospital stay. A higher risk of life-threatening bleeding and AKI was detected in the SAVR group, while the TAVR procedure was associated with a higher risk of VAC and paravalvular AR.

The increased risk of paravalvular AR with TAVR was noted in most included studies, as well as our meta-analysis. This finding can be attributed to multiple valvular and procedural factors, including native valve calcification, the angle of the left ventricle outflow tract to the proximal ascending aorta, inadequate balloon expansion, mismatch between the size of the aortic annulus and the TAVR device, and inadequate deployment technique [30]. However, the procedural limitations are expected to improve with the introduction of newer generation devices and increased TAVR experience among interventional practitioners [31]. Of note, several included trials used the 2-Dimensional echocardiography for valve sizing, which has been shown to cause systematic valve undersizing, leading to a higher incidence of AR, compared to multislice computed tomography (MSCT) [32]. Using MSCT to measure the valve size and the degree of native valve complications can reduce the risk of annulus rupture, coronary artery obstruction, and conduction abnormalities [33, 34].

In the 10 studies that compared both procedures regarding the incidence of stroke, neurological examination was clinically-based and imaging was only requested in patients with evident neurological manifestations. Because the main nuerological outcome was the occurrence of stroke, these studies did not assess for more subtle neurological sypmtoms. In a study by Rodes-Cabau et al., cerebral defects were detected in 70% of patients post-TAVR on magnetic resonance imaging [35]. Future studies should consider incorporating cognitive tests and neuroimaging techniques in their regular neurological evaluations.

As expected, our analysis showed a higher incidence of VAC in the TAVR group, compared to the SAVR group. This finding is commonly explained by the percutaneous nature of the procedure and using large-bore introducer sheaths. In a study by Mussardo et al. [36], a 60% reduction in the incidence of VAC was recorded following the introduction of catheter systems with smaller sheaths, such as the SAPIEN XT and the CoreValve systems. The vascular complications are expected to decrease with the continous improvement of catheter systems.

Although not assessed in this analysis, the PARTNER II trial [8] and SAPIEN III study [37] compared the echocardiographic findings in patients who underwent surgery or transcatheter replacement after 30 days of the procedure. These studies showed that both procedures significantly increased the left ventricular ejection fraction and decreased the mean aortic-valve gradients; however, the improvement was greater in the TAVR group at all time endpoints (up to 2 years following the procedure).

All included studies consistently used the logistic EuroSCORE or the STS risk models for operative risk calculation. However, these score are currently considered outdated and may overestimate the true individual risk [38]. Moreover, it does not consider several elderly-related risk factors, such as fraility, porcelain aorta, malnutrition, and chest deformities [39]. The transcatheter approach may be a better alternative for these patients because they may not be surgical candidates. However, this needs confirmation in future RCTs.

Our results are in accordance with a former meta-analysis of five clinical studies (3199 patients) by Kondur et al. [31]. However, they showed a comparable rate of AKI between both procedures. These differences can be attributed to the marked difference in study inclusion criteria. We believe our results are more credible because they are based on pooling a higher number of clinical trials, as well as observational studies. The low risk of bias in the majority of included studies adds to the credibility of our evidence. Additionally, we performed a subgroup analysis according to the time endpoint at which the outcome was measured (Up to 3 years).

Despite these strength points, our analysis is not without limitations. Observational studies are prone to the effect of unmeasured confounders, which may influence the accuracy of our results. Moreover, meta-analysis of relatively rare events, such as myocardial infarction after these procedures, has its limitations because the occurrence of few events can change the summary effect estimate [40]. Only one study (OBSERVENT) compared both techniques in terms of mortality rate at 3 years and showed a higher risk in the TAVR group; however, more data are needed to confirm this finding.

Future trials are advised to compare the durability of the implanted valves and surgical bioprostheses. Longer follow up periods would be of value because TAVR is likely to expand to younger patients with lower mortality risks. Osnabrugge et al. (2012) compared SAVR and TAVR techniques in terms of the procedural time and costs. Their analysis found a shorter procedural time and a higher cost in the TAVR group, compared to the SAVR group, mostly due to the use of more expensive TAVR devices. These costs were not compensated by the shorter hospital stay and reduced need for blood transfusion in the TAVR group according to their analysis [21].

Conclusion

In conclusion, our study shows comparable rates of mortality, stroke, and myocardial infarction between

SAVR and TAVR groups and a lower risk of life-threatening complications (major bleeding and AKI) in the TAVR group. Although the risks of paravalvular AR and VAC were higher in the TAVR group, these complications are expected to decrease with the continous improvement of catheter systems and TAVR experience among interventional cardiologists. Therefore, TAVR can be an acceptable alternative to SAVR in low-to-moderate risk patients with AS. Larger trials with longer follow-up periods are required to compare the long-term outcomes of both techniques.

Abbreviations

AR: Aortic regurgitation; AS: Aortic stenosis; MAACE: Major adverse cardiovascular and cerebrovascular events; SAVR: Surgical aortic valve replacement; TAVR: Transcatheter aortic valve replacement

Acknowledgements

None.

Funding

None.

Authors' contributions

AE: Participated in idea conception, literature search, screening records and writing. AI: Participated in screening records, data extraction and writing. AIA: Participated in data extraction, risk of bias assessment and writing. ME: Participated in data extraction, risk of bias assessment and writing. SS: Participated in data extraction and preparing supporting Tables AN: Participated in data extraction and manuscript writing. OMA: Participated in risk of bias assessment and writing. ARA: Participated in screening records and preparing supporting tables. AMAF: Participated in data extraction and preparing supporting tables. HMH: Participated in screening records and risk of bias assessment AGE: Participated in data extraction and preparing supporting Tables. MM: Participated in risk of bias assessment and writing. FA: Participated in data extraction and drafting the manuscript. MA: Participated in screening records and data analysis. AMA: Participated in data analysis and drafting the manuscript. All authors read and approved the final manuscript.

Competing interests

The authors declare that they have no competing interests.

Author details

[1]Faculty of Medicine, Al-Azhar University, Cairo, Egypt. [2]NovaMed Medical Research Association, Cairo, Egypt. [3]Faculty of Medicine, Ain Shams University, Cairo, Egypt. [4]Genetic Engineering & Biotechnology Research Institute (GEBRI), University of Sadat City, Sadat City, Egypt. [5]Faculty of Medicine, Tanta University, Tanta, Egypt. [6]Faculty of Medicine, Zagazig University, Zagazig, Egypt. [7]Ahmed Maher Teaching Hospital, Cairo, Egypt. [8]Faculty of Medicine, Benha University, Benha, Egypt. [9]Faculty of Medicine, Beni Suef University, Beni suef, Egypt. [10]Faculty of Medicine, Minoufia University, Shebin El-Kom, Egypt. [11]Faculty of Medicine, Misr University for science and technology (MUST), 6th of October City, Giza, Egypt. [12]Faculty of Medicine, Damascus University, Damascus, Syria.

References

1. Lindroos M, Kupari M, Heikkilä J, Tilvis R. Prevalence of aortic valve abnormalities in the elderly: an echocardiographic study of a random population sample. J Am Coll Cardiol. 1993;21:1220–5.
2. Nkomo VT, Gardin JM, Skelton TN, et al. Burden of valvular heart diseases: a population-based study. Lancet. 2006;368:1005–11.
3. Osnabrugge RLJ, Mylotte D, Head SJ, et al. Aortic stenosis in the elderly: disease prevalence and number of candidates for transcatheter aortic valve replacement: a meta-analysis and modeling study. J Am Coll Cardiol. 2013;62:1002–12.
4. Cribier A, Durand E, Eltchaninoff H. Patient selection for TAVI in 2014: is it justified to treat low-or intermediate-risk patients? The cardiologist's view. EuroIntervention: journal of EuroPCR in collaboration with the Working Group on Interventional Cardiology of the European Society of Cardiology. 2014;10:U16–21.
5. Oguri A, Yamamoto M, Mouillet G, et al. Clinical outcomes and safety of transfemoral aortic valve implantation under general versus local anesthesia. Circulation: Cardiovascular Interventions. 2014;7:602–10.
6. Rees CM, Eric HO. Should patients with low-moderate surgical risk be offered TAVI instead of conventional aortic valve replacement in the management of symptomatic aortic stenosis? Res Medica. 2015;23:15–21.
7. Tamburino C, Barbanti M, D'Errigo P, et al. 1-year outcomes after transfemoral transcatheter or surgical aortic valve replacement: results from the Italian OBSERVANT study. J Am Coll Cardiol. 2015;66:804–12.
8. Martin B. Leon, M.D. CR et cols (2016) Transcatheter or Surgical Aortic-Valve Replacement in Intermediate-Risk Patients. N Engl J Med 374:1609–1620. doi: 10.1056/NEJMoa1514616.
9. Thyregod HGH, Steinbrüchel DA, Ihlemann N, et al. Transcatheter versus surgical aortic valve replacement in patients with severe aortic valve stenosis: 1-year results from the all-comers NOTION randomized clinical trial. J Am Coll Cardiol. 2015;65:2184–94. doi: 10.1016/j.jacc.2015.03.014.
10. Reardon MJ, Adams DH, Kleiman NS, et al. 2-Year Outcomes in Patients Undergoing Surgical or Self-Expanding Transcatheter Aortic Valve Replacement. J Am Coll Cardiol. 2015;66:113–21. doi: 10.1016/j.jacc.2015.05.017.
11. Nielsen HH, Klaaborg KE, Nissen H, et al. A prospective, randomised trial of transapical transcatheter aortic valve implantation vs. surgical aortic valve replacement in operable elderly patients with aortic stenosis: the STACCATO trial. EuroIntervention. 2012;8:383–9. doi: 10.4244/eijv8i3a58.
12. D'Errigo P, Barbanti M, Ranucci M, et al. Transcatheter aortic valve implantation versus surgical aortic valve replacement for severe aortic stenosis: results from an intermediate risk propensity-matched population of the Italian OBSERVANT study. Int J Cardiol. 2013;167:1945–52.
13. Higgins JP, Green S (2008) Cochrane Handbook for Systematic Reviews of Interventions: Cochrane Book Series. Cochrane Handbook for Systematic Reviews of Interventions: Cochrane Book Series. doi: 10.1002/9780470712184.
14. Moher D, Liberati A, Tetzlaff J, Altman DG. Preferred reporting items for systematic reviews and meta-analyses: the PRISMA statement. PLoS Med. 2009;6:e1000097. doi:10.1371/journal.pmed.1000097.
15. Stang A. Critical evaluation of the Newcastle-Ottawa scale for the assessment of the quality of nonrandomized studies in meta-analyses. Eur J Epidemiol. 2010;25:603–5. doi: 10.1056/NEJMoa1400590.
16. Egger M, Davey Smith G, Schneider M, Minder C. Bias in meta-analysis detected by a simple, graphical test. BMJ (Clinical research ed). 1997;315:629–34.
17. Adams DH, Popma JJ, Reardon MJ, et al. Transcatheter Aortic-Valve Replacement with a Self-Expanding Prosthesis. N Engl J Med. 2014;370: 1790–8. doi: 10.1056/NEJMoa1400590.
18. Castrodeza J, Amat-Santos IJ, Blanco M, et al. Propensity score matched comparison of transcatheter aortic valve implantation versus conventional surgery in intermediate and low risk aortic stenosis patients: A hint of real-world. Cardiology Journal. 2016;23:541–51. doi: 10.5603/CJ.a2016.0051.
19. Latib A, Maisano F, Bertoldi L, et al. Transcatheter vs surgical aortic valve replacement in intermediate- surgical-risk patients with aortic stenosis: A propensity score-matched case-control study. Am Heart J. 2012;164:910–7. doi: 10.1016/j.ahj.2012.09.005.
20. Möllmann H, Bestehorn K, Bestehorn M, et al. In-hospital outcome of transcatheter vs. surgical aortic valve replacement in patients with aortic valve stenosis: complete dataset of patients treated in 2013 in Germany. Clin Res Cardiol. 2016;105:553–9. doi: 10.1007/s00392-016-0962-4.

21. Osnabrugge RLJ, Head SJ, Genders TSS, et al. Costs of transcatheter versus surgical aortic valve replacement in intermediate-risk patients. Ann Thorac Surg. 2012;94:1954–60. doi: 10.1016/j.athoracsur.2012.07.002.
22. Piazza N, Kalesan B, Van Mieghem N, et al. A 3-center comparison of 1-year mortality outcomes between transcatheter aortic valve implantation and surgical aortic valve replacement on the basis of propensity score matching among intermediate-risk surgical patients. J Am Coll Cardiol Intv. 2013;6: 443–51. doi: 10.1016/j.jcin.2013.01.136.
23. Rosato S, Santini F, Barbanti M, et al. Transcatheter aortic valve implantation compared with surgical aortic valve replacement in low-risk patients. Circulation: Cardiovascular Interventions. 2016;9:e003326. doi: 10.1161/ CIRCINTERVENTIONS.115.003326.
24. Schymik G, Heimeshoff M, Bramlage P, et al. A comparison of transcatheter aortic valve implantation and surgical aortic valve replacement in 1,141 patients with severe symptomatic aortic stenosis and less than high risk. Catheter Cardiovasc Interv. 2015;86:738–44. doi: 10.1002/ccd.25866.
25. Søndergaard L, Steinbrüchel DA, Ihlemann N, et al. Two-Year Outcomes in Patients With Severe Aortic Valve Stenosis Randomized to Transcatheter Versus Surgical Aortic Valve Replacement. Circulation: Cardiovascular Interventions. 2016;9(6):e003665.
26. Cribier A, Eltchaninoff H, Bash A, et al. Percutaneous transcatheter implantation of an aortic valve prosthesis for calcific aortic stenosis. Circulation. 2002;106:3006–8.
27. Nishimura RA, Otto CM, Bonow RO, et al (2014) 2014 AHA/ACC guideline for the management of patients with valvular heart disease. Circulation 129: CIR. 0000000000000031.
28. Vahanian A, Alfieri O, Andreotti F, et al. Guidelines on the management of valvular heart disease (version 2012). The Joint Task Force on the Management of Valvular Heart Disease of the European Society of Cardiology (ESC) and the European Association for Cardio-Thoracic Surgery (EACTS). G Ital Cardiol (2006). 2013;14:167–214.
29. Nishimura RA, Otto CM, Bonow RO, et al (2017) 2017 AHA/ACC focused update of the 2014 AHA/ACC guideline for the management of patients with valvular heart disease: a report of the American College of Cardiology/ American Heart Association Task Force on Clinical Practice Guidelines. Journal of the American College of Cardiology CIR.0000000000000503.
30. Détaint D, Lepage L, Himbert D, et al. Determinants of significant paravalvular regurgitation after transcatheter aortic valve implantation: impact of device and annulus discongruence. J Am Coll Cardiol Intv. 2009;2:821–7.
31. Kondur A, Briasoulis A, Palla M, et al. Meta-analysis of transcatheter aortic valve replacement versus surgical aortic valve replacement in patients with severe aortic valve stenosis. Am J Cardiol. 2016;117:252–7.
32. Mylotte D, Dorfmeister M, Elhmidi Y, et al. Erroneous measurement of the aortic annular diameter using 2-dimensional echocardiography resulting in inappropriate CoreValve size selection: a retrospective comparison with multislice computed tomography. J Am Coll Cardiol Intv. 2014;7:652–61.
33. Leipsic J, Gurvitch R, LaBounty TM, et al. Multidetector computed tomography in transcatheter aortic valve implantation. J Am Coll Cardiol Img. 2011;4:416–29.
34. Achenbach S, Delgado V, Hausleiter J, et al. SCCT expert consensus document on computed tomography imaging before transcatheter aortic valve implantation (TAVI)/transcatheter aortic valve replacement (TAVR). Journal of cardiovascular computed tomography. 2012;6:366–80.
35. Rodés-Cabau J, Dumont E, Boone RH, et al. Cerebral embolism following transcatheter aortic valve implantation: comparison of transfemoral and transapical approaches. J Am Coll Cardiol. 2011;57:18–28.
36. Mussardo M, Latib A, Chieffo A, et al. Periprocedural and short-term outcomes of transfemoral transcatheter aortic valve implantation with the Sapien XT as compared with the Edwards Sapien valve. J Am Coll Cardiol Intv. 2011;4:743–50.
37. Thourani VH, Kodali S, Makkar RR, et al. Transcatheter aortic valve replacement versus surgical valve replacement in intermediate-risk patients: a propensity score analysis. Lancet. 2016;387:2218–25.
38. Osswald BR, Gegouskov V, Badowski-Zyla D, et al. Overestimation of aortic valve replacement risk by EuroSCORE: implications for percutaneous valve replacement. Eur Heart J. 2008;30:74–80.
39. Wendt D, Osswald BR, Kayser K, et al. Society of Thoracic Surgeons score is superior to the EuroSCORE determining mortality in high risk patients undergoing isolated aortic valve replacement. Ann Thorac Surg. 2009;88:468–75.
40. Shuster JJ, Jones LS, Salmon DA. Fixed vs random effects meta-analysis in rare event studies: The Rosiglitazone link with myocardial infarction and cardiac death. Stat Med. 2007;26:4375–85.

7

Clinical outcomes of conventional surgery versus MitraClip® therapy for moderate to severe symptomatic mitral valve regurgitation in the elderly population

Anthony Alozie[1*], Liliya Paranskaya[2], Bernd Westphal[1], Alexander Kaminski[1], Mohammad Sherif[2], Magnus Sindt[1], Stephan Kische[4], Jochen Schubert[3], Doreen Diedrich[5], Hüseyin Ince[2], Gustav Steinhoff[1] and Alper Öner[2]

Abstract

Background: The aim of this study was to compare treatment of moderate to severe symptomatic mitral regurgitation (MR) with either conventional surgery or the mitral valve edge-to-edge device (MitraClip®) in very elderly patients. The newly introduced MitraClip device has demonstrated promising acute results in treating this patient cohort. Also noteworthy is the fact that patients who otherwise would have been denied surgery are increasingly referred for treatment with the MitraClip device. We sought to review our institutional experience, comparing outcomes in both surgical and MitraClip arms of treatment in the elderly population with symptomatic MR.

Methods: From October 2008 through October 2014, 136 consecutive patients aged ≥ 80 with moderate to severe symptomatic MR were scheduled for either conventional surgery or MitraClip intervention. 56 patients ≥ 80 were operated for symptomatic MR and 80 patients ≥ 80 were treated with the mitraClip device. Patients suitable for this study were identified from our hospital database. Patients ≥80 with moderate/severe symptomatic MR treated with either conventional surgery or the MitraClip device were eligible for our analysis. We compared the surgical patient cohort with the mitraClip patient cohort after eliminating patients that did not meet our inclusion criteria. Forty-two patients were identified from the conventional cohort who were then compared with 42 patients from the mitraClip cohort. Forty-two patients (50%) underwent mitral valve repair or replacement (40.5% functional MR, 59.5% organic/mixed MR) and 42 patients (50%) underwent MitraClip intervention (50% functional MR, 50% organic/mixed MR). Associated procedures in the conventional surgical group were myocardial revascularization 38%, pulmonary vein ablation 23.8%, left atrial appendage resection 52.4% and PFO occlusion 11.9%.

(Continued on next page)

* Correspondence: uju77de@yahoo.de
[1]Department of Cardiac Surgery, Heart Center Rostock, Schillingallee 35, 18057 Rostock, Germany
Full list of author information is available at the end of the article

(Continued from previous page)

Results: Patients who underwent MitraClip treatment were though slightly older but the differences did not attain statistical significance (mean, 82.2 ± 1.65 vs 81.7 ± 1.35 years, $p = 0{,}100$), had lower LVEF (mean, 47.6 ± 14.2 vs 53.4 ± 14.3, $p = 0.072$), lower logistic EuroScore II (mean, 11.3 ± 5.63 vs 12.1 ± 10.6, $p = 0.655$) but higher STS risk score (mean, 11.8 ± 6.7 vs 8.1 ± 5.6, $p = 0.008$) respectively compared to surgical patients. Procedural success was 100% vs 96% in surgery and MitraClip groups respectively. Thirty -day mortality was 7.1% vs 4.8% ($p = 1.000$) in surgery and MitraClip group respectively. Residual postoperative MR ≥2 at discharge was present in none of the patients treated surgically, whereas this was the case in 10 (23.8%) patients treated with the MitraClip device. At 1 year a cumulative number of four (9.52%) patients died in the surgical group vs 9 (21.4%) patients who died in the MitraClip group.

Conclusions: Elderly patients presenting with moderate to severe symptomatic MR may either be treated by conventional surgery or with the MitraClip device with acceptable acute outcomes. The decision for treatment with the MitraClip device should not depend on age alone rather on cumulative risk of conventional surgery. Concomitant cardiac pathologies, often times treated simultaneously during surgery for symptomatic MR may be omitted, if patients are scheduled outright to MitraClip treatment. The effect of concomitant cardiac pathologies left untreated at the time of interventional mitral valve repair on outcome after MitraClip therapy remain widely unknown.

Keywords: Mitral valve surgery, MitraClip therapy, Heart valve surgery, Mitral regurgitation

Background

More than 9% of patients ≥75 years have significant MR [1]. The proportion of individuals aged ≥75 with symptomatic MR is estimated to become a growing clinical problem. The decision whether to refer an elderly patient with symptomatic MR for mitral valve surgery and appropriate timing of referral is a highly debated issue. Age, severe MR and reduced left ventricular function amongst others have been identified as independent patient factors associated with non referal for mitral valve surgery [2]. Though, due to outstanding improvements in diagnostic modalities, patient selection criteria and operative techniques over the years, the operative mortality, in-hospital morbidity and long term outcomes associated with mitral valve surgery has significantly improved [3]. However, the benefit of surgery in the very elder population despite these significant improvements over the years has not been clearly documented. Increasing life expectancy and associated increase in the prevalence of valvular heart diseases, especially MR amongst the very elderly population is expected to become a rising clinical problem in the industrialized nations. Many patients at this advanced age will likely present with concomitant cardiac pathologies, necessitating surgical attention [4, 5]. The novel MitraClip device is anticipated to play a crucial role in addressing MR in this elderly patient population. In this context, staged percutaneous management of concomitant pathologies may be feasible in some cases. Coronary heart disease, aortic valve stenosis and certain pathologic rhythms may be treated in a staged total percutaneous manner. Data on the fate of moderate tricuspid regurgitation left untreated during conventional surgery remain insufficient and this is equally the case with percutaneous mitral valve repair. The impact of these residual pathologies on short and long term outcome has not been fully evaluated, leaving complete surgical intervention as gold standard [6]. Though there are indications that the novel MitraClip device may confer superior acute outcomes, with lower procedural mortality in symptomatic patients, however, long term outcomes, especially in the very elderly is not well known. The impact of residual MR, atrial septal defect, atrial fibrillation, incomplete revascularization and tricuspid valve disease in this patient population treated with the MitraClip device is not known. Despite higher mortality and morbidity in the acute phase post surgery, surgery in most cases offer complete repair of concomitant cardiac pathologies [7–10]. We sought to compare the overall outcome of conventional mitral valve surgery vs MitraClip treatment in a single center cohort of 84 patients.

Patient selection and methods

Patient selection

The criteria for selecting patients eligible for MitraClip intervention has been previously described by Paranskaya et al. [11]. We at first found 80 patients who underwent mitraClip intervention. Forty-two patients were found suitable for comparing with the surgical cohort. In the surgical arm, we retrospectively selected patients ≥80 years who presented with moderate/severe symptomatic MR and were treated with conventional surgery with the aim of comparing them with a similar MitraClip treatment population.

A team of experienced cardiac surgeons, cardiologists and anesthesiologists selected patients eligible for conventional surgery and decision was based on the guidelines as stipulated by the joint task force on the management of valvular heart diseases of the European Society of Cardiology [12]. Transthoracic echocardiography (TTE) followed by transoesophageal echocardiography (TEE) examination at baseline were applied for general screening purposes. A search into our department surgical database for patients ≥ 80 who received mitral valve surgery (repair or replacement) during this time frame yielded at first 56 patients. Forty-two patients suitable for our analysis were retained after excluding patients with concomitant tricuspid-, aortic valve surgeries, mitral valve stenosis, active endocarditis of any valve or intracardiac structures and emergency settings requiring hemodynamic or respiratory support prior to surgery (Table 1 depicts concomitant procedures in the surgical group). In-hospital data were retrospectively retrieved from each patient's personal file. Surgical patients who received concomitant myocardial revascularization were included because MitraClip patients with significant coronary stenosis received percutaneous coronary interventions prior to MitraClip therapy. All patients with justifiable EuroScore II and STS scores were referred for surgery after obtaining informed consent.

Table 1 Patients baseline demographics and clinical risk factors

	Surgery (*n* = 42)	MitraClip (*n* = 42)	*p*-value
Age (years), mean ± SD, (n)	81.7 ± 1.35, (42)	82.2 ± 1.65, (42)	0.100~
Female gender, n (%)	23 (54.8)	18 (42.9)	0.383*
BMI (kg/m^2), mean ± SD, (n)	26.3 ± 4.30, (42)	25.9 ± 3.96, (42)	0.682~
Previous cardiac surgery, n (%)	7 (16.7)	7 (16.7)	1.000*
Coronary artery disease, n (%)	31 (73.8)	26 (61.9)	0.350*
COPD, n (%)	10 (23.8)	14 (33.3)	0.469*
Atrial fibrillation, n (%)	23 (54.8)	29 (69.0)	0.261*
Pulmonary hypertension, n (%)	32 (76.2)	40 (95.2)	0.026*
Chronic renal disease, n (%)	26 (61.9)	32 (76.2)	0.238*
Arterial hypertension, n (%)	36 (85.7)	39 (92.9)	0.483*
Diabetes mellitus, n (%)	14 (33.3)	18 (42.9)	0.501*
Cardiac decompensation, n (%)	25 (59.5)	37 (88.1)	0.006*
Logistic Euroscore II, mean ± SD, (n)	12.1 ± 10.6, (42)	11.3 ± 5.63, (42)	0.655~
NYHA functional class, n (%)			
II	8 (19.0)	1 (2.4)	0.039**
III	27 (64.3)	30 (67.9)	
IV	7 (16.7)	11 (21.4)	
Operative Data			
Previous PCI, n (%)	-	7 (16.7)	
Concomitant CABG, n (%)	16 (38)	-	
Concomitant pulmonary vein ablation, n (%)	10 (23.8)	-	-
Concomitant LAA resection, n (%)	22 (52.4)	-	-
Concomitant PFO occlusion, n (%)	5 (11.9)	-	-

~ Student's unpaired *t*-test
* Fisher's exact Test for categorical data
** Chi-square test for categorical data

Methods

This study is based on our experience with very elderly patients with symptomatic moderate- severe MR, who underwent correction of this valve pathology during the period between October 2008 and October 2014.

Patients underwent surgical correction of MR with either mitral valve repair, replacement or placement of ≥1 MitraClip devices. A retrospective assessment was then perfomed after all follow-up data were retrieved. This was accomplished by obtaining all medical records from nursing home personnel, family physician or patient/ family members. Follow- up was obtained at different intervals post index procedure (last survey or death) in all 84 patients included in this study.

Follow-up

All patients were followed up after discharge by the family physicians and cardiologist with regular physical examination, including evaluation of NYHA score, ECG, TTE and TEE if need be. This was at first performed during the first 3 months post treatment and then dependent on clinical status at 6 months and on yearly basis there after. Two surgical patients were lost to follow-up. All other patients discharged alive from hospital were followed up at different intervals post index procedure.

Treatment procedures

Mitral valve surgery was performed via median sternotomy in all 42 surgical patients. Cardio pulmonal bypass was installed and valve repair or replacement with variable concomitant surgical procedures on the arrested heart under mild hypothermia (32 °C) performed. Access to mitral valve was gained either via a direct left atrial or trans septal incision depending on weather PFO occlusion was planned. Complete rigid or semi rigid annuloplasty rings or in case of valve replacement solely tissue prosthesis used. All procedures were quality controlled using intra operative TEE. MitraClip treatment was performed in the hybrid suit as previously described by *paranskaya* et al. [11].

Statistical analysis

Statistical analysis was conducted by using SPSS statistical package 22.0 (SPSS Inc. Chicago, Illinois, USA). Descriptive statistics were computed for continuous and categorical variables. The statistics computed included mean and standard deviations (SD) of continuous variables and are presented as mean ± SD, frequencies and relative frequencies of categorical factors. Testing for differences of continuous variables between the study groups was accomplished by the *t*-test for independent samples or the Mann-Whitney *U* test, as appropriate. Test selection was based on evaluating the variables for normal distribution employing the Kolmogorov-Smirnov test. Comparisons between the study groups for categorical variables were done using the chi-square test or the Fisher's exact test. For unbiased results the matched pairs method for the arrangement of statistical twins was used. For the matching process a correspondence of the parameters age, sex and MR Type was used. In specific, matching for age was performed using frequency matching to assure that cases and controls have similar distributions over strata defined by age. The matching on age involved the construction of three separate categories. The age categories were as follows: 80–82, 83–84 and ≥ 85 years respectively.

The period of time to death or last follow-up was estimated using the Kaplan-Meier method. Differences between curves were assessed by Mantel's log-rank test for censored survival data.

The Cox proportional hazards model was used to assess the independence of survival from prognostic factors. Univariate analyses were performed by computation of hazard ratios, 95% - confidence intervals and examination the significance by the Wald statistic to reveal unadjusted significant associations between prognostic variables and survival. Altogether, p-values ≤ 0.05 were considered to be statistically significant and all reported p-values resulted from two-sided statistical test.

Results

Patient baseline characteristics and risk profile

From October 2008 through October 2014, 84 consecutive patients aged ≥ 80 with moderate to severe symptomatic MR were scheduled for either conventional mitral valve surgery or MitraClip intervention. Patient data were analysed retrospectively. All patients suitable for our analysis were identified from our hospital database. Patients ≥ 80 with symptomatic MR treated with either conventional surgical or MitraClip intervention were eligible for our analysis. Patients with concomitant tricuspid-, aortic valve surgeries, mitral valve stenosis, active endocarditis of any valve or intracardiac structures and emergency settings requiring hemodynamic or respiratory support prior to surgery were excluded from this analysis. Patient baseline characteristics and risk factors are depicted in Table 1.

Forty-two patients (50%) underwent mitral valve surgery with mitral valve repair in 30 patients (71.4%) or replacement in 12 patients (28.6%). Of the 30 patients who received mitral valve repair, minimally invasive (MIC) mitral valve repair was performed in five (16.7%). Procedural success was similar (100%) in both repair and replacement groups respectively. There was no significant differences in both groups in terms of 30 day mortality (2 vs 1 patients). 40.5% of surgically treated patients had functional MR whereas 59.5% had organic/mixed MR. Forty-two patients (50%) underwent MitraClip implantation, 50% of which had functional MR whereas 50% had organic/mixed MR respectively. Seven patients (16.7%) in each group had previous cardiac surgery in the past. Associated procedures in the conventional surgical group were myocardial revascularization (38%), pulmonary vein ablation (23.8%), left atrial auriculum resection (52.4%) and PFO/ASD-closure (11.9%). All but a few important differences between patients in both arms of our analysis attained statistical significance. Patients in the MitraClip cohort had higher STS risk score (p = 0.008). They were though older, but the differences did not attain statistical difference (p = 0.100). MitraClip patients also had lower proportion of individuals in NYHA classes II (p = 0.039), had higher number of individuals with previous cardiac decompensation (p = 0.006). Patients in the conventional surgical cohort had higher mean logistic EUROSCORE II, but the differences did not attain statistical significance (p = 0.655). With regards to echocardiographic parameters, patients in the MitraClip cohort had higher proportion of individuals with functional MR, however this difference did not attain a statistical significance (p = 0.511). Table 2 shows further echocardiographic parameters.

Procedural and in-hospital outcomes

Procedural success was 100% in the conventional surgery group and 95.2% in the MitraClip group (p =0,494). In one MitraClip patient, MR grade was three at discharge. Another patient with symptomatic MR and significant inter atrial shunt was treated with mitral valve replacement and ASD closure prior to discharge. Thirty surgical patients (71.4%) received an annuloplasty

Table 2 Preoperative echocardiographic parameters

	Surgery (n = 42)	MitraClip (n = 42)	p-value
MR ≥ 3, n (%)	42 (100)	42 (100)	
LVEF, mean ± SD, (n)	53.4 ± 14.3, (38)	47.6 ± 14.2, (42)	0.072˜
LVEDD (mm), mean ± SD, (n)	55.3 ± 7.47, (30)	57.5 ± 9.54, (42)	0.296˜
LVESD (mm), mean ± SD, (n)	38.2 ± 6.81, (12)	44.1 ± 10.6, (42)	0.077˜
sPAP (mmHg), mean ± SD, (n)	47.2 ± 8.04, (13)	51.0 ± 12.2, (42)	0.212˜
MR Type			
Functional, n (%)	17 (40.5)	21 (50.0)	0.511*
Organic + mixed, n (%)	25 (59.5)	21 (50.0)	

˜ Student's unpaired t-test
* Fisher's exact Test for categorical data

using a complete rigid or semi rigid ring. Twelve patients received tissue valve replacement (28.6%). Nine patients in the MitraClip cohort were treated with one clip device, 22 patients with two clips, eight patients with three clips and the remaining three patients with four clips devices each. In-hospital- stay was significantly increased in the surgical group compared to the MitraClip group (18.0 ± 7.60 vs 8.81 ± 6.40, $p < 0.001$) as well as incidents of acute kidney injury (10 vs 2, $p = 0.026$) and pneumonia (12 vs 3, $p = 0.020$). Details of periprocedural characteristics of all patients are depicted in Table 3.

Follow- up, mortality and morbidity

Follow-up was performed at various intervals post index procedure in both surgical and the MitraClip cohort. Mean follow-up times were 2.08 ± 1.68 years for the surgical cohort and 0.75 ± 0.50 years for the MitraClip cohort respectively for a total of 87.53 and 31.57 patient years respectively. Overall early mortality and morbidity rates are shown in Table 3. Three patients (7.1%) in the mitral surgical cohort died within 30 days of the index procedure. At 1 year this number increased to four (9.5%). In the MitraClip cohort, two patients (4.8) died within 30 days of the index procedure and this number increased to nine (21.42%) at 1 year. Univariate analysis revealed that the only predictor of 30-day mortality was COPD in both the MitraClip and surgical cohort (HR 7.26, 95% CI 0.76–69.9, $p = 0.086$). None of the other preoperative variables was significantly associated with this outcome variable (Table 4). Ventilation time > 24 h was more frequent in the surgical group. ICU and in-hospital stays (18.0 ± 7.60 vs 8.81 ± 6.40, $p < 0.001$) were longer in the surgical cohort. In-hospital-death (3 vs 1, $p = 0.616$), acute kidney injury (10 vs 2, $p = 0.026$), need for dialysis (4 vs 1, $p = 0.202$), pneumonia (12 vs 3, $p = 0.02$) and need for permanent pacemaker implantation (9 vs 0) were more frequent in the surgical group (Table 3).

Table 3 Post operative results/characteristics

	Surgery (n = 42)	MitraClip (n = 42)	p-value
Procedure time (min), mean ± SD, (n)	214.1 ± 57.2, (42)	186.4 ± 73.7, (41)	0.059~
Ventilation time ≥ 24h, n (%)	8 (19.0)	1 (2.4)	0.029*
ICU stay(days), mean ± SD, (n)	3.71 ± 4.00, (41)	(0)	
In Hospital stay(days), mean ± SD, (n)	18.0 ± 7.60, (41)	8.81 ± 6.40, (42)	<0.001~
Procedural success, n (%)	42 (100)	40 (95.2)	0.494*
In-hospital-death, n (%)	3 (7.1)	1 (2.4)	0.616*
30-day-mortality, n (%)	3 (7.1)	2 (4.8)	1.000*
Major bleeding, n (%)	2 (4.8)	3 (7.1)	1.000*
Tracheotomy, n (%)	1 (2.4)	0 (0.0)	
Acute kidney injury, n (%)	10 (23.8)	2 (4.8)	0.026*
Dialysis post surgery, n (%)	4 (9.8)	1 (2.4)	0.202*
Pneumonia, n (%)	12 (28.6)	3 (7.1)	0.020*
Myocardial infarction, n (%)	1 (2.4)	0 (0.0)	
Permanent Pacemaker, n (%)	9 (21.4)	0 (0.0)	
Stroke, n (%)	4 (9.5)	0 (0.0)	0.116*
Predischarge MR Grades, n (%)			
MR 0	34 (82.9)	6 (14.3)	<0.001**
MR I	7 (17.1)	26 (61.9)	
MR II	0 (0.0)	9 (21.4)	
MR III	0 (0.0)	1 (2.4)	

~ Student's unpaired t-test
* Fisher's exact Test for categorical data
** Chi-square test for categorical data

Echocardiographic outcomes

Predischarge MR 0, I° and II° were found in 34, seven and zero patients versus six, 26 and nine patients in the mitral surgical and MitraClip groups respectively ($p <$ 001, Table 3). At follow up nine patients in the mitral surgical group had MR I°, one patient had MR II°. In the Mitraclip cohort, three patients remained at MR I°, 23 patients had MR I°, nine patients had MR II°, three patients had MR III°. One Patient had mitral stenosis II° post intervention in the Mitraclip cohort. In the surgical cohort, no mitral stenosis was recorded. In general, surgery was more effective in reducing the grade of MR acutely compared to MitraClip.

Discussion

Mitral valve surgery in the elderly oftentimes multi morbid population is a highly debated issue. Although more elderly patients with MR are increasingly being identified and referred for surgery, still as much as 50% are often denied surgery due to perceived higher risk and lower benefit expectation from surgical correction of MR [2]. This tendency is partly justifiable for secondary MR due to the fact that results of surgery are unpredictable in improving patient outcomes. Moreover surgery for secondary MR has never been compared with guidelines directed medical therapy (GDMT) alone for left ventricular dysfunction in a prospective randomized manner. Studies comparing outcomes of patients with secondary MR treated with mitral valve repair and those treated with GDMT are mostly retrospective in nature, using propensity score matching and have failed to demonstrate an advantage of surgery in improving survival [13]. However, results of surgical elimination of MR in primary (degenerative) MR on the other hand, especially reconstructive surgery are excellent.

Table 4 Predictors of 30- day Mortality in octogenarians treated with MVS vs. MC

	univariate Cox Regression								
	all Patients ($n = 84$)			MVS ($n = 42$)			MC ($n = 42$)		
Variable	Hazard Ratio	95%-CI	*p*-value	Hazard Ratio	95%-CI	*p*-value	Hazard Ratio	95%-CI	*p*-value
Logistic Euroscore									
> 10 vs. <=10[a]	**	**	**	**	**	**	**	**	**
NYHA baseline									
class 3/4 vs. class 1/2[a]	**	**	**	**	**	**	**	**	**
Baseline LVEF									
> 50% vs. <=50%[a]	1.07	0.07–17.1	0.963	**	**	**	1.18	0.07–18.9	0.905
Cardiac decompensation									
yes vs. no[a]	**	**	**	**	**	**	**	**	**
Age									
80–82 years vs. 83–85 years[a]	**	**	**	**	**	**	**	**	**
Sex									
female vs. male[a]	1.11	0.16–7.85	0.920	**	**	**	**	**	**
Coronary artery disease									
yes vs. no[a]	1.44	0.15–13.8	0.753	**	**	**	0.60	0.04–9.53	0.714
Diabetes mellitus									
no vs. yes[a]	1.82	0.19–17.5	0.604	**	**	**	0.77	0.05–12.3	0.851
COPD									
yes vs. no[a]	7.26	0.76–69.9	0.086	2.85	0.18–45.6	0.459	**	**	**
GFR ≤ 30									
yes vs. no[a]	**	**	**	**	**	**	**	**	**
GFR 30–50									
yes vs. no[a]	1.77	0.25–12.5	0.570	**	**	**	**	**	**
Atrial fibrillation									
yes vs. no[a]	1.68	0.17–16.1	0.655	0.71	0.04–11.4	0.810	**	**	**
Pulmonary hypertension									
yes vs. no[a]	**	**	**	**	**	**	**	**	**

**not determinable, because there are only censored times
[a]indicates reference category

Some studies provided insight into potential poorer prognosis for patients with functional MR and left ventricular dysfunction and this is especially true for patients with recent acute myocardial infarction and for patients with chronic ischemic and non ischemic cardiomyopathy [14]. It was shown that even with the current GDMT, there was always a tendency to adverse prognosis due to untreated ischemic functional MR. Therefore this category of patients who remain symptomatic despite GDMT and CRT may be a reasonable target for surgical or interventional therapy of functional MR. Swaans et al. recently reported mortality rates in patients receiving neither surgery nor percutaneous therapy for MR that even exceeded that of either surgical or interventional therapy [15]. This report provided new insights into the potential survival benefits of mitral valve intervention (both surgical and interventional) compared with GDMT alone in patients with LV dysfunction and secondary MR [15]. In the Survival and Ventricular Enlargement Trial (SAVE) patients with even mild functional MR after myocardial infarction were more likely to experience cardiovascular mortality (29% vs. 12%; $p < 0.001$), and severe heart failure (24% vs. 16%; $p < 0.0153$) than those without MR [16]. Trichon et al. reported 2057 patients with ischemic MR and chronic LV systolic dysfunction and showed residual MR to be an independent predictor of mortality. They also found significantly lower survival rates at 1, 3 and 5 years of heart failure patients with moderate to severe MR versus those without MR or with mild MR [17]. Hence, none referral of elderly symptomatic patients with MR for at least surgical evaluation, due to age alone is highly debatable. The optimal timing for surgery or percutaneous intervention is also critical in reducing mortality rates associated with both surgery and interventional therapy. The percutaneous edge-to-edge device has since its first application in human, continuously improved, and currently demonstrates superb acute interventional outcomes in the elderly population with MR classified as high surgical risk [18, 19]. Though operative risks of mitral valve surgery reduced significantly during the last decades [20], however quality of life after such surgical interventions, a factor of great importance in the elderly population has rarely been reported. Maissano et al [21] found that quality of life was suboptimal in more than half of elderly patients following mitral valve surgery and that surgical technique did not impact quality of life at follow up. They identified several factors significantly related to increased Minnesota Living With Heart Failure (MLHF) - score at follow-up after valve surgery in the elderly. Age, preoperative atrial fibrillation (or rhythm other than sinus rhythm at follow up), EuroSCORE, Charlson score and recurrent/residual MR at follow up amongst others were significantly associated with poorer quality of life at follow up. They suggested that quality of life should be a better indicator of successful surgery/intervention in this age group than survival alone. In our study, though the 30-day mortality was slightly higher in the surgical cohort, but there was equalization of mortality rates as time progressed, with even higher mortality rate in the MitraClip group (depicted in Fig. 1). At 1- year- follow up surgical patients had lower MR recurrence than found in the Mitraclip group. Kaneko et al in their recent study found that residual MR 2+ was associated with poorer prognosis in patients with impaired LV function, renal dysfunction, and severe heart failure. They suggested that the optimal endpoint of MC procedure should be individualized according to each patient's baseline characteristic [22].

The impact of tricuspid regurgitation left untreated at time of Mitraclip intervention was recently reported by ohno et al [23] who found that estimates for freedom from combined endpoint of death and rehospitalisation for heart failure were worse in moderate/severe tricuspid regurgitation group of patients treated with the MitraClip device compared with those with none/mild tricuspid regurgitation (67.7% vs 88.8% log-rank $p = 0.015$). Overall NYHA was also found to be worse in this group of patients with moderate/severe tricuspid regurgitation, despite improved LVEF and ventricular volumes at 12 month-follow-up. Since the current practice of Mitraclip intervention does not include concomitant cardiac interventions in the aortic valve, tricuspid valve, atrial fibrillation ablation or complete myocardial revascularisation, all of which have high prevalence in the elderly population, adequate patient selection should identify patients who would rather benefit from complete surgical intervention despite age.

Mitral valve surgical procedures in the very elderly with symptomatic MR is associated with profound operative morbidity and mortality rates, especially in deem of frequently associated comorbidities [10]. Mirabel et al [2] from the Euro Heart Survey on heart valve diseases reported that in a group of 396 patients with symptomatic MR, surgery was denied in 49%, with age, impaired LVEF and several comorbidities playing the main role in the decision not to offer surgery. However untreated symptomatic secondary MR seems to confer even higher mortality and morbidity. MitraClip therapy, though has acceptable procedural outcomes, but long term results are pending and the durability of acute reduction of MR in certain patients remains controversial. De Bonis et al.

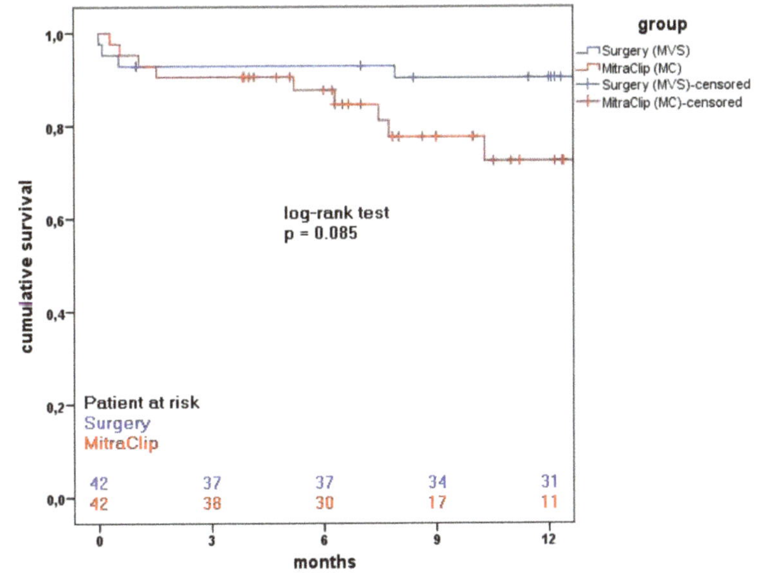

Fig. 1 Kaplan-Meier survival rate after MitraClip and surgery

recently failed to confirm the results of EVEREST II trial in which it was observed that the MItraClip results remained stable in the long term if initial therapy was successfull. Infact they found that patients with FMR, despite optimal initial results of MitraClip intervention had the tendency to develop recurrent MR. Whether FMR at this time can be seen as risk factor for recurrent MR after MitraClip therapy remain to be confirmed in a prospective randomized trial.

Treatment of concomitant cardiac pathologies, which have increased prevalence in this age group, is very limited. The impact of untreated concomitant cardiac pathologies, left untreated at the time of MitraClip therapy versus complete surgical interventions on the mid and long term outcomes should be the subject of future studies. Our acute procedural outcomes in the mitral surgical group is in line with published data on mortality and morbidity rates after mitral valve surgery in the very elderly, despite several concomitant surgical procedures and high EuroScore II values, and mid term outcomes are impressive.

As the number of elderly patients with mitral valve disease is expected to increase rapidly, there is need for data providing evidence on the benefits and harm of both conventional MV surgery and several percutaneous therapeutic options, being propagated for MR treatment in these high risk patients. As percutaneous mitral valve repair options are rapidly gaining ground as alternative option for mitral valve repair in these high risk surgical patients, at the same time some patients are reoperated successfully after failed interventions. However this is expected to decrease with perfection of this technology. Adequate patient selection prior to decision for either conventional surgery or MitraClip therapy should be pursued in the future. Age alone should at present not be a criterium for pro MitraClip therapy, rather comorbidities predisposing to high prohibitive risk of surgery and in those cases with ambiguous survival benefit of surgery. Benefit of surgery for MR due to ischemic cardiomyopathy remains a highly debated issue [24–26]. Multidisciplinary team approach is key to providing optimal individually tailored treatment for elderly patients with symptomatic MR. Primary and secondary MR are very different entities in terms of etiology, management and prognosis and these differences should be put into account during multidisciplinary decision pro or contra surgery or interventional treatment of symptomatic MR.

Study limitations

This is a retrospective, single-center observational study with a very limited number of observed patients. There may be some, unidentified confounding factors that might have influenced certain results, so strong conclusions from our study should not yet be deduced or generalized, until our results is confirmed by prospective and randomized clinical trials. Follow-up data were obtained by both facsimile questionnaire and telephone interviews with patients family practitioner and cardiologist. Hence, accuracy of grading NYHA functional class, MR grades may have been compromised by interobserver bias. Patient selection for the respective procedures did not follow standard operating procedures, but rather decisions were made after interdisciplinary consultation in each case within a heart team. The completely different burden of both treatment arms, with patients in the surgical arm receiving different and at times multiple concomitant procedures with subsequent impact on early clinical outcome is another important limitation.

In terms of quality of life, unfortunately due to the retrospective nature of our study, quality of life was not assessed preoperatively and therefore assessing quality of life during follow-up would not provide data usefull for any reasonable comparison.

Another important limitation is that the number of patients whose data were available for 1-year followed-up was less in the mitraClip group.

Conclusions

Elderly patients presenting with moderate to severe symptomatic MR may either be treated by conventional surgery or with the MitraClip device with acceptable acute outcomes. The decision for treatment with the MitraClip device should not depend on age alone rather on cumulative risk of conventional surgery. Concomitant cardiac pathologies, often times treated simultaneously during surgery for symptomatic MR may be omitted, if patients are scheduled outright to MitraClip treatment. The effect of concomitant cardiac pathologies left untreated at the time of interventional mitral valve repair on outcome after MitraClip therapy remain widely unknown.

Acknowledgement

We thank Dr. T. Najjar, Dr. B. Weiss and Dr. J. Wendeborn for taking care of the patients both during their hospital-stay and follow up.

Funding

None

Authors' contribution

AA, AÖ, BW, GS, AK, MS, LP, SK, JS, HI participated in treating the patients during surgery/intervention/ICU/hospital care. MS participated in data acquisation, DD performed statistical analysis. All authors wrote and approved the final manuscript.

Authors' information

Alozie Anthony

Competing interests
The authors declare that they have no competing interests.

Author details
[1]Department of Cardiac Surgery, Heart Center Rostock, Schillingallee 35, 18057 Rostock, Germany. [2]Department of Cardiology, Heart Center Rostock, Ernst-Heydemannstrasse 6, 18057 Rostock, Germany. [3]Department of Anesthesiology and Intensive Care Medicine, Heart Center Rostock, Schillingallee 35, 18057 Rostock, Germany. [4]Kardiologie und Konservative Intensivmedizin, Landsbergerallee 49, 10249 Berlin, Germany. [5]Institute For Biostatistics and Informatics in Medicine And Ageing Research, Ernst Heydemanstr. 8, 18057 Rostock, Germany.

References

1. Nkomo VT, Gardin JM, Skelton TN, Gottdiener JS, Scott CG, Enriquez-Sarano M. Burden of valvular heart diseases: a population-based study. Lancet. 2006;368:1005–11.
2. Mirabel M, Iung B, Baron G, Messika-Zeitoun D, Détaint D, Vanoverschelde JL, Butchart EG, Ravaud P, Vahanian A. What are the characteristics of patients with severe, symptomatic, mitral regurgitation who are denied surgery? Eur Heart J. 2007;28:1358–65.
3. Detaint D, Sundt TM, Nkomo VT, Scott CG, Tajik AJ, Schaff HV, Enriquez-Sarano M. Surgical correction of mitral regurgitation in the elderly: outcomes and recent improvements. Circulation. 2006;114:265–72.
4. Eurostat. Population structure and ageing. Available at: http://ec.europa.eu/eurostat/statistics-explained/index.php/Population_structure_and_ageing. Accessed 15 Mar 2017.
5. Alfieri O, Maisano F. Mitral valve surgery in the elderly: New insights and unanswered questions. Eur Heart J. 2011;32:535–6.
6. Paranskaya L, D'Ancona G, Bozdag-Turan I, Akin I, Kische S, Turan GR, Rehders T, Ortak J, Nienaber CA, Ince H. Residual mitral valve regurgitation after percutaneous mitral valve repair with the MitraClip® system is a risk factor for adverse one-year outcome. Catheter Cardiovasc Interv. 2013;81:609–17.
7. Neuhold S, Huelsmann M, Pernicka E, Graf A, Bonderman D, Adlbrecht C, Binder T, Maurer G, Pacher R, Mascherbauer J. Impact of tricuspid regurgitation on survival in patients with chronic heart failure: unexpected findings of a long-term observational study. Eur Heart J. 2013;34:844–52.
8. Alozie A, Westphal B, Kische S, Kaminski A, Paranskaya L, Bozdag-Turan I, Ortak J, Schubert J, Steinhoff G, Ince H. Surgical revision after percutaneous mitral valve repair by edge-to-edge device: when the strategy fails in the highest risk surgical population. Eur J Cardiothorac Surg. 2013;46:55–60.
9. Vahanian A, Baumgartner H, Bax J, Butchart E, Dion R, Filippatos G, et al. Task Force on the Management of Valvular Hearth Disease of the European Society of Cardiology; ESC Committee for Practice Guidelines. Guidelines on the management of valvular heart disease: the Task Force on the Management of Valvular Heart Disease of the European Society of Cardiology. Eur Heart J. 2007;28:230–68.
10. Biancari F, Schifano P, Pighi M, Vasques F, Juvonen T, Vinco GJ. Pooled estimates of immediate and late outcome of mitral valve surgery in octogenarians: a meta-analysis and meta-regression. Cardiothorac Vasc Anesth. 2013;27:213–9.
11. Paranskaya L, D'Ancona G, Bozdag-Turan I, Akin I, Kische S, Turan GR, Divchev D, Rehders T, Westphal B, Schubert J, Nienaber CA, Ince H. Percutaneous mitral valve repair with the MitraClip system: perioperative and 1-year follow-up results using standard or multiple clipping strategy. Catheter Cardiovasc Interv. 2013;81:1224–31.
12. Vahanian A, Alfieri O, Andreotti F, Antunes MJ, Barón-Esquivias G, Baumgartner H, Borger MA, Carrel TP, De Bonis M, Evangelista A, Falk V, Lung B, Lancellotti P, Pierard L, Price S, Schäfers HJ, Schuler G, Stepinska J, Swedberg K, Takkenberg J, Von Oppell UO, Windecker S, Zamorano JL, Zembala M. Guidelines on the management of valvular heart disease (version 2012): the Joint Task Force on the Management of Valvular Heart Disease of the European Society of Cardiology (ESC) and the European Association for Cardio-Thoracic Surgery (EACTS);.ESC Committee for Practice Guidelines (CPG); Joint Task Force on the Management of Valvular Heart Disease of the European Society of Cardiology (ESC); European Association for Cardio-Thoracic Surgery (EACTS). Eur J Cardiothorac Surg. 2012;42:S1–44.
13. Wu AH, Aaronson KD, Bolling SF, Pagani FD, Welch K, Koelling TM. Impact of mitral valve annuloplasty on mortality risk in patients with mitral regurgitation and left ventricular systolic dysfunction. J Am Coll Cardiol. 2005;45:381–7.
14. Benjamin MM, Smith RL, Grayburn PA. Ischemic and functional mitral regurgitation in heart failure: natural history and treatment. Curr Cardiol Rep. 2014;16:517.
15. Swaans MJ, Bakker AL, Alipour A, Post MC, Kelder JC, de Kroon TL, Eefting FD, Rensing BJ, Van der Heyden JA. Survival of transcatheter Mitral valve repair compared with surgical and conservative treatment in high-surgical-risk patients. JACC Cardiovasc Interv. 2014;7:875–81.
16. Lamas GA, Mitchell GF, Flaker GC, Smith Jr SC, Gersh BJ, Basta L, Moyé L, Braunwald E, Pfeffer MA. Clinical significance of mitral regurgitation after acute myocardial infarction. Survival and ventricular enlargement investigators. Circulation. 1997;96:827–33.
17. Trichon BH, Felker GM, Shaw LK, Cabell CH, O'Connor CM. Relation of frequency and severity of mitral regurgitation to survival among patients with left ventricular systolic dysfunction and heart failure. Am J Cardiol. 2003;91:538–43.
18. Glower DD, Kar S, Trento A, Lim DS, Bajwa T, Quesada R, Whitlow PL, Rinaldi MJ, Grayburn P, Mack MJ, Mauri L, McCarthy PM, Feldman T. Percutaneous mitral valve repair for mitral regurgitation in high-risk patients: results of the EVEREST II study. J Am Coll Cardiol. 2014;64:172–81.
19. Taramasso M, Maisano F, Denti P, Latib A, La Canna G, Colombo A, Alfieri O. Percutaneous edge-to-edge repair in high-risk and elderly patients with degenerative mitral regurgitation: Midterm outcomes in a single-center experience. J Thorac Cardiovasc Surg. 2014. doi: 10.1016/j.jtcvs.2014.03.036. [Epub ahead of print].
20. Gazoni LM, Kern JA, Swenson BR, Dent JM, Smith PW, Mulloy DP, Reece TB, Fedoruk LM, Lisle TC, Peeler BB, Kron IL. A change in perspective: results for ischemic mitral valve repair are similar to mitral valve repair for degenerative disease. Ann Thorac Surg. 2007;84:750–7.
21. Maisano F, Viganò G, Calabrese C, Taramasso M, Denti P, Blasio A, Guidotti A, Alfieri O. Quality of life of elderly patients following valve surgery for chronic organic mitral regurgitation. Eur J Cardiothorac Surg. 2009;36:261–6.
22. Kaneko H, Neuss M, Weissenborn J, Butter C. Impact of residual mitral regurgitation after MitraClip implantation. Int J Cardiol. 2017;227:813–819.
23. Ohno Y, Attizzani GF, Capodanno D, Cannata S, Dipasqua F, Immé S, Barbanti M, Ministeri M, Caggegi A, Pistritto AM, Chiarandà M, Ronsivalle G, Giaquinta S, Farruggio S, Mangiafico S, Scandura S, Tamburino C, Capranzano P, Grasso C. Association of tricuspid regurgitation with clinical and echocardiographic outcomes after percutaneous mitral valve repair with the MitraClip System: 30-day and 12-month follow-up from the GRASP Registry. Eur Heart J Cardiovasc Imaging. 2014;15:1246–55.
24. De Bonis M, Lapenna E, Buzzatti N, La Canna G, Denti P, Pappalardo F, Schiavi D, Pozzoli A, Cioni M, Di Giannuario G, Alfieri O. Optimal results immediately after MitraClip therapy or surgical edge-to-edge repair for functional mitral regurgitation: are they really stable at 4 years? Eur J Cardiothorac Surg. 2016;50:488–94.
25. Crabtree TD, Bailey MS, Moon MR, Munfakh N, Pasque MK, Lawton JS, Moazami N, Aubuchon KA, Al-Dadah AS, Damiano Jr RJ. Recurrent mitral regurgitation and risk factors for early and late mortality after mitral valve repair for functional ischemic mitral regurgitation. Ann Thorac Surg. 2008;85:1537–42.
26. Mihaljevic T, Lam BK, Rajeswaran J, Takagaki M, Lauer MS, Gillinov AM, Blackstone EH, Lytle BW. Impact of mitral valve annuloplasty combined with revascularization in patients with functional ischemic mitral regurgitation. J Am Coll Cardiol. 2007;49:2191–201.

8

An inappropriate pacing threshold increase after repeated electrical storm in a patient with implantable cardioverter defibrillator

Ye Zhu[1,2], Xiang Gu[1,2*] and Chao Xu[3]

Abstract

Background: Implantable cardioverter defibrillators (ICD) are capable of effectively terminating malignant ventricular arrhythmia and are the most effective way to prevent sudden cardiac death. However, some evidences demonstrated that both anti-tachycardia pacing (ATP) and ICD shock can also bring adverse prognosis.

Case presentation: A 66-year-old Han Chinese man with prior ICD implantation was admitted to our hospital because of frequent ICD shocks. Although intravenous amiodarone and esmolol succinate were administered daily, the patient suffered 155 episodes of VT/VF during 8 weeks after implantation. After repeated discharge of the device, the pacing threshold of the patient increased gradually. Considering the inappropriate increase of the pacing threshold, we decided to reposition the right ventricular (RV) lead with good sensing and threshold parameters confirmed. Subsequent 22 months interrogation follow-up revealed a stable lead position and electrical specifications. Furthermore, antiarrhythmic drugs were maximally increased, while ATP burst was remarkably decreased and the inappropriate ICD shock never occurred until now.

Conclusion: An inappropriate pacing threshold was increased secondary to repeated ICD electrical storm. A timely active lead position adjustment reduced the pacing threshold and eliminated the risk of premature battery depletion.

Keywords: Implantable cardioverter defibrillator, Anti-tachycardia pacing, Pacing threshold, Electrical storm

Background

Implantable cardioverter defibrillator (ICD) can effectively terminate malignant ventricular tachycardia (VT)/ ventricular fibrillation (VF) and prevent sudden death [1–3]. Electrical storm (ES), characterized by multiple attacks of VT or ventricular fibrillation (VF), is an unstable condition for which management and prevention are still a challenge. Whether ES is a causal factor or only an epiphenomenon remains unclear, although it is still a matter for debate that repeated shocks may provoke myocardial damage and result in further deterioration of the underlying disorders [4].

We report an ICD patient with severe ES caused by frequent VT/VF refractory to antiarrhythmic agents. The continuous discharge of the ICD might be related to an inappropriate increase of pacing threshold and it necessitated a repositioning of a lead.

Case presentation

A 66-year-old Han Chinese male was admitted after several VT attacks over the course of 1 month. The patient was diagnosed with rheumatic heart disease and impaired left ventricular ejection fraction (LVEF) of 42% in a functional New York Heart Association stage III, suffering from VT/VF and atrial fibrillation. He underwent surgery of the mitral valve and an aortic valve replacement 10 years ago. Electrolytic measurements showed sodium, calcium, and potassium values were within the normal range. He was treated with aldosterone antagonist, angiotensin converting enzyme inhibitor, lidocaine, β-blocker, and amiodarone, but VT recurred despite the optimized drug treatment. Additional doses of antiarrhythmic drugs were administered but unsuccessful. The

* Correspondence: guxiang@yzu.edu.cn
[1]Clinical Medical College, Yangzhou University, Yangzhou, Jiangsu 225001, China
[2]Department of Cardiology, Northern Jiangsu Province Hospital, Yangzhou, Jiangsu 225001, China
Full list of author information is available at the end of the article

patient was placed on amiodarone 200 mg orally once a day and metoprolol 25 mg orally four times a day. Attempts to reduce the frequency of VT using optimized antiarrhythmic drugs failed. VT could only be terminated by external cardioversion. The patient satisfied the requirement for ICD therapy according to the criteria of the Sudden Cardiac Death in Heart Failure Trial (SCD-HeFT), [5] so a single chamber ICD (Model 1231–40, St. Jude Medical Cardiac Rhythm Management, USA) was implanted with lead in the right ventricular (RV) apex after symptom stabilization (Fig. 1a). During the implantation, electrical specifications were confirmed, including the R-wave of 9.0 mV, the slew rate of 1.7 V/s, the impedance of 574 Ohm, and pacing threshold of 0.6 V/0.5 ms.

Two days later, the patient was abruptly awakened by an episode of VT/VF. The initial administration of the ATP therapy through the ICD was unsuccessful. VF was finally terminated by a 36 J ICD shock. Frequent ICD shocks were associated with anxiety and intolerance of ICD therapy. The patient was thin and weak. ATP and Low energy cardioversion (15/25 J) were successfully used to relieve the patient's pain, anxiety and possible myocardial injury (Fig. 2-a, b, c). Overall, the patient experienced 155 episodes of VT/VF and received a total of 27 shocks after the first implantation of ICD. The most severe attack was 34 VT/VF episodes within 24 h. Rarely, a 36.0 J shock at last reverted VT, which was not terminated by ATP burst and a 15.0 J/25 J shock (Fig. 2-d). Frequent ICD discharges depleted the battery life considerably. His treatment was aggressively escalated. Catheter ablation was contraindicated because of the patient's metal valve and multiple original VTs. Renal artery denervation was recommended but refused. Attempts to reduce the frequency of VT only using antiarrhythmic drugs, such as lidocaine, were unsuccessful. The combination of ATP and intravenous esmolol seemed to reduce, but did not fully eliminate the episodes of VT.

After repeated discharge of the device for 8 weeks, the capture threshold was gradually increased. Initial threshold of device interrogation was respectively 2.37 V/0.5 ms, 2.75 V/0.5 ms, and 3.75 V/1.0 ms in 2, 4 and 9 weeks post- implantation (Additional file 1). Thorax X-ray at 9 weeks post-implant did not show apparent dislocation of the lead (Fig. 1b). Considering the patient's reliance on the pacemaker, we decided to reposition the RV lead to better match the ventricular myocardium in the threshold field as a final alternative (Fig. 1c). Fortunately, this remedy did lower the pacing threshold. Lead measurements showed the ventricular sensing at 11.3 mV, a pacing threshold of 1.4 V/0.5 ms, and an impedance of 730 Ohms. The further clinical course of the patient was uncomplicated and he was discharged in good clinical status after the surgery. Recent device interrogation respectively showed a ventricular sensing of 8.9 mV, 7.9 mV and 9.1 mV, a pacing threshold of 1.75 V/0.5 ms, 1.5 V/1.0 ms and 1.5 V/1.0 ms at 13, 20, 24 months post-implantation follow-up (Additional file 1). Amiodarone 200 mg qd and metoprolol 25 mg q6h were given to enhance the efficacy of anti-arrhythmias. The patient's pacing threshold and ventricular arrhythmias have carefully being monitored in the long term. Until now, the shock never occurred again and ATP burst significantly decreased.

Discussion and conclusions

This case highlights a rare clinical situation: an increased pacing threshold may be increased by repeated ES in a patient with an ICD.

In the era of ICD therapy, ES has become increasingly common. It is generally defined as the occurrence of three or more obvious episodes of VT /VF in 24 h, separated by bouts of normal rhythm after successful therapy, either ATP burst or shock [6]. Previous studies have shown that ES occurs in about 10 – 28% of ICD recipients and is associated with increased mortality [7]. The

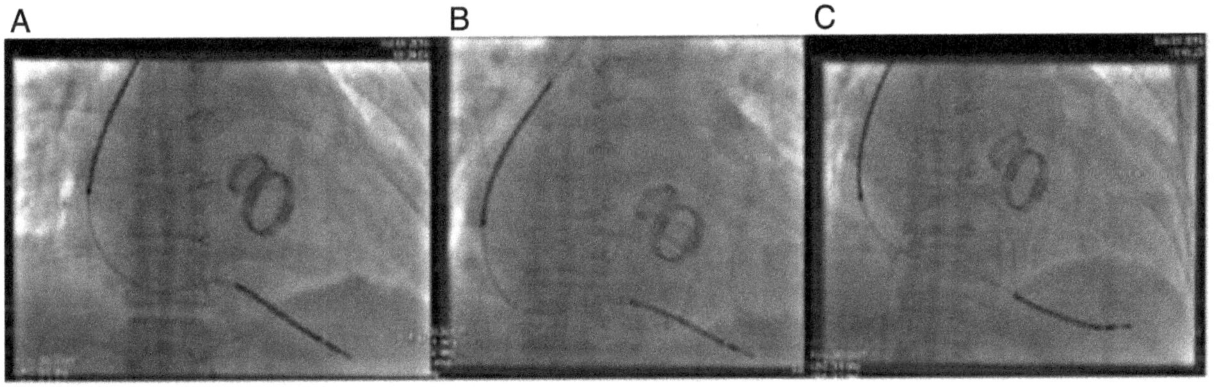

Fig. 1 Anteroposterior chest X-ray follow-up of the ICD lead position. **a** ICD lead position after first implant. **b** No apparent dislocation of the lead at 9 weeks post- first implant. **c** Chest X-ray image of lead reposition. ICD, implantable cardioverter-defibrillators

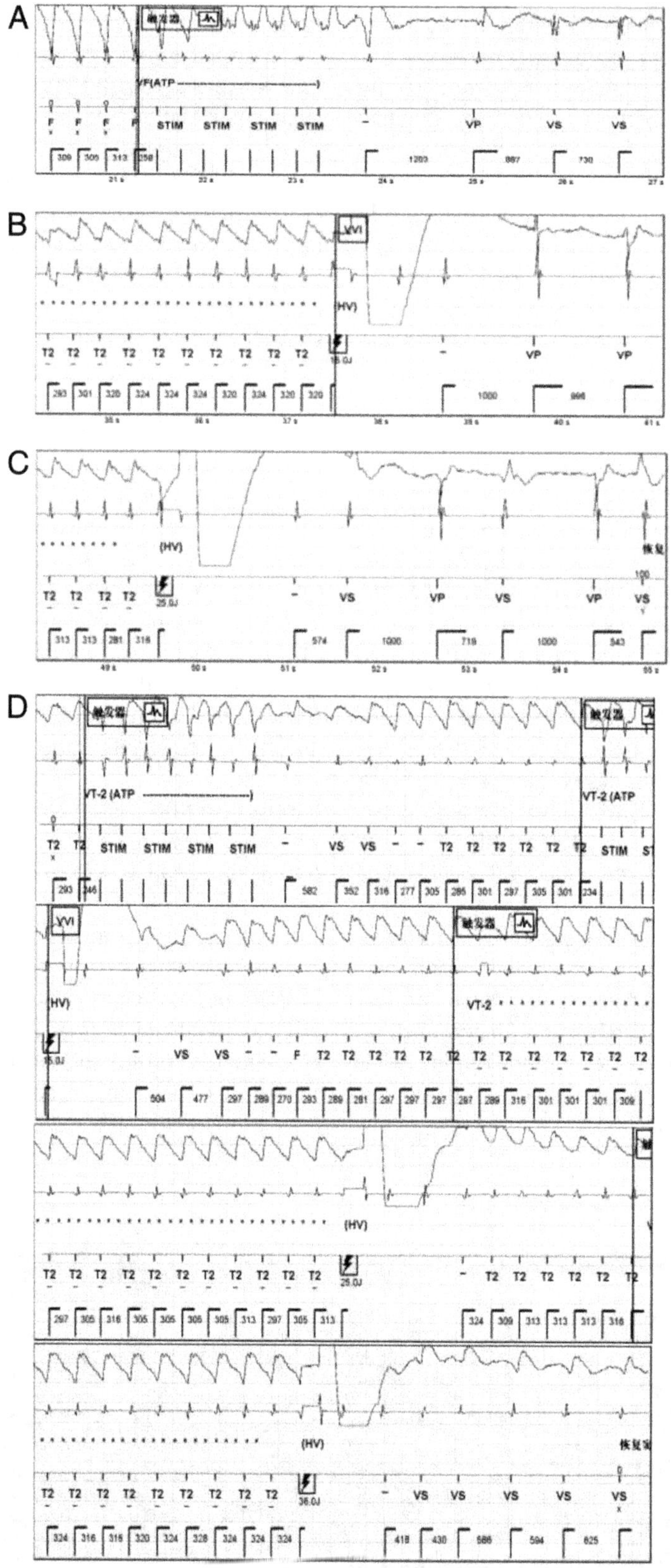

Fig. 2 ICD interrogation record of VT/VF and cardioversion. **a**, **b** and **c** representing a successful ATP burst, a 15.0 J shock and a 25.0 J shock cardioversion respectively. **d** A 36.0 J shock terminated VT after No successful ATP burst, a 15.0 J shock and a 25.0 J shock cardioversion. ICD, implantable cardioverter-defibrillators; VT, ventricular tachycardia; VF, ventricular fibrillation; ATP, anti-tachycardia pacing

first therapy for ES is eliminating the risk factors as soon as possible, then following a positive comprehensive management protocol [8]. Structural heart disease, electrolyte imbalance, myocardial infarction, inherited arrhythmic syndrome and other factors could all lead to ES [9]. In this case, VT was definitively identified on admission. The patient had a history of heart failure, rheumatic heart disease, and valve replacement surgery. He did not have diabetes, hyperlipidemia, a history of smoking or any other risk factors for coronary heart disease. Risk factors for acidosis and electrolyte disorders were also excluded [10]. The patient had considerable VTs during the perioperative period of ICD implantation. ES before ICD implantation may cause myocardial damage, and the placement of the ICD electrode may further damaged the local myocardium. The inappropriate discharge during 8 weeks after ICD implantation was attributed to myocardial injury caused by ES before ICD implantation. Additionally, the occurrence of ES seriously affected the patient's quality of life and induced psychological symptoms including anxiety and fear. This programming strategy should be minimal energy of the defibrillation and effectively terminate VT/VF. However, some patients at high risk for sudden cardiac death still require the maximum energy that ICDs can achieve. For such patients, a readjustment of the RV lead position is a successful strategy to lower the threshold [11].

Overdrive pacing, as implemented in this case, has been reported to stabilize an ES [12]. Comprehensive treatment of VT such as increasing the identifying frequency of VT, optimal medication, trigger or substrate ablation and denervation should be administered to reduce or eliminate false identification and inappropriate ICD discharges [13]. As illustrated in this case, the management of ES hinges on excluding every possible causative factor, no matter how rare. Catheter ablation appears to be effective in both short-term therapy and prevention of ES. Catheter ablation of the left ventricular was contraindicated because of the patient's metal valve. Renal artery denervation was offered but refused. Amiodarone and betablockers might lower the incidence of shock therapy in patients with ICD. Optimal programming aimed at reducing the burden of ICD therapy without an increase in adverse outcomes [14]. For this case, post-implantation inspection showed that the pacing threshold gradually increased. Thorax X-ray at 9 weeks post-implant did not show apparent dislocation of the lead. However, a lead tiny dislodgement seldom be excluded or confirmed. The repeated ES may have facilitated the development of heart failure and myocardium injury, which in turn increased the pacing threshold and shortened the life of the device. We took into consideration the fact that RV lead repositioning is a surgical procedure that exposes the patient to several risks. RV-ICD lead position adjustment can also be successfully performed to avoid the pacing threshold increase. Low pacing threshold is not only critical for the safety and effectiveness of the ICD therapy, but also can extend the life of the device. We made several efforts, invasively and noninvasively, to decrease this patient's pacing threshold, including lead repositioning and appropriate ICD adjustment [15]. Here, the positioning of the RV lead was used as a final remedy. The 22 months follow-up after the second ICD implantation showed a steady position of the RV lead and stable parameters for sensing and pacing. The inappropriate shock never occurred until now. However, lead repositioning may not lead to ES cessation. ES cessation was achieved by adjusting the administration and dosage of antiarrhythmic agents and myocardium rehabilitation.

In this case, the attack of VT/VF was safely terminated by maximal post-procedural administration of antiarrhythmic drugs, subsequent application of ATP and discharge by the ICD. The follow-up showed that an inappropriate pacing threshold by repeated ES could not be fully eliminated. A timely active lead position adjustment reduced the pacing threshold and eliminated the risk of premature battery depletion. A programmable strategy should be personally adjusted as the low, middle and high cardioversion energy for effectively terminating VT/VF and lessening myocardial injury secondary to ES.

Additional file

Additional file 1: I. 14 and 28 Oct, 2015 in 4 weeks post-first implantation follow-up. II.16, 18, 22, 24 and 30 Nov, 2015 in 2 months post- first implantation follow-up. III.1 and 3 Dec, 2015 in 2 months post- first implantation follow-up. IV.8, 9 and 16 Dec, 2015 in two weeks post- second implantation follow-up. V. 9 Mar and 13 Apr, 2016 in 3–4 months post- second implantation follow-up. VI. 9 Nov, 2016 in 9 months post- second implantation follow-up. VII. 14 Jun, 2017 in 18 months post- second implantation follow-up. VIII. 27 Sep, 2017 in 22 months post- second implantation follow-up. Initial threshold of device interrogation was respectively 2.37 V/0.5 ms, 2.75 V/0.5 ms, and 3.75 V/1.0 ms in 2, 4 and 9 weeks post- implantation. Recent device interrogation showed a ventricular sensing of 8.9 mV, 7.9 mV and 9.1 mV, a pacing threshold of 1.75 V/0.5 ms, 1.5 V/1.0 ms and 1.5 V/1.0 ms at 13, 20, 24 months post-implantation follow-up. (DOCX 902 kb)

Abbreviations

ATP: Anti-tachycardia pacing; ECG: Electrocardiogram; ES: Electrical storm; ICD: Implantable cardioverter-defibrillators; LVEF: Left ventricular ejection fraction; RV: Right ventricular; VF: Ventricular fibrillation; VT: Ventricular tachycardia

Acknowledgements

The authors would like to appreciate the assistance of Loula Burton, Office of Research at Tulane University, in polishing the English manuscript. We are grateful to Dr.Lei Sun, Dr.Yi Zhang, Dr. Zhengyu Bao and Dr. Jianhua Shen for their valuable advice on the management of the patient. We thank the editor and the reviewers whose comments/suggestions helped improve and clarify this manuscript.

Funding

This work was supported by funds from science and technology department of Jiangsu province, China (No. BL2013022).

Authors' contributions

YZ, XG, and CX were involved in identifying the literature, gathering the clinical data and editing the manuscript. All authors have read and approved the manuscript, and ensure that this is the case.

Competing interests

The authors declare that they have no competing interests.

Author details

[1]Clinical Medical College, Yangzhou University, Yangzhou, Jiangsu 225001, China. [2]Department of Cardiology, Northern Jiangsu Province Hospital, Yangzhou, Jiangsu 225001, China. [3]Department of Global Biostatistics and Data Science, School of Public Health and Tropical Medicine, Tulane University, New Orleans, LA 70112, USA.

References

1. Chang PM, Powell BD, Jones PW, Carter N, Hayes DL, Saxon LA. Implantable Cardioverter defibrillator programming characteristics, shocked rhythms, and survival among patients under thirty years of age. J Cardiovasc Electrophysiol. 2016;27(10):1183–90.
2. Jimenez-Candil J, Hernandez J, Martin A, Morinigo J, Perdiguero P, Bravo L, Ruiz S, Sanchez PL. Differences in ventricular tachyarrythmias and antitachycardia pacing effectiveness according to the ICD indication (primary versus secondary prevention): an analysis based on the stored electrograms. J Interv Card Electrophysiol. 2015;44(2):187–95.
3. Malagu M, Ferri A, Mancuso O, Trevisan F, Nardozza M, Bertini M. Implantable cardioverter defibrillator management: an update. Futur Cardiol. 2016;12(6):673–88.
4. Nedios S, Darma A, Stevanello C, Richter S, Doering M, Rolf S, Sommer P, Hindricks G, Bollmann A, Arya A. Electrical storm in patients with implantable cardioverter-defibrillator in the era of catheter ablation: implications for better rhythm control. Heart Rhythm. 2015;12(12):2419–25.
5. Au-Yeung WT, Reinhall PG, Poole JE, Anderson J, Johnson G, Fletcher RD, Moore HJ, Mark DB, Lee KL, Bardy GH. SCD-HeFT: use of R-R interval statistics for long-term risk stratification for arrhythmic sudden cardiac death. Heart Rhythm. 2015;12(10):2058–66.
6. Looi KL, Tang A, Agarwal S. Ventricular arrhythmia storm in the era of implantable cardioverter-defibrillator. Postgrad Med J. 2015;91(1079):519–26.
7. Ginwalla M, Battula S, Dunn J, Lewis WR. Termination of electrocution-induced ventricular fibrillation by an implantable cardioverter defibrillator. Pacing Clin Electrophysiol. 2010;33(4):510–2.
8. Hohnloser SH, Al-Khalidi HR, Pratt CM, Brum JM, Tatla DS, Tchou P, Dorian P. Electrical storm in patients with an implantable defibrillator: incidence, features, and preventive therapy: insights from a randomized trial. Eur Heart J. 2006;27(24):3027–32.
9. Camsari A, Yilmaz DC, Ozcan T. Inappropriate shock delivery by implantable cardioverter defibrillator due to electrical leak from bathroom tap. Clin Res Cardiol. 2010;99(11):761–3.
10. Lee WC, Chen HC, Chen YL, Tsai TH, Pan KL, Lin YS, Chen MC. Left ventricle remodeling predicts the recurrence of ventricular tachyarrhythmias in implantable cardioverter defibrillator recipients for secondary prevention. BMC Cardiovasc Disord. 2016;16(1):231.
11. Cesario D, Bhargava M, Valderrabano M, Fonarow GC, Wilkoff B, Shivkumar K. Azygos vein lead implantation: a novel adjunctive technique for implantable cardioverter defibrillator placement. J Cardiovasc Electrophysiol. 2004;15(7):780–3.
12. Kurisu S, Inoue I, Kawagoe T, Ishihara M, Shimatani Y, Mitsuba N, Hata T, Nakama Y, Kisaka T, Kijima Y. Temporary overdriving pacing as an adjunct to antiarrhythmic drug therapy for electrical storm in acute myocardial infarction. Circ J. 2005;69(5):613–6.
13. Gu X, Zhu Y, Sun L, Zhang Y, Cao K, Cheng J. Impact of rate control during atrial fibrillation on the proarrhythmic and antiarrhythmic effects of biventricular pacing. Int J Cardiol. 2012;159(2):162–3.
14. Tan VH, Wilton SB, Kuriachan V, Sumner GL, Exner DV. Impact of programming strategies aimed at reducing nonessential implantable cardioverter defibrillator therapies on mortality: a systematic review and meta-analysis. Circ Arrhythm Electrophysiol. 2014;7(1):164–70.
15. Grimard C, May MA, Mabo P, Babuty D. An original defibrillation lead implantation to avoid tricuspid prosthesis damage. Europace. 2010;12(4):589–90.

9

Alcohol consumption and mortality in patients undergoing coronary artery bypass graft (CABG)-a register-based cohort study

Mads Phillip Kofoed Grabas[1*], Steen Møller Hansen[2], Christian Torp-Pedersen[1,2], Henrik Bøggild[1], Line Rosenkilde Ullits[1], Ulrik Deding[1], Berit Jamie Nielsen[2], Per Føge Jensen[3] and Charlotte Overgaard[1]

Abstract

Background: Previous studies have shown that compared with abstinence and heavy drinking, moderate alcohol consumption is associated with a reduced risk of mortality among the general population and patients with heart failure and myocardial infarction. We examined the association between alcohol consumption and mortality in coronary artery bypass graft (CABG) patients.

Method: We studied 1,919 first-time CABG patients using data on alcohol consumption and mortality obtained from Danish national registers from March 2006 to October 2011. Alcohol consumption was divided into the following groups: abstainers (0 units/week), moderate consumers (1–14 units/week), moderate-heavy drinkers (15–21 units/week) and heavy drinkers (>21 units/week). Hazard ratios (HR) of all-cause mortality were calculated using Cox proportional hazard regression analysis.

Results: The median follow-up was 2.2 years [IQR 2.0]. There were 112 deaths, of which 96 (86 %) were classified as cardiovascular. Adjustments for age and sex showed no increased risk of all-cause mortality for the abstainers (HR 1.61, 95 % CI, 1.00–2.58) and moderate-heavy drinkers (HR 1.40, 95 % CI, 0.73–2.67) compared with moderate consumers. However, heavy drinkers had a high risk of all-cause mortality compared with moderate consumers (HR 2.44, 95 % CI, 1.47–4.04). A full adjustment showed no increase in mortality for the abstainers (HR 1.59, 95 % CI, 0.98–2.57) and moderate-heavy drinkers (HR 1.68, 95 % CI, 0.86–3.29), while heavy drinkers were associated with an increased mortality rate (HR 1.88, 95 % CI, 1.10–3.21). There was no increased risk of 30-day mortality for the abstainers (HR 0.74, 95 % CI, 0.23–2.32), moderate-heavy drinkers (HR 0.36, 95 % CI, 0.07–1.93) and heavy drinkers (HR 2.20, 95 % CI, 0.65–7.36).

Conclusion: There was no increased risk of mortality for abstainers (0 units/week) or moderate-heavy drinkers (15–21 units/week) following a CABG. Only heavy drinking (>21 units/week) were significantly associated with an increased mortality rate. These results suggest that only heavy drinking present a risk factor among CABG patients.

Keywords: CABG, Coronary artery bypass graft, Alcohol consumption, Mortality, Cox regression models

* Correspondence: madsgrabas@hotmail.com
[1]Department of Health Science and Technology, Public Health and Epidemiology Group, Aalborg University, Niels Jernes Vej 14, 9220 Aalborg Øst, Denmark
Full list of author information is available at the end of the article

Background

Alcohol consumption is associated with both harmful and beneficial health effects. Alcohol consumption increases the risk of death caused by oral cancer, cirrhosis and alcoholism [1], and heavy drinking increases the risk of all-cause mortality [2, 3]. In contrast, a beneficial effect of moderate alcohol consumption has been generally associated with reduced mortality, specifically for patients suffering from heart failure and acute myocardial infarction (AMI) [2–8].

Thus, while moderate alcohol consumption has beneficial effects in general, it is less certain how alcohol consumption influences patients with established coronary heart disease (CHD), particularly when surgical revascularization in the form of coronary artery bypass graft (CABG) [9] is needed. In terms of mortality, CHD is of considerable importance [9–11], and in cases of significant left main coronary artery stenosis, multi-vessel coronary disease or severe angina pectoris, CABG is recommended, which increases the blood supply to the heart, relieves pain and prolongs life [9].

In addition to established CHD, CABG patients often have several co-morbidities [12, 13] and high mortality rates. Consequently, it is important to determine whether strict recommendations regarding alcohol consumption also apply to this high-risk patient group.

A few studies have examined the influence of alcohol consumption on composite outcomes, including mortality, in CABG patients [14, 15]. In general, these studies have shown no harmful effects of alcohol consumption. As moderate alcohol consumption decreases the mortality risk in the general population, it is possible that moderate alcohol consumption may have beneficial effects or at least does not affect the risk of mortality in a high-risk population of CABG patients. Stroke, AMI, chronic obstructive pulmonary disease (COPD), liver disease, heart failure, renal failure, atrial fibrillation (AF), diabetes mellitus and hypertension have previously been identified as potential confounders in studies of mortality among CABG patients [12, 15]. Other potential risk factors are increased body mass index (BMI) [16–19], smoking [2, 17, 20], low household income [17], and low educational level [17]. However, previous studies of alcohol consumption and mortality in CABG patients [14, 15] were not able to account for the previously mentioned potential confounders, and furthermore, these studies had composite outcomes, including mortality. A more comprehensive investigation is needed to determine the influence of alcohol consumption on mortality in CABG patients.

The objective of this study was to examine the association between alcohol consumption and mortality among CABG patients, while considering a wide range of severe co-morbidities and other potential confounders.

Methods

Design and data sources

A nationwide register-based cohort study was conducted. The study included patients who underwent first-time CABG surgery between March 2006 and October 2011. We obtained data on alcohol consumption, mortality and covariates from seven administrative registers. From birth or at the time of immigration, all residents in Denmark are assigned a unique personal identification number (CPR-number), which enables linkage between national Danish registries [21].

The Danish National Patient Register, which contains information on all patients in Danish hospitals and diagnoses according to the International Classification of Diseases version 10 (ICD-10) [22], was one of the registers used. The Danish Anesthesia Database [23, 24] contains information on alcohol consumption, smoking status and BMI. This information is systematically registered by an anaesthesiologist with the aid of a standardized questionnaire prior to surgery; the questionnaire is filled in by the anaesthesiologist based on the information provided by the patient. The Danish Register of Causes of Death contains information on all-cause mortality and causes of death based on death certificates completed by a physician, according to the ICD-10 [25]. The Danish National Prescription Registry contains information on all redeemed prescriptions in Denmark, according to the Anatomical Therapeutic Chemical classification (ATC) [26], and the Income Statistics Register contains information on income and taxes for Danish residents [27]. The Population's Education Register contains information on completed education levels; it is approved by the Danish Ministry of Education [28].

Study population

All surgical procedures were registered according to the Nordic Medico-Statistical Committee (NOMESCO) classification of surgical procedures, which is used in Nordic countries [29]. The Danish National Patient Register was used to identify first-time CABG patients. Patients with the following surgical procedures were included (with related codes): connection to the coronary artery from the internal mammary artery (FNA), connection to the coronary artery from the gastroepiploic artery (FNB), aortocoronary venous bypass (FNC), aortocoronary bypass using a prosthetic graft (FND) (n = 1), coronary bypass using free arterial graft (FNE), coronary thromboendarterectomy (FNF) and repair of coronary artery (FNH). Patients were excluded if they also underwent other surgical procedures simultaneous, such as closure of coronary fistula (FNJ), repair of anomalous origin of a coronary artery (FNK), right ventricle and pulmonary valve (FJ), mitral valve (FK), aortic valve (FM), transplantation of heart or heart and lung (FQ), arrhythmias and disturbances of impulse propagation (FP), pulmonary artery with branches (FB) and thoracic and thoracoabdominal aorta, excluding malformations (FC). Patients were also excluded if they were diagnosed with cancer (ICD-10 C00-C97) prior to baseline.

Exposure measure

The CABG operation dates, which were obtained from the Danish National Patient Register, were used as the date of entry. Patients were excluded if they not met the inclusion criteria in the study population section described above or did not have data on alcohol consumption registered. The alcohol consumption measurement date was obtained from the Danish Anesthesia Database, and only patients for whom alcohol consumption was measured less than three days before the operation date were included in the final study population. Alcohol consumption was divided into four groups: 0 units/week (abstainers), 1–14 units/week (moderate consumers), 15–21 units/week (moderate-heavy drinkers), >21 units/week (heavy drinkers). One unit of beer, wine or liquor contains approximately the same amount of alcohol, and alcohol consumption is often considered in units rather than in grams or millilitres of alcohol [30–32]. One standard unit of alcohol contain 12 g of alcohol [33], and moderate consumption is regarded as 1–2 units of alcohol per day [7].

Outcomes measured

Information on mortality was obtained from the Danish Register of Causes of Death. Patients were followed until death or the end of follow-up, which was December 31, 2011 (censoring), whichever was first. In addition to all-cause mortality, we also examined cardiovascular mortality, which was followed up in the same manner, except that death from causes other than cardiovascular mortality was censured at the date of death. ICD-10 I00-I99 was used to define cardiovascular mortality. All-cause mortality also included cardiovascular death, and 30-day mortality was defined as patients dying within 30 days after the CABG operation date.

Covariates

Stroke, liver disease, heart failure, renal failure, COPD, AMI, AF, hypertension and diabetes mellitus [12, 15] were included as potential confounders. Apart from hypertension and diabetes mellitus, diagnoses registered in the Danish National Patient Registry were used to determine whether the patients suffered from one or more of these diseases prior to the CABG operation. Redeemed prescriptions were used as a proxy for hypertension and diabetes mellitus prior to baseline [26]. Patients suffering from hypertension were identified by combination treatment with at least two classes of antihypertensive drugs, as previously described elsewhere [34]. If the patients claimed prescriptions for glucose-lowering medications (ATC A10) prior to baseline, then they were considered to have diabetes mellitus.

Information on BMI and smoking status was obtained from the Danish Anesthesia Database. BMI was divided into three groups: underweight (<18.5) or normal weight (18.5–24.9), overweight (25–29.9) and obese (>30). The grouping follows the BMI definition from the World Health Organization (WHO): <18.5 is underweight, 18.5–24.9 is normal weight, 25–29.9 is overweight and >30 is obese [35]. Smoking status was registered as never smoked, previous smoker or current smoker. Household income in Danish kroner (DKK) was divided into quartiles: quartile 1 (<218,122), quartile 2 (218,123–286,685), quartile 3 (286,686–418,426), and quartile 4 (>418,426). Education levels were obtained from the Danish Education Registers [28]. According to the United Nations Educational, Scientific and Cultural Organization's (UNESCO) guidelines for classifying education (the International Standard Classification of Education 2011), the levels for highest completed education at baseline were classified as follows: basic school, high school education, vocational education, short or medium higher education and long higher education [36].

Ethics

This study was approved by the Danish Data Protection Agency (Ref.GEH-2014-014). All data were linked and stored in computers held by Statistics Denmark and made available with encrypted CPR-numbers to ensure that no individuals were identified. In agreement with the Act on Processing of Personal Data, only aggregated statistical analysis and results are published [37, 38]. Written informed consent or ethical approval is not required for register-based studies in Denmark [37, 38].

Statistical analysis

Analyses of variance (ANOVA) for continuous variables and Chi-squared (x^2) tests for categorical variables were used to test for between-group differences in weekly alcohol consumption. Survival analysis was performed, with Cox proportional hazard models. Hazard ratios (HR) and 95 % confidence interval (95 % CI) were estimated. Model 1 in the Cox regression was adjusted for age and sex, and the full adjustment in model 2 further included smoking status, BMI, household income, educational level, CABG after 2008 (time), hypertension, diabetes mellitus, COPD, AMI, AF, heart failure, liver disease, stroke and renal failure. P-values < 0.05 were considered to be statistically significant. Survival was estimated by the Kaplan-Meier method, and group differences were assessed with the log-rank test to examine the between-group differences. The analyses were performed with multivariate imputations using chained equations (MICE) on missing covariates (education level, smoking status and BMI) [39], as they increase the size of the study population and are typically more efficient than complete cases analyses [40, 41]. Thus, the main results are presented with the imputed data. For sensitivity analysis, the analyses were also conducted on the population with complete data. Tests for the interaction between alcohol consumption and covariates were conducted, and none were found. Data management was performed using SAS software, version 9.4 (SAS institute Inc. Cary, North Carolina, USA). Statistical analysis was performed using the R statistical software package, version 3.2.2 (R Development Core Team).

Result

In total, 3,821 first-time CABG patients were identified; however, 280 patients were excluded due to having cancer at baseline, and 1,622 patients were excluded due to missing alcohol consumption data. The final sample size was 1,919 (Fig. 1).

Baseline and demographic characteristics stratified by alcohol consumption are reported in Table 1. The patients had a median age of 67, and 83.4 % were males. The median follow-up was 2.2 years [IQR 2.0], (range 0–5.8 years). Of the 1,919 patients, 554 (28.8 %) reported alcohol consumption of 0 units/week, 783 (40.8 %) reported 1–14 units/week, 296 (15.4 %) reported 15–21 units/week, and 286 (14.9 %) reported >21 units/week. Of the study population of 1,919 patients, 99 had missing smoking status data, 54 had missing educational level data, and two patients had missing BMI data.

Compared to the other alcohol groups, abstainers (0 units/week) were characterized by a high proportion of obesity (28.4 %), diabetes mellitus (26.6 %), and more had basic school education (49.0 %) as their highest educational level. Moderate consumers (1–14 units/week) had a higher proportion of former smoking (58.1 %) and underweight or normal weight (35.8 %). Moderate-heavy drinkers (15–21 units/week) had higher rates of overweight (47.0 %), household income in the highest quartile (quartile 4) (46.3 %), vocational education (46.9 %), and heart failure (78.0 %). Heavy drinkers (>21 units/week) had a higher proportion of smoking (28.2 %) and short or medium-length higher education levels (20.1 %). In the lowest income quartile (quartile 1), there was a higher proportion of abstainers (25.6 %), while in the highest income quartile (quartile 4) there was a higher proportion of moderate-heavy drinkers. The majority of those with basic school as the highest educational level consisted of abstainers, while those with long higher education as the highest educational level were more likely to be moderate-heavy drinkers (8.3 %) (Table 1).

Figure 2 shows the Kaplan-Meier survival estimates for all-cause mortality stratified by weekly alcohol consumption. A total of 112 (5.84 %) patients died from all-cause mortality. The curves show the different mortality rates for the four alcohol groups (log-rank p-value = 0.02).

All-cause mortality

The most frequent cause of death was from a cardiovascular cause (96 patients, 86 % of all deaths). Other causes of death (in all cases $n <= 3$) were sepsis, pneumonia, COPD, diverticular disease with perforation and

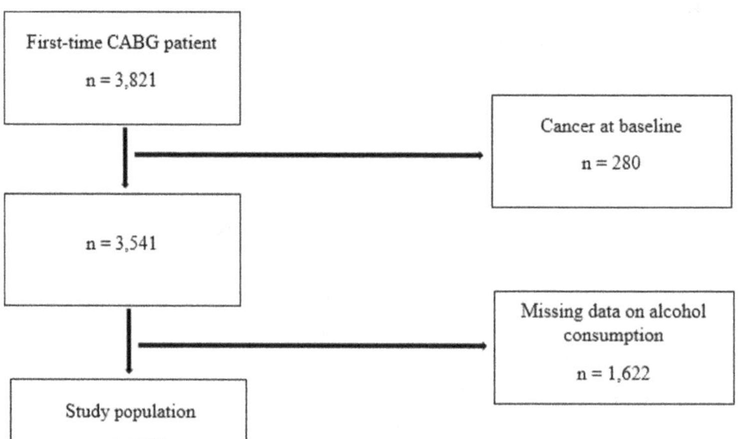

Fig. 1 A flow chart of the exclusion process for the study population. CABG patients were identified in the Danish National Patient Register and from information in the Danish Anesthesia Database (3,821) between March 2006 and October 2011. Missing values for the following covariates were included due to the application of MICE: *99 patients were included with missing smoking status data, 54 patients were included with missing educational level data, and 2 patients were included with missing BMI data

Table 1 Baseline characteristics of CABG patients by weekly alcohol consumption

Characteristics	Level	0 units (*n* = 554)	1–14 units (*n* = 783)	15–21 units (*n* = 296)	>21 units (*n* = 286)	Total (*n* = 1,919)	*P*-value
Sex	Male	394 (71.1)	647 (82.6)	291 (98.3)	267 (93.4)	1599 (83.3)	<0.0001
Age	median [IQR]	66.9 [13.1]	68.1 [13.1]	65.3 [10.6]	66.2 [11.8]	67.0 [12.5]	0.0039
Smoking status	Never smoked	158 (30.2)	186 (24.4)	58 (20.5)	36 (14.3)	438 (24.1)	
	Former smoker	255 (48.8)	443 (58.1)	147 (51.9)	145 (57.5)	990 (54.4)	
	Smoking	110 (21.0)	133 (17.5)	78 (27.6)	71 (28.2)	392 (21.5)	< 0.0001
	Missing	31	21	13	34	99	
BMI	Underweight or normal weight	149 (26.9)	280 (35.8)	86 (29.1)	82 (28.8)	597 (31.1)	
	Overweight	247 (44.7)	349 (44.6)	139 (47.0)	137 (48.1)	872 (45.5)	
	Obese	157 (28.4)	154 (19.7)	71 (24.0)	66 (23.2)	448 (23.4)	0.0019
	Missing[a]	.	.	.	.	< 3	
Household income[b]	Quartile 1	142 (25.6)	155 (19.8)	41 (13.9)	52 (18.2)	390 (20.3)	
	Quartile 2	118 (21.3)	140 (17.9)	44 (14.9)	60 (21.0)	362 (18.9)	
	Quartile 3	141 (25.5)	178 (22.7)	74 (25.0)	54 (18.9)	447 (23.3)	
	Quartile 4	153 (27.6)	310 (39.6)	137 (46.3)	120 (42.0)	720 (37.5)	< 0.0001
Educational level	Basic school	258 (49.0)	289 (37.6)	80 (27.6)	85 (30.5)	712 (38.2)	
	High school education	14 (2.7)	14 (1.8)	10 (3.4)	5 (1.8)	43 (2.3)	
	Vocational education	190 (36.1)	330 (42.9)	136 (46.9)	118 (42.3)	774 (41.5)	
	Short or medium higher education	47 (8.9)	96 (12.5)	40 (13.8)	56 (20.1)	239 (12.8)	
	Long higher education	18 (3.4)	40 (5.2)	24 (8.3)	15 (5.4)	97 (5.2)	< 0.0001
	Missing	27	14	6	7	54	
CABG after 2008		387 (69.9)	534 (68.2)	244 (82.4)	144 (50.3)	1309 (68.2)	< 0.0001
Hypertension		319 (57.6)	433 (55.3)	149 (50.3)	174 (60.8)	1075 (56.0)	0.0632
Diabetes		147 (26.5)	129 (16.5)	56 (18.9)	51 (17.8)	383 (20.0)	< 0.0001
COPD		33 (6.0)	42 (5.4)	17 (5.7)	16 (5.6)	108 (5.6)	0.9737
Heart failure		391 (70.6)	590 (75.4)	231 (78.0)	201 (70.3)	1413 (73.6)	0.0371
Liver disease		10 (1.8)	9 (1.1)	10 (3.4)	< 3 (< 0.9)	< 32 (<1.7)	0.0172
Stroke		62 (11.2)	68 (8.7)	31 (10.5)	31 (10.8)	192 (10.0)	0.4444
AMI		208 (37.5)	268 (34.2)	119 (40.2)	106 (37.1)	701 (36.5)	0.2845
Renal failure		26 (4.7)	21 (2.7)	6 (2.0)	10 (3.5)	63 (3.3)	0.1180
AF		43 (7.8)	56 (7.2)	15 (5.1)	34 (11.9)	148 (7.7)	0.0164

BMI Body mass index, *COPD* chronic obstructive pulmonary disease, *AMI* acute myocardial infarct, *AF* atrial fibrillation, *CABG after 2008* number of patients who underwent CABG surgery after 2008 (time)

[a]< 3 observations in some rows

[b]Household income is reported in Danish Kroner (DKK)

abscess, unknown cause of mortality, traffic accident, and malignant neoplasm: colon, prostate, bladder and primary site unspecified. The risk of all-cause mortality, according to alcohol consumption in model 1 (adjusted for age and sex), was not increased for the abstainers (HR 1.61, 95 % CI, 1.00–2.58) and moderate-heavy drinkers (HR 1.40, 95 % CI, 0.73–2.67) compared with the moderate consumers. However, the heavy drinkers had a high risk of all-cause mortality compared with the moderate consumers (HR 2.44, 95 % CI, 1.47–4.04) (Fig. 3, model 1). Likewise, in the fully adjusted model 2, the abstainers and moderate-heavy drinkers did not have an increased risk of all-cause mortality (HR 1.59, 95 % CI, 0.98–2.57) and (HR 1.68, 95 % CI, 0.86–3.29), respectively, while the heavy drinkers remained highly associated with increased all-cause mortality rate (HR 1.88, 95 % CI, 1.10–3.21) (Fig. 3, model 2).

Cardiovascular mortality

The risk of cardiovascular mortality according to alcohol consumption in model 1 (adjusted for age and sex) was not increased for the abstainers (HR 1.44, 95 % CI, 0.87–2.40) and moderate-heavy drinkers (HR 1.45, 95 % CI, 0.74–2.85). However, the heavy drinkers had a high

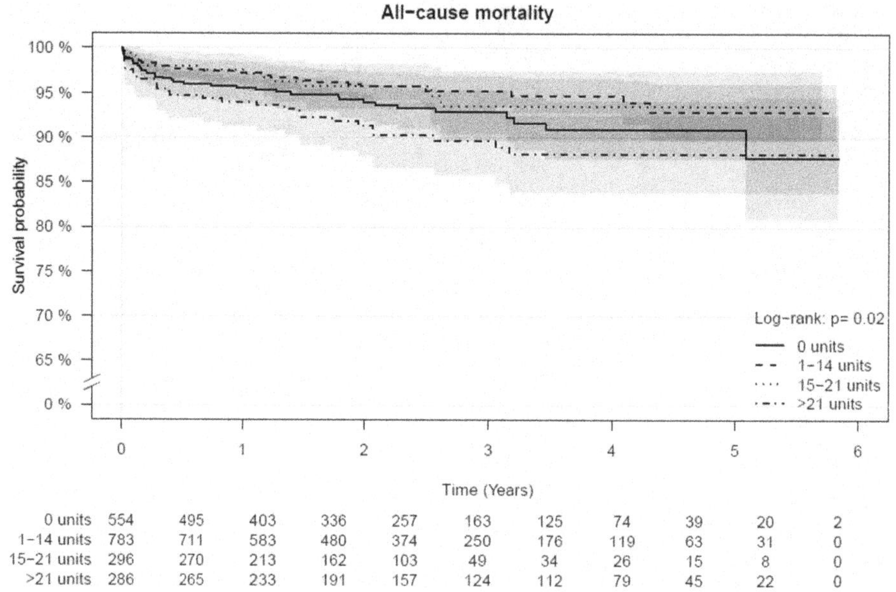

Fig. 2 Kaplan-Meier survival estimates for all-cause mortality stratified by weekly alcohol consumption

risk of cardiovascular mortality compared with the moderate consumers (HR 2.24, 95 % CI, 1.30–3.87) (Fig. 4, model 1). In the fully adjusted model 2, there was no increased risk of cardiovascular mortality for the abstainers (HR 1.42, 95 % CI, 0.84–2.38), moderate-heavy drinkers (HR 1.63, 95 % CI, 0.80–3.29) and heavy drinkers (HR 1.70, 95 % CI, 0.94–3.06) (Fig. 4, model 2).

30-day mortality

Twenty-two patients died within 30 days. In a fully adjusted model, the hazard ratio for 30-day mortality was 0.74 (95 % CI, 0.23–2.32) for the abstainers, 0.36 (95 % CI, 0.07–1.93) for the moderate-heavy drinkers and 2.20 (95 % CI, 0.65–7.36) for the heavy drinkers.

Other analyses

Complete case analyses were performed for comparisons with primary analyses on imputed data. No increased risk was observed in model 1 for all-cause mortality among the abstainers (HR 1.57, 95 % CI, 0.95–2.57) and moderate-heavy drinkers (HR 1.32, 95 % CI, 0.66–2.65). The heavy drinkers had a high risk of all-cause mortality compared with the moderate consumers (HR 2.42, 95 % CI, 1.40–4.20). The fully adjusted model showed a risk of all-cause mortality for the abstainers (HR 1.69, CI, 1.02–2.81) and heavy drinkers (HR 2.18, CI, 1.23–3.88) but not for the moderate-heavy drinkers (HR 1.63, CI, 0.78–3.36).

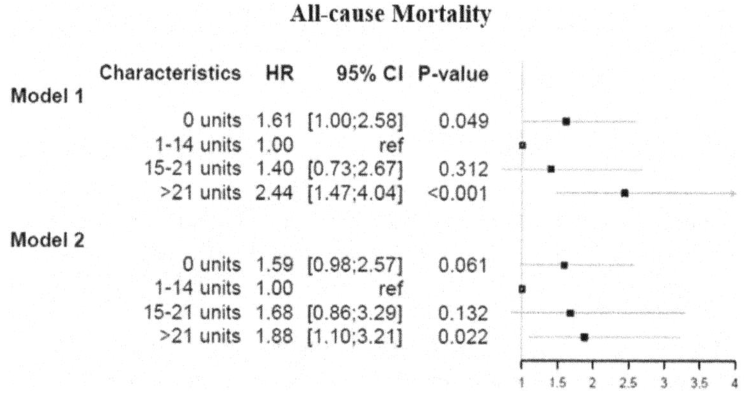

Fig. 3 Hazard ratios and 95 % confidence intervals for all-cause mortality, as calculated by Cox regression models on the imputed data. Model 1: Adjusted for age and sex. Model 2: Adjusted for age, sex, smoking status, body mass index, educational level, household income, coronary artery bypass graft after 2008 (time), chronic obstructive pulmonary disease, acute myocardial infarction, atrial fibrillation, hypertension, liver disease, stroke, diabetes mellitus, heart failure and renal failure

Cardiovascular Mortality

	Characteristics	HR	95% CI	P-value
Model 1				
	0 units	1.44	[0.87;2.40]	0.158
	1-14 units	1.00	ref	
	15-21 units	1.45	[0.74;2.85]	0.283
	>21 units	2.24	[1.30;3.87]	0.004
Model 2				
	0 units	1.42	[0.84;2.38]	0.187
	1-14 units	1.00	ref	
	15-21 units	1.63	[0.80;3.29]	0.178
	>21 units	1.70	[0.94;3.06]	0.078

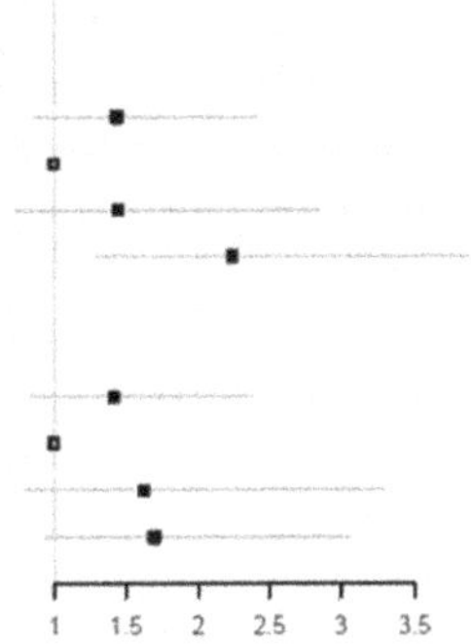

Fig. 4 Hazard ratios and 95 % confidence intervals for cardiovascular mortality, as calculated by Cox regression models on the imputed data. Model 1: Adjusted for age and sex. Model 2: Adjusted for age, sex, smoking status, body mass index, educational level, household income, coronary artery bypass graft after 2008 (time), chronic obstructive pulmonary disease, acute myocardial infarction, atrial fibrillation, hypertension, liver disease, stroke, diabetes mellitus, heart failure and renal failure

In model 1, no increased risk of cardiovascular mortality was observed for the abstainers (HR 1.48, 95 % CI, 0.87–2.52) and moderate-heavy drinkers (HR 1.35, 95 % CI, 0.65–2.81). The heavy drinkers had a high risk of cardiovascular mortality (HR 2.22, 95 % CI, 1.22–4.02) compared with the moderate consumers. The fully adjusted model showed no risk of cardiovascular mortality for the abstainers (HR 1.60, 95 % CI, 0.93–2.75) and moderate-heavy drinkers (HR 1.54, 95 % CI, 0.71–3.31), while the heavy drinkers had an increased risk (HR 1.98, 95 % CI, 1.05–3.73).

This study had missing alcohol consumption data for 1,622 patients (45.8 %). Of these 1,622 patients, 466 underwent acute CABG. The x^2 tests showed no difference between the population with complete data and the group of missing alcohol consumption on education (p-value 0.57), diabetes mellitus (p-value 0.12), stroke (p-value 0.40), renal failure (p-value 0.11), liver disease (p-value 0.08), COPD (p-value 0.53) and AF (p-value 0.24) data.

Discussion

This study examined the association between alcohol consumption and mortality among CABG patients. The primary result was that among CABG patients, only heavy drinkers (>21 units/week) were significantly associated with an increased risk of all-cause mortality. The risk of dying did not differ between the abstainers and moderate consumers.

Interpretation

Our results are comparable with those of previous studies that investigated the influence of alcohol consumption on composite outcomes, including mortality, among CABG patients [14, 15]. Likewise, these studies showed no risk of increased mortality with moderate alcohol consumption. In addition, our results aligned with those from other studies, that did not target CABG patients; in these studies, moderate alcohol consumption did not adversely affect all-cause mortality and cardiovascular mortality [2–8].

In contrast to comparable studies [14, 15], our results showed an increased risk of all-cause mortality for heavy drinkers. One of these studies was not able to distinguish between heavy drinking and moderate alcohol consumption, and the other study used a lower threshold to define the highest alcohol use (≥14 units/week) than our study, thus limiting knowledge concerning heavy drinkers (>21 units/week). The different definition of heavy alcohol consumption and the lack of examining heavy drinkers might explain why our results reveal an increased risk for all-cause mortality for this specific patient group. The results of an increased risk of all-cause mortality for heavy drinkers aligned with the results of other studies not targeting CABG patients [2, 3]. Thus, our study extends this observation to include CABG patients who, consequently, do not seem to differ from the general population in terms of alcohol consumption and mortality, even though the burden of co-morbidities for CABG patients has increased over time [12, 13].

The fully adjusted model examining the association of alcohol consumption and cardiovascular mortality showed an increased cardiovascular mortality rate among heavy drinkers, but this result was not statistically significant. As shown in the forest plots (Figs. 3 and 4), the results from model 1 and model 2 for all-cause mortality and cardiovascular mortality illustrate J-shaped curves, which indicate higher mortality rates for the heavy drinkers, as reported elsewhere [3, 7, 32, 42]; thus, these results indicate an increased mortality rate among heavy drinkers. The pattern for all-cause mortality and cardiovascular mortality is nearly identical, as 86

% of all deaths are ascribed to cardiovascular causes. This majority of deaths attributable to cardiovascular mortality calls for separate investigation of this specific cause of death. However, as alcohol consumption may be related to other not-cardiovascular related causes of death (e.g. cancer), all-cause mortality is the most important outcome and the cardiovascular mortality results should be interpreted with caution. Conclusively, this result does not alter the finding that alcohol consumption seems to have little influence on mortality among CABG patients, except for heavy drinkers.

Other studies have found beneficial effects of moderate alcohol consumption on all-cause mortality and cardiovascular mortality [2–8]. The beneficial effect of alcohol is generally ascribed to increased plasma high-density lipoprotein (HDL) [43] and antithrombotic effects [44], where increased HDL levels are best established [30]. No beneficial effects of moderate alcohol consumption were observed in our study. For the sensitivity analysis, analyses were also conducted on the population with complete data. Conclusively, no major differences were observed between the analyses on the imputed data and the population with complete data; however, the risk estimates were generally slightly attenuated. Our results showed no harm for moderate-heavy drinkers regardless of whether the analysis was performed as complete cases or with multivariate imputation, thereby indicating that CABG patients do not need stricter advice to abstain from alcohol consumption, other than heavy drinking.

Previously comparable studies [14, 15] have examined alcohol consumption and composite outcomes, including mortality, for CABG patients. Therefore, our results most likely reflect a fairer examination between alcohol consumption and mortality for CABG patients because we did not use composite outcomes.

Strength and limitations

A major limitation of our study is the observational design, which does not eliminate unmeasured confounders. Residual confounding may, therefore, be present. Due to the study design, our results should only be considered as associations and not as causal relationships.

Although this study had missing data on alcohol consumption for 1622 patients, there was no difference in relation to educational level, diabetes mellitus, stroke, renal failure, liver disease, COPD and AF between the population with complete data and the group with missing data, which decreases the possibility that the missing data introduced selection bias in the study. Of the 1622 patients, 466 underwent acute CABG, which might explain the missing information on alcohol consumption (i.e., the condition of the patient may have been too severe to report the amount of weekly alcohol consumption). Multivariate imputation was performed on the missing covariates. This technique has the advantage of increasing the size of the study population and is typically more efficient than complete cases analysis [40, 41]. Analysis with complete cases only could lead to over-or underestimation of the effect sizes [41]; thus, multivariate imputation is seen as a strength. However, the multivariate imputation did only increase the study population with 155 patients with missing values on covariates, and the high number of missing data should be recognized as a limitation.

We have adjusted for a wide range of potential confounders, which have been possible due to national registers and increases the strength of the analysis. In general, the information of the robust data obtained from the registers is regarded as high quality, and it is one of the main strengths of this study [21, 22, 27, 28, 38]. The data obtained from the national registers are collected independently of this study and, therefore, decrease the possibility of both selection and information bias. The use of the registers further adds to the strength of the study because complete follow-up data are available for all CABG patients.

The amount of alcohol consumption reported tends to be underestimated, particularly among heavy drinkers [45], and the validity of the amount of moderate alcohol consumption is more stable than heavy drinking [42]. An underestimation where some heavy drinkers by mistake is classified as moderate-heavy drinkers would probably lead to a lower association between alcohol consumption and mortality for heavy drinkers. This could also lead to an elevated risk for moderate-heavy drinkers. However, no increased risk was found for this group. Thus, underestimation of alcohol consumption for moderate-heavy drinkers would probably have little impact on the results. Nevertheless, newer studies consider the measurement of alcohol consumption as valid [46, 47]. In this study, alcohol consumption was measured as a part of the anaesthesiologist anamnesis prior to the operation because alcohol consumption can impact the administration of anaesthesia. The measurement of alcohol consumption obtained in connection with the comprehensive CABG procedure is, therefore, expected to be reliable.

We were not able to identify the different types of alcohol that could have potentially influenced the results if one type of alcohol is more harmful or beneficial than another. Compared to a moderate intake of beer or liquor, moderate wine drinking has been associated with reduced mortality [48] and higher socioeconomic position [49]. We have adjusted for income and educational level as a proxy for socioeconomic position. The reduced association between moderate wine drinking and mortality may, however, be ascribed to more favourable drinking habits and socioeconomic position than wine *per se*

[49]. Nevertheless, it would have been favourable to have access to separate information on wine, beer and liquor. It has been proposed that it is alcohol *per se* that has a protective effect on mortality rather than different types of alcohol [5, 30, 50]. In this study, we found no beneficial effect of moderate alcohol consumption, and the lack of separating different types of alcohol should, therefore, not affect the results crucially.

The use of all-cause mortality as an outcome had the advantage that it requires no further ascertainment than the time of death, and therefore, it will tend to eliminate the possibility of information bias for the outcomes. However, this issue could occur depending on the cardiovascular mortality because the correctness of cause-specific mortality depends on an individual physician's registration of the death certificate, which might lead to misclassification and possible bias if the specific cause of death registration was dependent on alcohol consumption. Nevertheless, there seems to be a high validity of causes of death compared to clinical records [25].

Conclusion

Only heavy drinking (>21 units/week) was significantly associated with increased mortality among CABG patients. The risk of dying did not differ between the abstainers and moderate consumers. Alcohol consumption seems to have little influence on mortality among CABG patients, except for heavy drinkers. Given the wide confidence intervals, other than to abstain from heavy drinking, further studies are necessary to justify advising patients regarding alcohol consumption.

Abbreviations

AF: Atrial fibrillation; AMI: Acute myocardial infarction; ANOVA: Analyses of variance; ATC: Anatomical therapeutic chemical classification; BMI: Body mass index; CABG: Coronary artery bypass graft; CHD: Coronary heart disease; COPD: Chronic obstructive pulmonary disease; CPR-number: Personal identification number; DKK: Danish kroner; HDL: Plasma high-density lipoprotein; ICD-10: International classification of diseases, version 10; MICE: Multivariate imputation by chained equations; NOMESCO: Nordic medico-statistical committee; UNESCO: United Nations Educational, Scientific and Cultural Organization

Acknowledgments

The authors wish to express their gratitude for the assistance and support received from the Public Health and Epidemiology Group at the Department of Health Science and Technology at Aalborg University.

Funding

No specific funding was provided for this study.

Authors' contributions

CTP and MG conceived the idea for this study. MG performed data management and statistical analysis with help and advice from CTP, UD, HB, SMH and BJN. MG was the main author of this manuscript with guidance and advice from UD, CTP, SMH, PFJ, HB, BJN, LRU and CO. All authors contributed to the interpretation of results, manuscript revisions and revised and approved the final manuscript.

Competing interest

The authors declare that they have no competing interests.

Author details

[1]Department of Health Science and Technology, Public Health and Epidemiology Group, Aalborg University, Niels Jernes Vej 14, 9220 Aalborg Øst, Denmark. [2]Department of Clinical Epidemiology, Aalborg University Hospital, Sdr. Skovvej 15, DK-9000 Aalborg, Denmark. [3]Department of Anaesthesiology, Næstved Hospital, Ringstedgade 61, DK-4700 Næstved, Denmark.

References

1. Thun MJ, Peto R, Lopez AD, Monaco JH, Henley SJ, Heath CW, et al. Alcohol Consumption and Mortality among Middle-Aged and Elderly U.S. Adults. New Engl J Med. 1997;337:1705–14.
2. Klatsky AL, Armstrong MA, Friedman GD. Alcohol and Mortality. Ann Intern Med. 1992;117:646–54.
3. Fuller TD. Moderate alcohol consumption and the risk of mortality. Demography. 2011;48:1105–25.
4. Mukamal KJ, Maclure M, Muller JE, Sherwood JB, Mittleman MA. Prior alcohol consumption and mortality following acute myocardial infarction. JAMA. 2001;285:1965–70.
5. Mukamal KJ, Conigrave KM, Mittleman MA, Camargo CA, Stampfer MJ, Willett WC, et al. Roles of drinking pattern and type of alcohol consumed in coronary heart disease in men. New Engl J Med. 2003;348:109–18.
6. Faris RF, Henein MY, Coats AJS. Influence of gender and reported alcohol intake on mortality in nonischemic dilated cardiomyopathy. Heart Dis. 2003;5:89–94.
7. Fagrell B, De Faire U, Bondy S, Criqui M, Gaziano M, Gronbaek M, et al. The effects of light to moderate drinking on cardiovascular diseases. J Intern Med. 1999;246:331–40.
8. Gisbertz SS, Derksen WJM, de Kleijn DPV, Vink A, Bots ML, de Vries J-PPM, et al. The effect of alcohol on atherosclerotic plaque composition and cardiovascular events in patients with arterial occlusive disease. J Vasc Surg. 2011;54:123–31.
9. Hall S, Lorenc T. Secondary prevention of coronary artery disease. Am Fam Physician. 2010;81:289–96.
10. Murray CJ, Lopez AD. Mortality by cause for eight regions of the world: Global Burden of Disease Study. Lancet. 1997;349:1269–76.
11. Kaski JC, Fernandez-Berges D. Secondary Prevention After Acute Myocardial Infarction and Coronary Revascularisation: Focus on Angiotensin Converting Enzyme Inhibitors. Cardiovasc Drug Ther. 2008;22:185–91.
12. Thorsteinsson K, Fonager K, Mérie C, Gislason G, Køber L, Torp-Pedersen C, et al. Age-dependent trends in postoperative mortality and preoperative comorbidity in isolated coronary artery bypass surgery: a nationwide study†. Eur J Cardio-Thorac. 2015:1-7
13. Ferguson Jr TB, Hammill BG, Peterson ED, DeLong ER, Grover FL. A decade of change—risk profiles and outcomes for isolated coronary artery bypass grafting procedures, 1990–1999: a report from the STS National Database Committee and the Duke Clinical Research Institute. Ann Thorac Surg. 2002;73:480–9.
14. Maheshwari A, Dalton JE, Yared J-P, Mascha EJ, Kurz A, Sessler DI. The Association Between Alcohol Consumption and Morbidity and Mortality in Patients Undergoing Coronary Artery Bypass Surgery. J Cardiothor Vasc An. 2010;24:580–5.
15. Mukamal KJ, Girotra S, Mittleman MA. Alcohol consumption, atherosclerotic

progression, and prognosis among patients with coronary artery bypass grafts. Am Heart J. 2006;151:368–72.
16. Yuan J-M, Ross RK, Gao Y-T, c Yu M. Body weight and mortality: a prospective evaluation in a cohort of middle-aged men in Shanghai, China. Int J Epidemiol. 1998;27:824–32.
17. Schrijvers CT, Stronks K, van de Mheen HD, Mackenbach JP. Explaining educational differences in mortality: the role of behavioral and material factors. Am J Public Health. 1999;89:535–40.
18. Calle EE, Thun MJ, Petrelli JM, Rodriguez C, Heath CW. Body-mass index and mortality in a prospective cohort of U.S. adults. New Engl J Med. 1999;341:1097–105.
19. Stevens J, Cai J, Evenson KR, Thomas R. Fitness and Fatness as Predictors of Mortality from All Causes and from Cardiovascular Disease in Men and Women in the Lipid Research Clinics Study. Am J Epidemiol. 2002;156:832–41.
20. Lindsay G, Tolmie E, Martin W, Hutton I, Belcher P. Smoking after Coronary Artery Bypass: High Three-Year Mortality. Thorac Cardiov Surg. 2009;57:135–40.
21. Pedersen CB. The Danish Civil Registration System. Scand J Public Healt. 2011;39:22–5.
22. Lynge E, Sandegaard JL, Rebolj M. The Danish National Patient Register. Scand J Public Healt. 2011;39:30–3.
23. Vester-Andersen M, Lundstrøm LH, Møller MH, Waldau T, Rosenberg J, Møller AM, et al. Mortality and postoperative care pathways after emergency gastrointestinal surgery in 2904 patients: a population-based cohort study. Brit J Anaesth. 2014;112:860–70.
24. Lund CA, Møller AM, Wetterslev J, Lundstrøm LH. Organizational factors and long-term mortality after hip fracture surgery. A cohort study of 6143 consecutive patients undergoing hip fracture surgery. PLoS One. 2014;9, e99308.
25. Helweg-Larsen K. The Danish Register of Causes of Death. Scand J Public Healt. 2011;39:26–9.
26. Kildemoes HW, Sørensen HT, Hallas J. The Danish National Prescription Registry. Scand J Public Healt. 2011;39:38–41.
27. Baadsgaard M, Quitzau J. Danish registers on personal income and transfer payments. Scand J Public Healt. 2011;39:103–5.
28. Jensen VM, Rasmussen AW. Danish Education Registers. Scand J Public Healt. 2011;39:91–4.
29. NOMESCO Classification of Surgical Procedures, 2009 [Internet]. Available from: http://www.nordclass.se/NCSP_1_16.pdf. Accessed 10 Nov 2016.
30. Klatsky AL. Alcohol and cardiovascular diseases: where do we stand today? J Intern Med. 2015;278:238–50.
31. Bovet P, Paccaud F. Commentary: Alcohol, coronary heart disease and public health: which evidence-based policy. Int J Epidemiol. 2001;30:734–7.
32. Klatsky AL. Epidemiology of Coronary Heart Disease—Influence of Alcohol. Alcohol Clin Exp Res. 1994;18:88–96.
33. Tolstrup J, Jensen MK, Tjønneland A, Overvad K, Mukamal KJ, Grønbaek M. Prospective study of alcohol drinking patterns and coronary heart disease in women and men. BMJ. 2006;332:1244–8.
34. Olesen JB, Lip GYH, Hansen ML, Hansen PR, Tolstrup JS, Lindhardsen J, et al. Validation of risk stratification schemes for predicting stroke and thromboembolism in patients with atrial fibrillation: nationwide cohort study. BMJ. 2011;342:d124.
35. World Health Organization. Obesity: preventing and managing the global epidemic. Report of a WHO Consultation (WHO Technical Report Series 894). Geneva: ISBN; 2000. 92 4 120894 5 [Internet]. Available from: http://whqlibdoc.who.int/trs/WHO_TRS_894.pdf?ua=1. Accessed 10 Nov 2016.
36. United nation educational scientific and cultural organisation (UNESCO), Institute for Statistics. International Standard Classification of Education (ISCED) 2011. [Internet]. Available from: http://www.uis.unesco.org/Education/Documents/isced-2011-en.pdf. Accessed 10 Nov 2016.
37. The Danish Data Protection Agency, Datatilsynet: Compiled version of the Act on Processing of Personal Data [Internet]. Available from: http://www.datatilsynet.dk/english/the-act-on-processing-of-personal-data/read-the-act-on-processing-of-personal-data/compiled-version-of-the-act-on-processing-of-personal-data. Accessed 10 Nov 2016.
38. Thygesen LC, Daasnes C, Thaulow I, Brønnum-Hansen H. Introduction to Danish (nationwide) registers on health and social issues: structure, access, legislation, and archiving. Scand J Public Healt. 2011;39:12–6.
39. Buuren S van, Groothuis-Oudshoorn K. mice: Multivariate Imputation by Chained Equations in R. J Stat Softw [Internet]. 2011;45. Available from: http://www.jstatsoft.org/v45/i03. Accessed 10 Nov 2016.
40. White IR, Royston P. Imputing missing covariate values for the Cox model. Stat Med. 2009;28:1982–98.
41. Newman DA. Missing Data Five Practical Guidelines. Organ Res Methods. 2014;17:372–411.
42. Doll R, Peto R, Hall E, Wheatley K, Gray R. Mortality in relation to consumption of alcohol: 13 years' observations on male British doctors. BMJ. 1994;309:911–8.
43. Hines LM, Stampfer MJ, Ma J, Gaziano JM, Ridker PM, Hankinson SE, et al. Genetic Variation in Alcohol Dehydrogenase and the Beneficial Effect of Moderate Alcohol Consumption on Myocardial Infarction. New Engl J Med. 2001;344:549–55.
44. Lacoste L, Hung J, Lam JYT. Acute and delayed antithrombotic effects of alcohol in humans. Am J Cardiol. 2001;87:82–5.
45. Orrego H, Blake JE, Blendis LM, Kapur BM, Israel Y. Reliability of assessment of alcohol intake based on personal interviews in a liver clinic. Lancet. 1979;2:1354–6.
46. Del Boca FK, Darkes J. The validity of self-reports of alcohol consumption: state of the science and challenges for research. Addiction. 2003;98 Suppl 2:1–12.
47. Lang I, Guralnik J, Wallace RB, Melzer D. What level of alcohol consumption is hazardous for older people? Functioning and mortality in U.S. and English national cohorts. J Am Geriatr Soc. 2007;55:49–57.
48. Grønbaek M, Deis A, Sørensen TI, Becker U, Schnohr P, Jensen G. Mortality associated with moderate intakes of wine, beer, or spirits. BMJ. 1995;310:1165–9.
49. Mortensen EL, Jensen HH, Sanders SA, Reinisch JM. Better psychological functioning and higher social status may largely explain the apparent health benefits of wine: a study of wine and beer drinking in young Danish adults. Arch Intern Med. 2001;161:1844–8.
50. Rimm EB, Klatsky A, Grobbee D, Stampfer MJ. Review Of Moderate Alcohol Consumption And Reduced Risk Of Coronary Heart Disease: Is The Effect Due To Beer, Wine, Or Spirits? BMJ. 1996;312:731–6.

Self-rated health is associated with the length of stay at the intensive care unit and hospital following cardiac surgery

Zsuzsanna Cserép[1,2], Eszter Losoncz[3], Roland Tóth[1,4], Attila Tóth[3], Boglárka Juhász[4], Piroska Balog[5], Péter Vargha[6], János Gál[2], Richard J Contrada[7], Paul RJ Falger[8] and Andrea Székely[2,3*]

Abstract

Background: Recently, a considerable amount of evidence suggested that anxiety, depression and other psychosocial variables might influence the outcomes of cardiac surgery. This study investigated the relationship between length of stay at the intensive care unit (ICU) and hospital after surgery and different psychosocial variables (e.g. depression, anxiety, self rated health, happiness, satisfaction).

Methods: We enrolled prospective patients who were waiting for elective cardiac surgery (N = 267) and consented to take part in the study. We collected data of sociodemographic, medical and perioperative factors as well as psychosocial questionnaires completed 1.56 days (standard deviation [SD] = 0.7) before surgery. The primary clinical endpoint was an ICU stay of at least 3 days and the secondary was hospital stay of at least 10 days.

Results: Two hundred sixty-seven patients participated in this study. Four patients (1.5%) died in the hospital and 38 patients (14.5%) spent more than 3 days in the ICU and 62 patients (23.2%) spent more than 10 days in the hospital. After controlling for medical and sociodemographic factors, lower self rated health (Adjusted Odds Ratio [AOR]: 0.51, 95% confidence interval [CI]: 0.28-0.95; $p = 0.03$), lower rate of happiness (AOR: 0.76, 95% CI: 0.59-0.97, $p = 0.03$), postoperative cardiac failure (AOR: 7.09, 95% CI:1.21-41.54; $p = 0.03$) and postoperative complications (AOR: 9.52, 95% CI: 3.76-24.11; $p < 0.001$) were associated with longer ICU stay. More than 10 days of hospital stay was associated with higher occurrence of COPD (AOR 4.56, CI: 1.95-10.67, $p < 0.001$), NYHA stage (AOR 6.76, CI: 2.57-17.79, $p < 0.001$), operation time (AOR 1.45, CI: 1.19-1.76, $p < 0.001$), female gender (AOR 2.16, CI: 1.06-4.40, $p = 0.034$) and lower self-rated health (AOR 0.63, CI: 0.41-0.99, $p = 0.044$).

Conclusions: Lower happiness and self-rated health may influence the outcome of cardiac surgery. Therefore, these variables should be assessed in patients.

Keywords: ICU stay, Happiness, Self-rated health, Cardiac surgery, Risk stratification

Background

Coronary artery bypass grafting (CABG), with or without heart valve surgery is a safe and effective intervention for patients with symptomatic coronary artery disease. Although surgical techniques and perioperative care continue to improve, there is still a significant risk of death or major morbidity after surgery. Therefore, the accurate prediction of risk plays a pivotal role in clinical practice. The widely used EUROSCORE risk assessment system covers only medical variables; however, medical factors alone do not fully explain short- and long-term physical health outcomes, including postoperative length of hospital stay, recurrent cardiac events and CABG-related mortality [1]. Prolonged intensive care unit (ICU) stay does not only mean a significant use of hospital resources [2] but is also a risk factor for death within 60 days of hospital discharge [3]. Despite the increasing recognition of psychosocial factors in cardiovascular morbidity and mortality, CABG patients do not routinely

* Correspondence: szekelya@kardio.hu
[2]The Department of Anesthesia and Intensive Care, Semmelweis University, Budapest, Hungary
[3]The Department of Anesthesia and Intensive Care, Gottsegen György Hungarian Institute of Cardiology, Budapest, Hungary
Full list of author information is available at the end of the article

receive psychosocial screening. However, identification of preoperatively existing psychosocial risk factors might improve clinical risk stratification, decision-making and the ultimate success of surgery. Although depressed and anxious mood states [4,5] are perhaps the most strongly established psychosocial variables linked to cardiovascular outcomes, other characteristics may also be important. For example, we found that poor social support and self-rated health predict poor health outcomes in CABG patients [6].

The purpose of this study was to investigate the possible association of prolonged ICU and hospital stay following CABG and valve surgery with psychosocial factors after adjustment for medical factors. Little evidence is available about potential predictors. Moreover, psychosocial variables that are possible predictors of prolonged ICU and hospital stay have not yet been adequately controlled for biomedical and other psychosocial factors. Furthermore, identification of these predictors may help to assess risks for extended ICU and hospital after cardiac surgery.

Methods

Participants

Six hundred forty-four consecutive patients awaiting elective CABG, combined CABG/valve, or valve surgery only at Gottsegen Hungarian Institute of Cardiology were eligible to participate between November 1, 2006 and October 31, 2007. We considered all patients eligible to participate regardless of age, sex, cardiac condition or on- versus off-pump surgical procedures. The only exclusion criterion was severe psychological/ psychiatric comorbidity, because these patients were unable to answer our questionnaires. The patients in the study were admitted to the surgical ward at least 2 days before surgery.

After admission, we invited patients to participate in our study. Patients completed baseline questionnaires 1.56 days (standard deviation (SD) = 0.7) before surgery. Tests were fulfilled by the patients. Two hundred sixty-seven (41.5%) patients agreed to participate and provided informed consent. Surgery was cancelled for 4 patients and 3 patients had non-CABG surgery (2 pericardectomy, 1 porcelain aorta). Nineteen patients were unable to complete the psychological tests for various reasons (e.g., mental disabilities and dysgraphia). If patients refused or were unable to participate (n = 370; 57.5%), we used only their medical data from the institutional database. The participation of patients with neuropsychiatric disorders was very low, only 2 patients had treated depression, 1 patient had major depressive psychosis, 2 patients had preoperative stroke. In the postoperative period, 10 patients (3.7% of 267) had neurological complications, and at 9 patients were started antidepressant treatment in the postoperative period. The Institutional Medical Ethics Committee approved this study, file number: EKB 625-1/2006.

Written informed consent was obtained from every patient for the publication of this report.

Clinical factors

We assessed a wide range of demographic, medical and psychosocial factors as potential predictors of length of ICU and hospital stay. Medical factors included previous myocardial infarction, previous CABG or valve surgery, history of arrhythmia, congestive heart failure, diabetes mellitus, hypercholesterolemia, cerebrovascular disease, chronic renal insufficiency, hypertension, chronic obstructive pulmonary disease, gastrointestinal disease, peripheral arterial disease, pulmonary hypertension, stroke and previous psychiatric hospitalization. Detailed definitions of these variables can be accessed at the Society of Thoracic Surgeons' homepage [7]. Also smoking was evaluated, we categorized patients into two groups: those who quitted smoking before operation (previously smoking group) and those who did not (right before operation group). In addition, we examined specific aspects of the surgical procedure. Finally, we noted the responsible surgeon, whether an intraoperative intraaortic balloon pump was used and whether a heart-lung machine was used (i.e., an on/off pump procedure). Continuous variables from patient medical charts included the number of grafts, cardiopulmonary bypass time, aortic cross clamp time and total duration of surgery (in minutes).

The Society of Thoracic Surgeons Database [8] defines the key outcomes of postoperative complications, such as permanent stroke (new-onset cerebrovascular accident persisting for more than 72 hours), reoperation for any reason, serious infection (e.g., positive blood culture, deep sternal wound infection and catheter-related infection), prolonged mechanical ventilation (ventilation support for more than 48 hours), renal failure requiring dialysis and myocardial infarction. A diagnosis of acute heart failure required the use of an intra-aortic balloon pump or continuous intravenous inotropic support for at least 48 hours. These postoperative complications were added together and the number of postoperative complications was created as a continuous variable (postoperative complication score). We also measured the duration of ICU and total hospital stay.

Potential covariates

We investigated eight demographic variables (age, sex, marital status, current living/working arrangements, number of children and siblings, and years of education completed) as potential covariates. We used several validated psychosocial tests with Cronbach's alfa for study population. Self-rated health (SRH) was measured with the question: "How do you rate your health in general?"

There were five possible responses: very good, good, fair, poor and very poor (1 = very poor, 5 = excellent) [9]. Cronbach's alpha for the studied population is not available as it was single question.

The question "How happy are you in general?" assessed happiness. The answer was rated from unhappy (0) to happy (10). The same question was used in Hungarostudy [10].

General satisfaction was measured by a single question "How satisfied are you?"

The trait scores of the Spielberger State-Trait Anxiety Inventory (STAI-T) characterized the patients' anxiety symptoms. STAI-T scores reflect relatively enduring traits with regard to anxiety. STAI-T scores range from 0–70; scores of 0–48 indicate no psychiatric disorder; 48–52 indicate mild/transient symptoms and scores above 52 suggest the presence of a psychiatric disorder. The validity and reliability of the full version of STAI-T has been well documented in the Hungarian population [11,12]. Cronbach's alpha was calculated for the studied population as 0.81. The STAI-T has been used in more than 3000 studies and has been translated into over 30 languages. Since Spielberger's review more than 1000 articles contain the test according to recent PubMed search, suggesting the measure continues to be very popular in psychological research. However, the test has been criticized for its inability to adequately discriminate between anxiety and depression symptoms [13].

The full version of the Beck Depression Inventory (BDI) is a self-report checklist that assesses cognitive, affective, behavioural and physiological symptoms of depression. Scores from 0–9 are normal, 10–18 indicate mild to moderate depression, 19–25 suggest moderate to severe depression and scores above 26 indicate severe depression [14]. Cronbach's alpha was calculated for the studied population as 0.80. In case of BDI, the way the instrument is administered can have an effect on the final score. If a patient is asked to fill out the form in front of other people in a clinical environment, for instance, social expectations have been shown to elicit a different response compared to administration via a postal survey [15]. In participants with concomitant physical illness the BDI's reliance on physical symptoms such as fatigue may artificially inflate scores due to symptoms of the illness, rather than of depression [16].

Cronbach's alfa provides a measure of the internal consistency of a test or scale; it is expressed as a number between 0 and 1 [17].

Outcome assessment

The clinical outcomes were length of ICU and hospital stay (i.e., the number of days from the date of surgery to the date of ICU discharge). We defined extended postoperative ICU stay as a length of at least 3 days for patients who were alive at discharge. The mean ICU stay was 5.7 days (median = 1 day 95% C.I.: 1–6 days) with a skew of 4.6. Previous literature has transformed or dichotomized skewed length of stay data [18]. There is no consensus in the definition of a prolonged ICU stay; it extended from 1 to 10 days depending on the authors' choice. In accordance with Bucerius et al. who defined extended ICU stay as ≥3 days in the conviction that it includes almost all patients suffering postoperative complications [19] we chose to dichotomize this variable at 3 days because this definition identified a clinically meaningful subset of patients (14.3%) with a higher incidence of post-procedure events.

Statistical analyses

We described the data in terms of the mean and SD or the median and the interquartile range for continuous variables, and as frequencies and percentages for categorical variables. We used different variables from EUROSCORE and those showing $p < 0.20$ in the univariate analysis were entered into a multivariable logistic regression model (e.g. gender, COPD, diabetes, pulmonary hypertension).

To create a base model, a multivariate analysis used medical record predictors including age, sex, preoperative clinical variables and intraoperative surgical factors. To minimize collinearity, we used the length of the operation instead of cardiopulmonary bypass time and aorta cross-clamp time, because they were highly correlated.

Next, we developed a patient survey model using patient survey data predictors (socioeconomic questions and psychosocial measures) to determine the predictors that were associated with extended ICU stay and hospital stay after adjusting for the base variables. In the patient survey model, univariate analysis analyzed the relationship between extended ICU stay and the psychosocial test scores.

The multivariable model combined the base model with the patient survey model to determine the psychosocial predictors that were independently related to extended ICU stay after controlling for sociodemographic and medical predictors. Again, we entered all predictors ($p < 0.2$) into the model. We assessed the fit of the logistic models using the Hosmer-Lemeshow Goodness-of-Fit test. Bootstrapping method was used to examine the discriminating power of the logistic model using the area under the receiver operating characteristic (AUC-ROC) curve. We performed all analyses using SPSS 16.0 (SPSS Inc., Chicago, IL).

Results

Of the 644 eligible patients, we analyzed the data of 267 (41.5%). The mean age was 60.3 years (SD: 8.9 years) and 73% of the patients were male. The most common preoperative conditions were hypertension, hyperlipidemia, previous myocardial infarction, diabetes and arrhythmia (Table 1).

Table 1 Pre- and perioperative characteristic of participants

	N = 267	
	Number/median/ mean	%/(IQR)/SD
Preoperative factors		
Age (years)	60.3	8.9
Male	194	73%
Female	73	27%
Body weight (kg)	81.9	14.5
BMI (kg/m2)	27.9	4.3
Medical history		
Hypertension	204	76.4%
Diabetes	66	24.7%
Myocardial infarction	84	31.5%
Arrhythmia	62	23.2%
Hyperlipidemia	156	58.4%
Kidney failure	25	9.3%
COPD	37	13.8%
Gastrointestinal disease	57	21.3%
NYHA III/IV	30	11.2%
Atrial fibrillation	39	14.6%
Stroke	8	3.0%
Peripheral arterial disease	23	8.6%
Pulmonary hypertension	17	6.4%
Perioperative factors		
Valve	101	37.8%
CABG	174	61.4%
Complex procedure	21	7.9%
Operation time	133	(110–160)
Cardiopulmonary bypass time	37	(0–71)
Off-pump procedure	147	55.1%
Surgeon A	24	9.8
B	13	5.9
C	39	15.1
D	13	4.8
E	87	26.1
F	37	17.3
G	13	6.8
H	33	11.1
I, J, K	9	2.6
Postoperative complication		
Sepsis	7	2.6%
Death	4	1.5%
Dialysis	6	2.2%
Intra-aortic balloon pump	11	4.1%
	12	4.5%
Mechanical ventilation more than 48 hours		
Bleeding	20	7.5%
Acute myocardial infarction	7	2.6%
Sepsis	9	3.4%
Liver failure	9	3.4%
Multiple organ failure	5	1.9%
Neurological disorder	10	3.7%
Hospital days	9.5	6.2

IQR: Interquartile range; SD: standard deviation; BMI: body mass index; COPD: Chronic obstructive pulmonary disease; NYHA: New York Heart Association; CABG: Coronary artery bypass grafting; ASA: American Society of Anesthesiologists risk score. Data are described as the mean and standard deviation (SD) or the median and interquartile range (25th–75th percentile) for continuous variables and as counts and percentages for categorical variables.

The median length of ICU stay was 1 day (range = 0-46 days). Those who spent 3 or more days in the ICU were treated for 839 days of the total of 1,437 (58.4%).

The mean hospital stay was 9.55 days (SD: 6.22) and 62 patients (23.3%) spent more than 10 days in the hospital. There was no significant difference in terms of age and BMI between the two groups; patients with long hospital stay had longer operation time, longer ICU stay and more complications in the ICU. These patients were more likely to have preoperative arrhythmia, COPD, heart failure functional class III/IV, and they had more postoperative complications, like need for IABP, respiratory failure, neurological disorder (any new neurological deficit after surgery), sepsis and need for antidepressant use. There were more female patients among them (Table 2).

We also investigated the relationship between the psychosocial tests. BDI and STAI-T scores correlated to each other (r: 0.24, $p < 0.001$) BDI and happiness exhibited inverse correlation (r:-0.21, $p < 0.001$). Satisfaction and happiness correlated strongly (r: 0.72, $p < 0.001$) and satisfaction and STAI-T correlated inversely (r: −0.47, $p < 0.001$). Similarly, there was an inverse correlation between happiness and STAI-T scores (r: −0.51, $p < 0.001$). SRH showed no correlation with any tests.

Patients with ICU stay equal or longer than 3 days had lower self-rated health and lower happiness scores, but higher BDI scores. Smoking before surgery, level of education and living alone did not influence the length of ICU stay. After controlling for medical and sociodemographic factors, lower self rated health, lower happiness, longer operation time, higher NYHA stages and the occurrence of severe COPD were independently associated with long ICU stay (Table 3). We adjusted for medical factors including age, gender, NYHA class, diabetes, complex surgery, operation time. The c-index of the multivariate model was 0.72 and the Hosmer-Lemeshow

Table 2 Hospital stay

	Hospital stay <10 days n/mean (%/SD)	Hospital stay ≥10 days n/mean (%/SD)	p-value
Age	59.8 (9.3)	62.1 (7.2)	0.39
Female	49 (23.9%)	24 (38.7%)	**0.02**
BMI	28.0 (4.2)	27.5 (4.5)	0.43
Hypertension	160 (78.4%)	44 (71.0%)	0.22
Diabetes mellitus	52 (25.4%)	14 (22.6%)	0.66
Arrhythmia	41 (20.0%)	21 (33.9%)	**0.02**
Hyperlipidemia	122 (59.5%)	34 (54.8%)	0.51
Renal failure	18 (8.8%)	7 (11.3%)	0.55
COPD	19 (9.3%)	18 (29.0%)	**<0.001**
NYHA III/IV	14 (6.8%)	16 (25.8%)	**<0.001**
Stroke	6 (2.9%)	2 (3.2%)	0.90
Perioperative factors			
Operation time	134.0 (40.2)	166.9 (74.6)	**0.001**
Off pump	118 (80.0%)	29 (19.7%)	0.14
CABG	137 (78.7%)	37 (21.3%)	0.30
Valve surgery	72 (71.3%)	29 (28.7%)	0.10
Postoperative factors			
ICU days	1.46 (3.00)	5.54 (9.16)	**0.001**
Respiratory failure	4 (2.0%)	8 (12.9%)	**<0.001**
Bleeding	12 (5.9%)	8 (12.9%)	0.07
Neurological disorder	3 (1.5%)	7 (11.3%)	**<0.001**
Sepsis	2 (1.0%)	5 (8.1%)	**0.002**
Antidepressant therapy	3 (1.5%)	6 (9.7%)	**0.002**

SD: standard deviation; BMI: body mass index; COPD: Chronic obstructive pulmonary disease; NYHA: New York Heart Association; CABG: Coronary artery bypass grafting; IABP: intraaortic balloon pump.
Bold values represent statistical significance.

chi-square test = 5.3, p = 0.72. Adding psychosocial factors (BDI, STAI-T, somatic severity, self rated health and happiness) to the model improved the c-index to 0.77.

Long hospital stay (longer than or equal to 10 days) was associated with NYHA severity, COPD, longer operation time and female gender. Among psychosocial factors, self-rated health remained a predictor (Table 4). Adding psychosocial factors (BDI, STAI-T, somatic severity, self rated health and happiness) to the final multivariate model improved the c-index from 0.74 to 0.76 and the Hosmer-Lemeshow chi-square test = 6.8, p = 0.55.

Discussion

We have found that long operation time, high NYHA levels and severe COPD were significantly associated with ICU stay equal to or longer than three days after cardiac surgery. After adjusting for medical factors, lower self-rated health and low level of happiness were

Table 3 Multivariable model for ICU stay

	AOR	95% CI		p-value
COPD	3.34	1.30	8.56	**0.012**
NYHA	2.99	1.06	8.42	**0.038**
Operation time (30 min)	1.41	1.14	1.75	**0.001**
Self-rated health (points)	0.60	0.36	0.99	**0.045**
Happiness (points)	0.84	0.71	0.98	**0.032**

OR: odds ratio; CI: confidence interval; AOD: adjusted odds ratio; COPD –chronic aspecific pulmonary disease; NYHA: New York Heart Association heart failure severity class. P < 0.05 indicates significance and is highlighted bold.

Table 4 Multivariable model for hospital stay longer than 10 days

	AOR	95% CI		p-value
COPD	4.56	1.95	10.67	**<0.001**
NYHA	6.76	2.57	17.79	**<0.001**
Operation time (30 min)	1.45	1.19	1.76	**<0.001**
Female gender	2.16	1.06	4.40	**0.03**
Self-rated health	0.63	0.41	0.99	**0.04**

OR: odds ratio; CI: confidence interval; AOD: adjusted odds ratio; COPD chronic obstructive pulmonary disease; NYHA New York Heart Association heart failure severity class. P < 0.05 indicates significance and is highlighted bold.

also independently associated with length of ICU stay. Long hospital stay was associated with the same clinical factors and female gender but only self-rated health predicted it among the psychosocial factors after adjusting for depression and anxiety.

Since the in-hospital mortality after cardiac surgery is generally low (between 2% and 6.6% among studies) [20,21], several studies have been attempted to investigate the role of medical and psychosocial variables in the length of ICU or hospital stay or postoperative complications. Many authors have tried to develop a scoring system to better predict extended ICU stay and obtained different results. These medical factors included several risk factors for cardiac surgery (congestive heart failure, sepsis, renal failure, respiratory insufficiency, and cardiac arrest), major cardiovascular events or both [22,23]. Risk scoring algorithms exclusively for the prediction of ICU stay can emphasize objective, patient-specific estimation of early risk and short-term prognosis. However, many of these algorithms have not been validated in multi-institutional, international studies and in different patient populations. Interpretation of these algorithms can be difficult, since all risk systems evaluate different patient populations and types of cardiac surgical interventions [24].

In our study, severe COPD, cardiac failure and long operation time were associated with prolonged ICU stay. Patients with preoperative CHF often have pulmonary edema, which deteriorates the ventilation/blood flow ratio, thus resulting in postoperative hypoxemia [25]. In addition, long-term respiratory muscle overwork may result in postoperative respiratory failure [26]. In a study about need for re-intubation and therefore extended ICU stay, preoperative congestive heart failure and severe COPD were important associated factors following CABG. The investigators observed small airway obstruction and larger physiological dead space in patients suffering from COPD. Furthermore, CABG surgery with cardiopulmonary bypass reduced the volumes and capacities of the lung [27]. The association between lower left ventricular ejection fraction and longer ICU stay and hospitalization was also observed by other authors [22,28]. Consistent with previous findings, female gender was found to be an independent risk factor. Although the explanation is controversial [29,30], it has been suggested that a greater mortality among women may be a reflection of their greater severity of illness, increased morbidity at presentation, smaller body surface area, and smaller coronary vessels [31].

This study's main finding is that low self-rated health and lower happiness significantly predicted prolonged ICU stay. Low self-rated health was also associated with longer hospitalization. Assessment of both variables before surgery is a quick and non-invasive, easy tool for clinicians, since each consists of one question and takes only short time to answer. Self-rated health was associated with mortality, even after controlling for a wide range of health measurements and mortality risk factors in accordance with previous findings [32-34]. In our study, self-rated health was an independent but not an exclusive predictor of longer ICU and hospital stay. In a previous study, we found that lower self-rated health was associated with an increased risk of major cardiac and cerebral events five years after cardiac surgery, even after adjusting for biomedical and psychosocial factors [6].

Predicting whether a critically ill patient will need a long ICU and hospital stay (thus having a greater risk of morbidity and mortality) remains difficult and the advantages of identifying patients who do not benefit from ICU treatment are evident. SRH is an individual and subjective conception that is related to death, and builds a connection from the social and psychological approach to the biological world. Therefore the answer to the SRH question may summarize the dimensions of health that are most important and determinant for each individual [35]. SRH has been described as one of the most important health outcomes available and recommended as a tool for disease risk screening, as an outcome indicator in the primary care, and standard part of clinical trials [36]. Therefore, we recommend that self-rated health score should be a complementary outcome measure in clinical trials and clinical practice. Besides its important predictive value, SRH provides possibilities for intervention. In an interventional study about the effect of telephone based counselling on self rated health of cardiac patients the authors found that the intervention made a significant improvement on patient SRH among distressed patients hospitalized for cardiac disease. The authors suggested that this treatment might be an effective additional disease management program [37].

Negative emotional states (e.g., depressed and anxious mood and anger) are proven risk factors for cardiovascular disease [38]; however, much less is known about the association between positive emotional states (e.g., happiness and optimism) and cardiovascular health. Steptoe et al. have suggested that positive emotions may have a direct and beneficial effect on physiological processes including those involving neuroendocrine, inflammatory, immunological and cardiovascular systems [39]. The association between positive psychological well-being and mortality could be mediated in part via behavioural pathways. For example, positive dispositions are related to predictors of prolonged survival, such as not smoking, exercising regularly, reduced alcohol consumption, and better sleep quality. Psychologically balanced persons might have increased adherence to medical regimens as inverse associations between adherence and depression have been described. However, the protective effect of positive emotions on mortality in healthy population studies persisted even after fully controlling for behavioural covariates, suggesting that other pathways may also be involved. Direct physiological pathways might also contribute to associations. Positive psychological well-being could alter the disease susceptibility of people via the attenuation of sympathetic nervous system activity and the enhancement of parasympathetic activation. Positive affects may reduce stress-induced elevations of inflammatory and coagulation factors, such as fibrinogen and interleukin-6, which are crucial in cardiovascular diseases, and reduce vulnerability to infectious illness. Positive psychological well-being was associated with reduced cardiovascular mortality in healthy population studies, with a near significant effect in patients with established cardiovascular disease [40]. Optimism was associated with better recovery from CABG surgery within 6 months [41]. We showed that a lower rating of happiness significantly predicted longer ICU stay. Low level of positive emotions does not necessary mean depression and vice versa, since we found only moderate correlation between depression and happiness; however, the inverse correlation was stronger between anxiety and happiness.

Anxiety, which is an established risk factor for cardiac mortality [42,43] increases sympathetic activity with its known cardiovascular adverse affects (e.g. abnormally increased production of catecholamines, which can result in increased myocardial oxygen demand due to elevations in heart rate, blood pressure, and the rate of ventricular contraction) [44], so it has the opposite effect as happiness. The relationship between a higher level of depression (BDI > 10 points) and longer post-operative length of hospital stay in univariate analysis is consistent with the relationships shown in previous cardiac research [45-49], however this could not be detected in multivariable analysis using continuous variables and adjusted for postoperative complications. It can be speculated that the role of depression need a longer period to cause adverse event after cardiac surgery like 5 year or after [50].

This study has certain limitations; the most important one being that 42% of the population refused participation and small sample size. Non-participants were more likely to be female and had higher incidences of hypertension, diabetes, arrhythmia, gastrointestinal diseases and stroke and higher risk scores. Thus, the present results may actually underestimate the importance of SRH and happiness since these may be thought to have been lower in non-participants. Psychological factors predicting length of ICU stay may have been somewhat biased by institutional factors (number of beds, surgery case load, insurance, etc.). Therefore, our sample may not have been representative of the entire cardiac surgery population. Our single-center findings need further investigation in a larger, multicentre population. Furthermore, patients with severe psychological/psychiatric comorbidities could not be enrolled in our study, due to inability to fill out questionnaires. We enrolled patients who underwent CABG surgery, valve surgery or both. Not differentiating between these types of surgeries in our analyses may have influenced our results, although previous reports did not find significant differences with regard to mortality and morbidity [51]. Interpretation and integration of our results can be difficult, since all prior ICU and hospital and prediction studies evaluate different patient populations and types of cardiac surgical interventions. We used a rather extensive set of biomedical and psychosocial variables to cover as much predictors as possible in a mixed cardiac population. We could not rule out that the preoperative scores of individual tests were influenced by acute changes in the health status or conversely long duration of a disease modified the score. Finally, we could not establish causal relationships because our study was purely observational, e.g. we had only one measurement point.

All questionnaires used share the same problems as other self-report inventories, in that scores can be easily exaggerated or minimized by the person completing them. However, they are widely used in clinical studies, generally among similar circumstances (e.g. before and after difficult life-situations, like in this case before and after surgery) and accepted in psychological research.

Self-rating about general health is influenced by several clinical factors, e.g. it is a better predictor of mortality among men than among women, which suggests men evaluate their health status differently. Obese patients may incorporate their information about health risk associated with obesity in their assessments independent from signs and symptoms. Individuals with high cholesterol are also influenced by the diagnosis, although the disorder is asymptomatic [52].

A study about pre- and postoperative depression revealed that depressed individuals tend to be physically and emotionally vulnerable to the stresses of surgical interventions. The catastrophic thinking before operation could heighten depressive symptoms due to the uncertain outcomes (i.e. survival vs. death). Conversely, improvement in physical functioning seen in many patients following CABG may have the added effect of elevating mood [48].

Conclusion

We found that assessing particular psychosocial factors might predict the likelihood of longer ICU and hospital stay. Long hospital stay was associated only with self-rated health after adjusting for medical variables. Lower scores of self-rated health and happiness were independently associated with longer ICU stay after adjusting for the most relevant medical factors. These tests are easy to perform, and do not take long time. Measures of self-rated health, happiness, and depressed and anxious moods have not previously been studied simultaneously; thus, this study may fill a gap in the field of emotional factors and chronic stressors of cardiac surgery.

Abbreviations

AOR: Adjusted odds ratio; ASA: American Society of Anesthesiologists risk score; BDI: Beck depression inventory; BMI: Body mass index; CABG: Coronary artery bypass grafting; CI: Confidence interval; COPD: Chronic obstructive pulmonary disease; CU: Intensive care unit; IQR: Interquartile range; N: Number; NYHA: New York Heart Association; OR: Odds ratio; ROC: Receiver operating characteristic; SD: Standard deviation; SRH: Self-rated health; STAI-T: Spielberger state-trait anxiety inventory.

Competing interest

None of the authors are affiliated or involved with any organization or entity with a direct financial interest in this manuscript; thus, the authors declare that they have no competing interests.

Authors' contributions

AS and PB designed the study. AS, ZC, RT, AT and EL collected the clinical data. AS, ZC analysed and interpreted the data. AS BJ and ZC drafted the manuscript. AS, JG, RJC and PRJF made critical revision of the manuscript for important intellectual content. PV, AS and ZC performed the statistical analysis. All authors read and approved the final manuscript.

Acknowledgments

The administrative staff of the Department of Anesthesia and Intensive Care, Gottsegen György Hungarian Institute of Cardiology supported this manuscript.

Author details

[1]The School of Ph.D. Studies, Semmelweis University, Budapest, Hungary. [2]The Department of Anesthesia and Intensive Care, Semmelweis University, Budapest, Hungary. [3]The Department of Anesthesia and Intensive Care, Gottsegen György Hungarian Institute of Cardiology, Budapest, Hungary. [4]The Department of Cardiac Surgery of Gottsegen György Hungarian Institute of Cardiology, Budapest, Hungary. [5]The Institute of Behavioral Sciences, Semmelweis University, Budapest, Hungary. [6]The Hungary Heart Center, Semmelweis University, Budapest, Hungary. [7]The Department of Psychology, Rutgers the State University of New Jersey, New Brunswick, New Jersey, USA. [8]Department of Psychiatry and Neuropsychiatry, Faculty of Health Medicine and Life Sciences, Maastricht University, Maastricht, The Netherlands.

References

1. Roques F, Nashef SA, Michel P, Gauducheau E, de Vincentiis C, Baudet E, Cortina J, David M, Faichney A, Gabrielle F, Gams E, Harjula A, Jones MT, Pintor PP, Salamon R, Thulin L: **Risk factors and outcome in European cardiac surgery: analysis of the EuroSCORE multinational database of 19030 patients.** *Eur J Cardiothorac Surg* 1999, **15:**816–822.
2. Csomós A, Hoffer G, Fülesdi B, Ludwig E: **The incidence and cost of severe sepsis in intensive care units.** *Orv Hetil* 2005, **146:**1543–1547.
3. Cowper PA, Peterson ED, DeLong ER, Jollis JG, Muhlbaier LH, Mark DB: **Impact of early discharge after coronary artery bypass graft surgery on rates of hospital re-admission and death.** *J Am Coll Cardiol* 1997, **30:**908–913.
4. Andrew MJ, Baker RA, Kneebone AC, Knight JL: **Mood state as a predictor of neuropsychological deficits following cardiac surgery.** *J Psychosom Res* 2000, **48:**537–546.
5. Tully PJ, Baker RA, Turnbull D, Winefield H: **The role of depression and anxiety symptoms in hospital readmissions after cardiac surgery.** *J Behav Med* 2008, **31:**281–290.
6. Cserép Z, Baloq P, Székely J, Treszl A, Kopp MS, Thayer JF, Székely A: **Psychosocial factors and major adverse cardiac and cerebrovascular events after cardiac surgery.** *Interact Cardiovasc Thorac Surg* 2010, **11:**567–572.
7. STS National Database, data collection STS Adult Cardiac Database v2.52.1. http://www.sts.org/sections/stsnationaldatabase/datamanagers/adultcardiacdb/datacollection/index.html]
8. Ferguson TB Jr, Dziubian SW, Edwards FH: **Committee to establish a national database in cardiothoracic surgery. The society of thoracic surgeons. The STS database. Current changes and challenges for the new millennium.** *Ann Thorac Surg* 2000, **69:**680–691.
9. Kopp MS, Skrabski Á, Réthelyi J, Kawachi I, Adler N: **Self Rated Health, Subjective Social Status and Middle Aged Mortality in a Changing Society.** *Behav Med* 2004, **30:**65–70.
10. Perczel Forintos D, Rózsa S, Pilling J, Kopp M: **Proposal for a short version of the beck hopelessness scale based on a national representative survey in Hungary.** *Community Ment Health J* 2013, **49**(6):822–830.
11. Spielberger CD, Gorsuch A, Lushane R, Vagg PR, Jacobs GA: *Manual for the State-Trait Anxiety Inventory.* Palo Alto, California: Consulting Psychologists Press; 1970.
12. Sipos K, Sipos M: **The development and validation of the Hungarian form of Spielberger State Trait Anxiety Inventory.** In *Cross-Cultural Anxiety. Volume 2.* Edited by Spielberger CD, Dia-Guerrero R. Washington, New-York, London: Hemisphere Publishing Corporation; 1983:27–39.
13. Grös DF, Antony MM, Simms LJ, McCabe RE: **Psychometric properties of the State-Trait Inventory for Cognitive and Somatic Anxiety (STICSA): comparison to the State-Trait Anxiety Inventory (STAI).** *Psychol Assess* 2007, **19**(4):369–381.
14. Beck AT, Steer RA, Brown GK: *Beck Depression Inventory-Second Edition Manual.* San Antonio, Texas: The Psychological Corporation; 1996.
15. Bowling A: **Mode of questionnaire administration can have serious effects on data quality.** *J Public Health (Oxf)* 2005, **27**(3):281–291.
16. Moore MJ, Moore PB, Shaw P: **Mood disturbances in motor neurone disease.** *J Neurol Sci* 1998, **160**(Suppl 1):S53–S56.
17. Tavakol M, Dennick R: **Making sense of Cronbach's alpha.** *Int J Med Educ* 2011, **2:**53–55.
18. Johnston G, Goss JR, Malmgren JA, Spertus JA: **Health status and social risk correlates of extended length of stay following coronary artery bypass surgery.** *Ann Thorac Surg* 2004, **77:**557–562.
19. Bucerius J, Gummert JF, Walther T, Doll N, Falk V, Schmitt DV, Mohr FW: **Predictors of prolonged ICU stay after on-pump versus off-pump coronary artery bypass grafting.** *Intensive Care Med* 2004, **30:**88–95.
20. Hannan EL, Racz M, Culliford AT, Lahey SJ, Wechsler A, Jordan D, Gold JP, Higgins RS, Smith CR: **Risk Score for Predicting In-Hospital/30-Day Mortality for Patients Undergoing Valve and Valve/Coronary Artery Bypass Graft Surgery.** *Ann Thorac Surg* 2013, **95**(4):1282–1290.
21. Sabzi F, Moradi GR, Dadkhah H, Poormotaabed A, Dabiri S: **Low dose aprotinin increases mortality and morbidity in coronary artery bypass surgery.** *J Res Med Sci* 2012, **17:**74–82.
22. Hein OV, Birnbaum J, Wernecke K, England M, Konertz W, Spies C: **Prolonged intensive care unit stay in cardiac surgery: Risk factors and long-term-survival.** *Ann Thorac Surg* 2006, **81:**880–885.
23. Ghotkar SV, Grayson AD, Fabri BM, Dihmis WC, Pullan DM: **Preoperative calculation of risk for prolonged intensive care unit stay following coronary artery bypass grafting.** *J Cardiothorac Surg* 2006, **1:**14.
24. Messaoudi N, De Cocker J, Stockman B, Bossaert LL, Rodrigus IE: **Prediction of prolonged length of stay in the intensive care unit after cardiac surgery: the need for a multi-institutional risk scoring system.** *J Card Surg* 2009, **24:**127–133.
25. Kjaergaard S, Rees SE, Grønlund J, Nielsen EM, Lambert P, Thorgaard P, Toft E, Andreassen S: **Hypoxaemia after cardiac surgery: clinical application of a model of pulmonary gas exchange.** *Eur J Anaesthesiol* 2004, **21:**296–301.
26. van Hees HW, Li YP, Ottenheijm CA, Jin B, Pigmans CJ, Linkels M, Dekhuijzen PN, Heunks LM: **Proteasome inhibition improves diaphragm function in congestive heart failure rats.** *Am J Physiol Lung Cell Mol Physiol* 2008, **294:**L1260–L1268.
27. Jian L, Sheng S, Min Y, Zhongxiang Y: **Risk factors for endotracheal re-intubation following coronary artery bypass grafting.** *J Cardiothorac Surg* 2013, **8:**208.
28. Oliveira EK, Turquetto AL, Tauil PL, Junqueira LF Jr, Porto LG: **Risk factors for prolonged hospital stay after isolated coronary artery bypass grafting.** *Rev Bras Cir Cardiovasc* 2013, **28**(3):353–363.
29. Blankstein R, Ward RP, Arnsdorf M, Jones B, Lou YB, Pine M: **Female gender is an independent predictor of operative mortality after coronary artery**

bypass graft surgery: contemporary analysis of 31 Midwestern hospitals. *Circulation* 2005, **112**(9 Suppl):I323–I327.

30. Koch CG, Khandwala F, Nussmeier N, Blackstone EH: **Gender and outcomes after coronary artery bypass grafting: a propensity-matched comparison.** *J Thorac Cardiovasc Surg* 2003, **126**(6):2032–2043.
31. Edwards FH, Carey JS, Grover FL, Bero JW, Hartz RS: **Impact of gender on coronary bypass operative mortality.** *Ann Thorac Surg* 1998, **66**(1):125–131.
32. Schroeder S, Baumbach A, Herdeg C, Oberhoff M, Buchholz O, Kuettner A, Hanke H, Karsch KR: **Self-rated health and clinical status after PTCA: results of a 4-year follow-up in 500 patients.** *Eur J Intern Med* 2001, **12**:101–106.
33. Norekvål TM, Fridlund B, Rokne B, Segadal L, Wentzel-Larsen T, Nordrehaug JE: **Patient-reported outcomes as predictors of 10-year survival in women after acute myocardial infarction.** *Health Qual Life Outcomes* 2010, **8**:140.
34. Oxlad M, Wade TD: **Longitudinal risk factors for adverse psychological functioning six months after coronary artery bypass graft surgery.** *J Health Psychol* 2008, **13**:79–92.
35. Jylhä M: **What is self-rated health and why does it predict mortality? Towards a unified conceptual model.** *Soc Sci Med* 2009, **69**:307–316.
36. Arnadottir SA, Gunnarsdottir ED, Stenlund H, Lundin-Olsson L: **Determinants of self-rated health in old age: a population-based, cross-sectional study using the International Classification of Functioning.** *BMC Public Health* 2011, **11**:670.
37. Bambauer KZ, Aupont O, Stone PH, Locke SE, Mullan MG, Colagiovanni J, McLaughlin TJ: **The effect of a telephone counseling intervention on self-rated health of cardiac patients.** *Psychosom Med* 2005, **67**(4):539–545.
38. Rozanski A, Blumenthal JA, Kaplan J: **Impact of psychological factors on the pathogenesis of cardiovascular disease and implications for therapy.** *Circulation* 1999, **99**:2192–2217.
39. Steptoe A, Wardle J, Marmot M: **Positive affect and health-related neuroendocrine, cardiovascular, and inflammatory processes.** *Proc Natl Acad Sci U S A* 2005, **102**:6508–6512.
40. Steptoe A, Dockray S, Wardle J: **Positive affect and psychobiological processes relevant to health.** *J Pers* 2009, **77**:1747–1776.
41. Scheier MF, Matthews KA, Owens JF, Schulz R, Bridges MW, Magovern GJ, Carver CS: **Optimism and rehospitalization after coronary artery bypass graft surgery.** *Arch Intern Med* 1999, **159**:829–835.
42. Kawachi I, Sparrow D, Vokonas PS, Weiss ST: **Symptoms of anxiety and risk of coronary heart disease.** *Normative Aging Study Circulation* 1994, **90**:2225–2229.
43. Rosenbloom JI, Wellenius GA, Mukamal KJ, Mittleman MA: **Self-reported anxiety and the risk of clinical events and atherosclerotic progression among patients with Coronary Artery Bypass Grafts (CABG).** *Am Heart J* 2009, **158**:867–873.
44. Krantz D, Helmers K, Bairey CN, Nebel L, Hedges S, Rozanski A: **Cardiovascular reactivity and mental stress-induced myocardial ischemia in patients with coronary artery disease.** *Psychosom Med* 1991, **53**:1–12.
45. Pirraglia PA, Peterson JC, Williams-Russo P, Gorkin L, Charlson ME: **Depressive symptomatology in coronary artery bypass graft surgery patients.** *Int J Geriatr Psychiatry* 1999, **14**:668–680.
46. Contrada RJ, Goyal TM, Cather C, Rafalson L, Idler EL, Krause TJ: **Psychosocial factors in outcomes of heart surgery: The impact of religious involvement and depressive symptoms.** *Health Psychol* 2004, **23**:227–238.
47. Oxlad M, Stubberfield J, Stuklis R, Edwards J, Wade TD: **Psychological risk factors for increased post-operative length of hospital stay following coronary artery bypass graft surgery.** *J Behav Med* 2006, **29**:179–190.
48. Horne D, Kehler S, Kaoukis G, Hiebert B, Garcia E, Duhamel TA, Arora RC: **Depression before and after cardiac surgery: do all patients respond the same?** *J Thorac Cardiovasc Surg* 2013, **145**:1400–1406.
49. Poole L, Leigh E, Kidd T, Ronaldson A, Jahangiri M, Steptoe A: **The combined association of depression and socioeconomic status with length of post-operative hospital stay following coronary artery bypass graft surgery: data from a prospective cohort study.** *J Psychosom Res* 2014, **76**:34–40.
50. Majed B, Arveiler D, Bingham A, Ferrieres J, Ruidavets JB, Montaye M, Appleton K, Haas B, Kee F, Amouyel P, Ducimetiere P, Empana JP, PRIME Study Group: **Depressive symptoms, a time-dependent risk factor for coronary heart disease and stroke in middle-aged men: the PRIME Study.** *Stroke* 2012, **43**(7):1761–1767.
51. Jenkins CD, Jono RT, Stanton BA: **Predicting completeness of symptom relief after major heart surgery.** *Behav Med* 1996, **22**:45–57.
52. Goldman N, Glei DA, Chang MC, Glei DA, Chang MC: **The role of clinical risk factors in understanding self-rated health.** *Ann Epidemiol* 2004, **14**(1):49–57.

11

Effects of angiotensin receptor blockers on neointimal characteristics in angina patients requiring stent implantation: optical coherence tomography analysis

Jae Young Cho, Soon Jun Hong and Do-Sun Lim*

Abstract

Background: Angiotensin receptor blockers (ARBs) are known for its anti-inflammatory and anti-proliferative effects. The aim of the study was to evaluate long-term effects of ARBs on morphologic characteristics of stent restenosis in patients with coronary artery disease requiring stent implantation by optical coherence tomography (OCT).

Methods: Patients with coronary artery disease having history of drug-eluting stent implantation ($n = 407$) were analyzed on the basis of ARB therapy as the ARB group ($n = 162$) and the non-ARB group ($n = 245$). Neointimal characterizations were performed at lesions with diameter stenosis >30% with OCT in each group. Major adverse cardiovascular events (MACEs), lumen area, stent area, neointimal area, neointimal thickness, nonapposed struts, uncovered struts, and intraluminal mass between two groups were also observed.

Results: More patients in the ARB group revealed homogeneous and layered neointimal pattern (44.9% vs. 35.6%, $P < 0.001$, and 16.8% vs. 10.6%, $P < 0.001$, respectively), and whereas patients in the non-ARB group revealed heterogeneous neointimal pattern (1.1% vs. 7.6%, $P < 0.001$). Mean neointimal area (1.09 ± 1.00 mm2 vs. 1.38 ± 1. 24 mm2) and mean neointimal thickness (140.6 ± 112.0 μm vs. 189.6 ± 423.1 μm) with OCT were smaller in the ARB group when compared to the non-ARB group. Percentage of covered stents was significantly higher in the ARB group when compared to the Non-ARB group (97.3% vs. 92.6%, $P = 0.015$). Other factors such as follow-up % diameter stenosis, late lumen loss, binary restenosis, MACEs, various neointimal characteristics analyzed by image analyzing software did not show significant differences.

Conclusion: The use of ARBs after drug-eluting stent implantation demonstrated difference in neointimal characteristics, less amount of neointimal area and fewer number of uncovered stent struts during the follow-up OCT, indicating the anti-proliferative and anti-inflammatory effects of ARBs.

Keywords: Angiotensin receptor blockers, Neointima, Drug-eluting stents, Optical coherence tomography

Background

Angiotensin receptor blockers (ARBs) have been widely used in hypertensive patients with coronary artery disease (CAD) requiring stent implantation. In addition to its antihypertensive effect, ARBs are also known for their anti-inflammatory and anti-proliferative effects. The renin–angiotensin system has been implicated in the pathogenesis of restenosis and acute coronary syndrome [1–6] and, thus, may be a potential target for the prevention of in-stent restenosis and atherothrombotic events in patients who have CAD. It is well known that direct vascular effects of angiotensin II include vasoconstriction, inflammation, endothelial dysfunction, and stimulation of growth processes and remodeling, which are mediated by type 1 receptors [3, 7]. The single-center VALsartan for Prevention of REstenosis after Stenting of Type B2/C lesions (VAL-PREST) trial documented the remarkable therapeutic effects of the ARB valsartan on restenosis after stenting in complex coronary lesions [8]. In that trial, the ARB was more effective than

* Correspondence: dslmd@kumc.or.kr
Department of Cardiology, Korea University Anam Hospital, Inchon-ro 73, Seongbuk-gu, Seoul, South Korea

placebo for preventing in-stent intimal proliferation and its superiority over an angiotensin-converting enzyme (ACE) inhibitor can be predicted from the result that 68% of patients in the placebo group were taking an ACE inhibitor.

Optical coherence tomography (OCT) is an emerging intracoronary diagnostic modality that provides high-resolution images of coronary artery in vivo [9]. In addition to tissue characterization in native coronary plaques, OCT has been applied to characterize neointima after stent implantation [10]. Indeed, several OCT studies revealed the development of lipid-laden neointima inside the stents, and OCT has become the modality of choice to study atherosclerotic change of neointima [11–13]. However, correlation between anti-proliferative effect of ARB and change of neointimal characterization has not been studied yet. We investigated and compared the long-term effects of ARBs on neointimal characteristics in patients with CAD requiring stent implantation by OCT image analysis.

Methods

Study design and patients

This study was based on a retrospective observational data on patients who underwent OCT in Korea university Anam hospital between January 2011 and December 2012. Patients with CAD having history of drug-eluting stent (DES) implantation were analyzed on the basis of ARB therapy. Type of ARB or DES was not limited and administering other medications such as aspirin, β-blocker, calcium channel blocker for angina was not prohibited. Patients were divided in terms of taking ARBs as the ARB group and the non-ARB group. Inclusion criteria were: age between 40 to 75 years, CAD requiring drug-eluting stent implantation, diagnosed with hypertension or under antihypertensive medications, and OCT measurements during the follow-up. Patients with left main CAD, previous history of coronary artery bypass graft, acute myocardial infarction (MI), chronic total occlusion, ejection fraction <50%, unsuccessful reperfusion after coronary stent implantation, and liver or renal dysfunction were excluded from this study. Age and risk factor matching (diabetes, hyperlipidemia, smoking, family history of CAD) was performed. Major adverse cardiovascular events (MACEs) such as all-cause death, non-fatal MI, stroke, and target lesion revascularization (TLR) were compared between the two groups during the follow-up.

Quantitative coronary angiography

Offline quantitative coronary angiography (QCA) was conducted using the view that revealed the highest degree of stenosis. Severity of coronary stenosis was measured using the Cardiovascular Measurement System (MEDIS Medical Imaging System; Leiden, The Netherlands). For every patient, angiograms were analyzed at the time of OCT examination. Lesion length, reference diameter, minimal luminal diameter, and percent diameter stenosis were calculated by a single operator who was blinded to clinical characteristics. Analysis of angiographic frames was performed in the end-diastolic stage. Angiographic restenotic lesion type was classified as follows: focal restenosis, <10 mm in length (A) (articulation or gap [IA], margin [IB], focal body [IC], multifocal [ID]), or diffuse intrastent restenosis (B), >10 mm in length (intrastent [II], proliferative [III]) [14].

OCT examination and analysis

OCT examination and analysis was performed during the follow-up (LightLab Imaging Inc., Ilumien Offline review workstation, Ver D.O 2, MA, USA). Under guidance of a 0.014 in. angioplasty wire, OCT imaging catheter (C7 DragonflyTM, LightLab Imaging Inc., MA, USA) was advanced into the distal end of the DES implantation site. The entire length of the stent was imaged with an automatic pullback device moving at 15 mm/s and the OCT image clearly visualized the stent cross-section.

Neointimal characterizations were performed with OCT images at lesions of diameter stenosis >30% and were analyzed into two groups with same lesions by experienced observers using established criteria [10, 15]. The first group was categorized simply with patterns defining neointimal tissue structure of homogeneous, heterogeneous or layered (Fig. 1). Another group was classified into seven categories using densitometric analysis with image analyzing software (Image Pro Plus 7.0, Media cybernetics Inc., Bethesda, MD, USA): (1) macrophage, (2) cholesterol plaque, (3) fibrous plaque, (4) proteoglycan rich plaque, (5) calcified plaque, (6) lipid plaque, and (7) neovascularization. With densitometry, ranging from contrast of minimum 0(darkest) to maximum 255(brightest), lipid or calcified plaque or neovascularization was set to 0–69 (purple), proteoglycan plaque to 70–108 (yellow), fibrous plaque to 109–194 (orange) and macrophage or cholesterol crystal to 195–255 (red) (Fig. 2). Overlapping categories (macrophage or cholesterol crystal and lipid plaque or calcified plaque or neovascularization) could not be differentiated by densitometry; therefore, setting

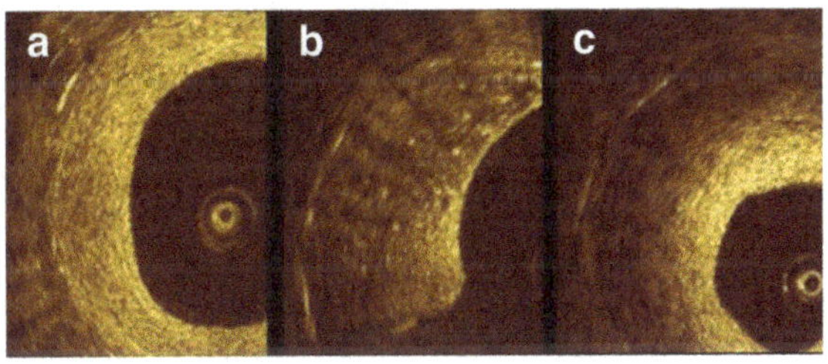

Fig. 1 Neointimal characterizations. **a** Homogeneous **b** Heterogeneous **c** Layered

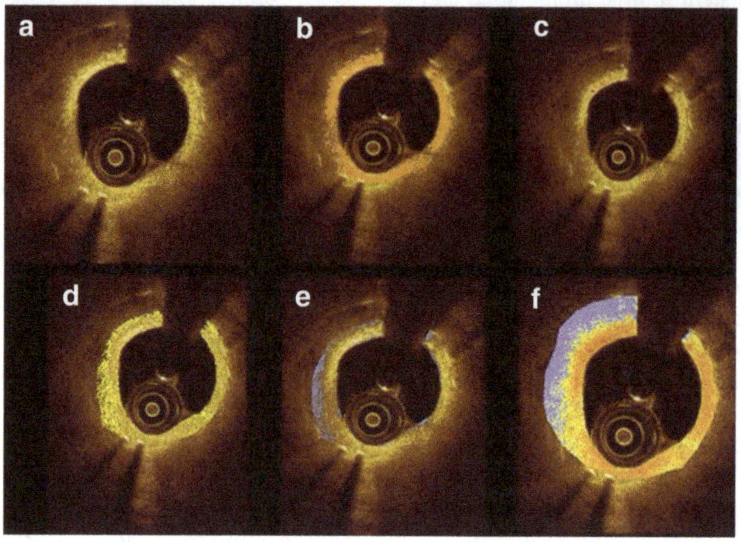

Fig. 2 Neointimal characterizations categorizing by contrast-color matching. **a** Original OCT finding **b** Macrophage or cholesterol crystal **c** Fibrous plaque **d** Proteoglycan plaque **e** Lipid or calcified plaque or neovascularization **f** Whole image of analysis

boundaries manually between overlapping categories and calculating ratio with pixels was done manually (Fig. 3). Lumen area, stent area, neointimal area, neointimal thickness, nonapposed struts, uncovered struts, and intraluminal mass were also observed.

Study endpoints

Primary end point was to compare neointimal characteristics and neointimal area with OCT during the follow-up. The secondary end point was to compare major adverse cardiovascular events (MACEs defined as non-fatal MI, death, stroke, and TLR) and late lumen loss, diameter stenosis, in-stent restenosis (defined according to the Academic Research Consortium criterion) [16] during the follow-up.

Statistical analysis

Categorical variables are expressed as numbers and percentages. Continuous variables are expressed as mean ± SD. Comparisons between groups were performed with 2-tailed Student t test for continuous variables and with $\chi 2$ or Fisher exact test for categorical variables. The reproducibility of qualitative variables was assessed with κ test. A $P < 0.05$ was considered statistically significant. All statistical analyses were performed using SPSS (SPSS 12.0; Chicago, IL) software.

Results

Participant characteristics and baseline assessments

In total, we included 407 patients who were diagnosed as CAD having history of DES implantation and underwent OCT. Of these patients, 162 (39.8%) were in ARB group and 245 (60.2%) were in non-ARB group. Patient baseline characteristics were well matched in the study groups except sex. In the ARB group, fewer patients were male compared with the non-ARB group (66.0% vs. 79.6%, $P = 0.002$). Regarding as a retrospective data, various types of ARB were used in this study but difference of other medication use for angina was not statistically significant except CCB (24.1% vs. 68.9%, $P < 0.001$) (Table 1).

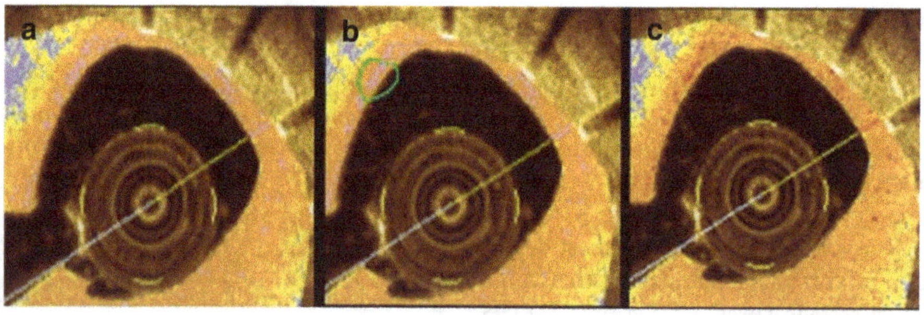

Fig. 3 Neointimal characterizations categorizing by contrast-color matching. **a** original OCT finding filled with contrast-color category **b** Count whole contrast-color pixels (color pink) **c** Set boundary of corresponding lesion (green)

Table 1 Baseline patient characteristics

Variable	ARB Group ($n = 162$)	Non-ARB Group ($n = 245$)	P value
Age (years)	60.8 ± 9.5	60.5 ± 10.1	0.751
Men	107 (66.0%)	195 (79.6%)	0.002
Body mass index (kg/m^2)	24.7 ± 4.3	24.9 ± 4.2	0.372
Risk factors			
Diabetes	55 (34.0%)	68 (28.1%)	0.21
Hyperlipidemia	64 (39.5%)	101 (41.2%)	0.119
Current smoker	38 (23.9%)	67 (27.7%)	0.208
Family History of CAD	4 (2.5%)	5 (2.1%)	0.766
History of CVA	3 (1.9%)	4 (1.6%)	1
LVEF (%)	55 ± 5	54 ± 4	0.673
Mean follow-up duration (months)	19.0 ± 11.4	20.3 ± 14.1	0.523
ARBs			
Candesartan	34 (21.0%)		
Valsartan	29 (17.9%)		
Irbesartan	34 (21.0%)		
Telmisartan	10 (6.2%)		
Losartan	31 (19.1%)		
Olmesartan	15 (9.3%)		
Eprosartan	10 (6.2%)		
Medications			
Aspirin	160 (98.8%)	235 (95.9%)	0.859
Clopidogrel	106 (65.4%)	169 (69.0%)	0.582
Statins	153 (94.4%)	237 (96.7%)	0.775
Beta blocker	34 (21.0%)	51 (20.8%)	0.218
Calcium channel blockers	39 (24.1%)	169 (68.9%)	<0.001
Diuretics	17 (10.5%)	27 (11.0%)	0.947

CAD coronary artery disease, *CVA* cerebrovascular accident, *LVEF* left ventricular ejection fraction, *ARBs* angiotensin receptor blockers
Values are expressed as mean ± SD for quantitative variables or as n (%) for qualitative variables

Target lesion characteristics and QCA analysis

Target arteries or types of target lesion did not differ within both groups (Table 2). Atherosclerotic lesions were located in left anterior descending artery (LAD) mainly (72.8% vs. 68.7%, $P = 0.129$), and angiographic restenotic lesion type C took the largest portion in both groups (44.1% vs. 43.3%, $P = 0.939$). Although several types of DES used in the study, there was no significant difference. Also, QCA findings on baseline, postprocedure and OCT follow-up revealed no significant differences in any parameters between the 2 groups (Table 3).

Endpoints

Descripted above, neointimal characteristics obtained by OCT were analyzed in two different methods, three patterns of homogenous, heterogeneous or layered and seven categories of using image analyzing software. As we analyzed with former method, all three patterns were differed with statistical significance between two groups (Table 4). Homogeneous and layered pattern existed more in the ARB group (44.9% vs. 35.6%, $P < 0.001$ and 16.8% vs. 10.6%, $P < 0.001$, respectively), whereas heterogeneous pattern was more seen in the non-ARB group (1.1% vs. 7.6%, $P < 0.001$). By using latter method, both groups were statistically similar (Table 4), but macrophage seemed to be lower in the ARB group (0.98% vs. 1.23%, $P = 0.225$). Secondary endpoints consist with comparing major adverse cardiovascular events and late lumen loss, diameter stenosis, in-stent restenosis during the follow-up did not show any statistical significance, although patients in the ARB group were more likely to occur TLR than the non-ARB group (15.4% vs. 9.4%, $P = 0.077$). In quantitive OCT findings, stent struts were covered more likely in the ARB group than the non-ARB group (97.3% vs. 92.6%, $P = 0.015$) (Table 5).

Discussion

Stent restenosis is an infrequent but poorly understood clinical problem in the drug-eluting stent era and its

Table 2 Target lesion characteristics

Variable	ARB Group ($n = 162$)	Non-ARB Group ($n = 245$)	P value
Number of lesions stented	195	307	
Target coronary artery	142 (72.8%)	211 (68.7%)	
LAD	31 (15.9%)	49 (16.0%)	0.129
LCX	22 (11.3%)	47 (15.3%)	0.91
RCA			0.104
Type of lesion (%)	5 (2.6%)	11 (3.6%)	
A	35 (17.9%)	56 (18.2%)	0.636
B1	69 (35.4%)	107 (34.9%)	0.877
B2	86 (44.1%)	133 (43.3%)	0.945
C	121 (62.1%)	175 (57.0%)	0.939
Stent type			
EES	105 (64.8%)	147 (60.0%)	0.288
BES	29 (17.9%)	47 (19.2%)	0.768
ZES	16 (9.9%)	32 (13.1%)	0.342
SES	11 (6.8%)	20 (8.2%)	0.622

LAD left anterior descending artery, *LCX* left circumflex artery, *EES* everolimus-eluting stent, *BES* Biolimus A9-eluting stent, *ZES* zotarolimus-eluting stent, *SES* sirolimus-eluting stent
Values are expressed as mean ± SD for quantitative variables or as n (%) for qualitative variables

treatment is challenging. Experimental and clinical studies have identified excessive neointimal hyperplasia as leading cause of stent restenosis [17–19]. Neointima was composed of various characteristic lesions, such as fibrous tissue, proteoglycan-rich tissue, approved by pathologic examination of restenosis in bare-metal stent (BMS) and in DES in tissue samples obtained by atherectomy [20]. In the other hand, ARBs inhibit atherosclerosis as reduced plaque burden in atherosclerotic vessels and reduced incidence of in-stent restenosis [21]. In this concept of anti-inflammatory and anti-proliferative effect of ARBs toward atherosclerosis and neointimal growth, our present study assessed difference of neointimal characterization in use of long term ARBs by OCT. Furthermore, we tried to discover changes of specific neointimal component related to ARBs use.

Neointimal characterization in OCT was analyzed into two groups: a group which is classified conventionally into three patterns of homogeneous, heterogeneous and layered, and another group of specific neointimal component described above in methods. Considering former group, although currently no OCT criteria have been validated with histology for the identification of these tissue types, there are consumptions of each pattern correlating

Table 3 QCA Measurements at baseline

Variable	ARB Group ($n = 162$)	Non-ARB Group ($n = 245$)	P value
Baseline			
RD (mm)	2.54 ± 0.21	2.58 ± 0.16	0.454
MLD (mm)	0.63 ± 0.25	0.58 ± 0.31	0.323
% stenosis	75 ± 6	78 ± 8	0.401
Mean lesion length (mm)	19.5 ± 8.5	22.2 ± 10.4	0.287
Postprocedure			
RD (mm)	2.65 ± 0.28	2.68 ± 0.32	0.128
MLD (mm)	2.53 ± 0.27	2.52 ± 0.29	0.323
% stenosis	5 ± 4	6 ± 4	0.709
Acute gain (mm)	1.9 ± 0.3	1.9 ± 0.4	0.892
Mean stent length (mm)	23.1 ± 7.9	25.0 ± 7.5	0.564
Mean stent diameter (mm)	2.64 ± 0.37	2.65 ± 0.36	0.768

QCA quantitative coronary angiography, *RD* reference diameter, *MLD* minimal lumen diameter
Values are expressed as mean ± SD for quantitative variables or as n (%) for qualitative variables

Table 4 Primary endpoint. Neointimal characterization by OCT

	ARB Group (n = 162)	Non-ARB Group (n = 245)	P value
Analyzing patterns			
Number of lesions analyzed	89	132	
Homogenous pattern	40 (44.9%)	47 (35.6%)	<0.001
Layered pattern	15 (16.8%)	14 (10.6%)	<0.001
Heterogeneous pattern	1 (1.1%)	10 (7.6%)	<0.001
Analyzing with Image Pro			
Number of lesions analyzed	57	81	
Macrophage (%)	0.98	1.23	0.225
Cholesterol plaque (%)	0.01	0.00	0.355
Fibrous plaque (%)	55.63	58.36	0.479
Proteoglycan rich plaque (%)	26.4	25.7	0.705
Calcified plaque (%)	0.21	0.11	0.568
Lipid plaque (%)	16.73	13.28	0.198
Neovascularization (%)	0.04	0.19	0.217

OCT optical coherence tomography
Values are expressed as mean ± SD for quantitative variables or as n (%) for qualitative variables

with neointimal characteristics. Homogeneous pattern is regarded identical to fibrous plaque, which was shown predominance in DES comparing with BMS [20]. Heterogeneous pattern is believed to be a mixture of various neointimal components within whole portion of neointimal growth that might result to show different optical properties [10]. Layered pattern could be visualized in OCT based on pathologic examinations that have demonstrated the density and orientation of smooth muscle cells vary within restenotic tissue compared to the inner luminal

Table 5 Secondary endpoint. Cardiovascular events, QCA measurements and quantitative OCT findings during the follow-up period

Cardiovascular events	ARB Group (n = 162)	Non-ARB Group (n = 245)	P value
Cardiovascular Events			
Non-fatal MI	3 (1.9%)	2 (0.8%)	0.354
Cardiac death	1 (0.6%)	0	0.319
Stroke	0	0	1.000
TLR	25 (15.4%)	23 (9.4%)	0.077
QCA measurements			
Angiographic follow-up duration (months)	19.0 ± 11.4	20.3 ± 14.1	0.523
RD (mm)	2.66 ± 0.30	2.68 ± 0.34	0.543
MLD (mm)	2.24 ± 0.29	2.21 ± 0.27	0.648
% stenosis	16 ± 8	19 ± 12	0.321
Late lumen loss (mm)	0.29 ± 0.28	0.32 ± 0.36	0.196
Binary restenosis	14 (8.6%)	22 (9.0%)	0.465
Quantitative OCT findings			
Mean lumen area, mm^2	6.40 ± 2.49	6.74 ± 2.18	0.318
Mean neointimal area, mm^2	1.09 ± 1.00	1.38 ± 1.24	0.096
Mean neointimal thickness, μm	140.6 ± 112.0	189.6 ± 423.1	0.217
Malapposed strut No, %	0.70%	1.00%	0.322
Exposed strut No, %	0.80%	1.10%	0.372
Covered strut No, %	97.30%	92.60%	0.015

MI myocardial infarction, *TLR* target lesion restenosis, *QCA* quantitative coronary angiography, *RD* reference diameter, *MLD* minimal lumen diameter, *OCT* optical coherence tomography, *No* numbers
Values are expressed as mean ± SD for quantitative variables or as n (%) for qualitative variables

border and tissue located far from the lumen [22]. In the current study, homogeneous and layered pattern of neointima were more likely to be present in use of ARBs. Considering an experimental data that ARBs increased the thickness of the fibrous cap and collagen content in the plaque resulting in reduce of plaque vulnerability [23] and homogeneous pattern is identical to fibrous plaque, our result suggests neointimal change seen in OCT by ARBs may have correlation histopathology. As layered pattern is known to be divided into the inner luminal border, which the smooth muscle cells are more compact and show a homogeneous concentric orientation, whereas the density of cells decreases and the orientation becomes more heterogeneous in the tissue located far from the lumen, it can be assumed that stabilized neointima by ARBs can be explained as homogeneous portion. In contrast, heterogeneous pattern was more appeared in the non-ARB group. This can mean in an opposite view that anti-inflammatory effect of ARBs play a role for less appearing of heterogeneous pattern in long-term ARBs use.

Another goal was to objectify and quantify specific neointimal component by using image analyzing software, so as to classify lesions easily. However, an attempt to discover changes of specific neointimal component related to ARBs use has failed, although macrophage seemed to be lower in the ARB group (0.98% vs. 1.23%, $P = 0.225$), but in other hand, recent study showed decreased plaque macrophages after use of ARBs in histological evaluation [23]. Main cause of the difference between histological finding and result OCT analysis by densitometry can be thought as the measurement bias, as lesions were defined not by characteristic morphology but brightness.

Interestingly, stent struts were covered more likely in the ARB group than the non-ARB group (97.3% vs. 92.6%, $P = 0.015$). Degree of reendothelialization, which is identical with coverage of stent struts, is regarded as the most powerful predictor of stent thrombosis proven by an autopsy or animal study [24, 25]. ARBs attenuate in-stent neointima formation by inhibiting inflammation and progenitor cells, and in other hand, angiotensin II is known to exert an inhibitory effect on thrombolysis, stimulating thrombus formation, suggesting that ARBs may have an anti-thrombotic effect also [26, 27]. Contradiction of opposing effects of ARBs may have caused the situation that there was no difference of cardiovascular event including thrombotic diseases between the ARB and non-ARB group.

Study limitations

Present study has several limitations. Unlike prior studies that revealed ARBs reduced incidence of in-stent restenosis, difference of TLR between two groups in our result did not show any statistical significance. It may be because of the retrospective character, the limited sample size, or different types of ARBs were used in this study. Available data suggest that the beneficial effects of ARBs on atherosclerosis cannot be considered a class effect. Losartan and candesartan have not shown any effect on atherosclerosis or on in-stent restenosis, but valsartan, olmesartan and telmisartan appear to have a significant beneficial effect [21]. Also, various types of DES were used, from first generation (SES) to second generation (EES, BES, ZES), limiting this study that second-generation DES lead to a lower percentage of uncovered and malapposed struts, as well as a lower incidence of intra-stent thrombi, compared with first-generation DES [28, 29]. Measurement bias in analyzing densitometry with image analyzing software was described above in discussion.

Conclusions

In conclusion, the use of ARBs after DES implantation demonstrated different neointimal characteristics when compared with the non-ARB group, and stent struts were covered more likely with the use of ARBs during the follow-up OCT, indicating the anti-inflammatory effects of ARBs. For more definite conclusions, long-term clinical and serial OCT follow-up with a larger population will be needed in the future.

Abbreviations

ACE: Angiotensin converting enzyme; ARB: Angiotensin receptor blocker; BMS: Bare-metal stent; CAD: Coronary artery disease; DES: Drug-eluting stent; MACE: Major adverse cardiovascular event; OCT: Optical coherence tomography; QCA: Quantitative coronary angiography; TLR: Target lesion revascularization; VAL-PREST: Valsartan for prevention of restenosis after Stenting of Type B2/C lesions trial

Acknowledgments

Not applicable.

Funding

This research received no specific grant from any funding agency in the public, commercial, or not-for-profit sectors.

Authors' contributions

All named authors were involved in this project. SJH and DSL conceived and designed the study, provided methodological advice, participated in data interpretation and provided guidance and revisions for final draft of the manuscript. JYC assisted with study design and data analysis, performed literature study and wrote the first several drafts of the manuscript. All authors have read and approved the final draft of this manuscript.

Competing interests

The authors declare that they have no competing interests.

References

1. Bell L, Madri JA. Influence of the angiotensin system on endothelial and smooth muscle cell migration. Am J Pathol. 1990;137(1):7–12.

2. Daemen MJ, Lombardi DM, Bosman FT, Schwartz SM. Angiotensin II induces smooth muscle cell proliferation in the normal and injured rat arterial wall. Circ Res. 1991;68(2):450–6.
3. Gibbons GH, Dzau VJ. The emerging concept of vascular remodeling. N Engl J Med. 1994;330(20):1431–8.
4. Prasad A, Koh KK, Schenke WH, Mincemoyer R, Csako G, Fleischer TA, Brown M, Selvaggi TA, Quyyumi AA. Role of angiotensin II type 1 receptor in the regulation of cellular adhesion molecules in atherosclerosis. Am Heart J. 2001;142(2):248–53.
5. Tharaux PL, Chatziantoniou C, Fakhouri F, Dussaule JC. Angiotensin II activates collagen I gene through a mechanism involving the MAP/ER kinase pathway. Hypertension (Dallas, Tex: 1979). 2000;36(3):330–6.
6. Wolf G. Free radical production and angiotensin. Curr Hypertens Rep. 2000; 2(2):167–73.
7. Dzau VJ. Theodore Cooper lecture: tissue angiotensin and pathobiology of vascular disease: a unifying hypothesis. Hypertension (Dallas, Tex: 1979). 2001;37(4):1047–52.
8. Peters S, Gotting B, Trummel M, Rust H, Brattstrom A. Valsartan for prevention of restenosis after stenting of type B2/C lesions: the VAL-PREST trial. The Journal of invasive cardiology. 2001;13(2):93–7.
9. Yabushita H, Bouma BE, Houser SL, Aretz HT, Jang IK, Schlendorf KH, Kauffman CR, Shishkov M, Kang DH, Halpern EF, et al. Characterization of human atherosclerosis by optical coherence tomography. Circulation. 2002;106(13):1640–5.
10. Gonzalo N, Serruys PW, Okamura T, van Beusekom HM, Garcia-Garcia HM, van Soest G, van der Giessen W, Regar E. Optical coherence tomography patterns of stent restenosis. Am Heart J. 2009;158(2):284–93.
11. Habara M, Terashima M, Nasu K, Kaneda H, Inoue K, Ito T, Kamikawa S, Kurita T, Tanaka N, Kimura M, et al. Difference of tissue characteristics between early and very late restenosis lesions after bare-metal stent implantation: an optical coherence tomography study. Circulation Cardiovascular interventions. 2011;4(3):232–8.
12. Kang SJ, Mintz GS, Akasaka T, Park DW, Lee JY, Kim WJ, Lee SW, Kim YH, Whan Lee C, Park SW, et al. Optical coherence tomographic analysis of in-stent neoatherosclerosis after drug-eluting stent implantation. Circulation. 2011;123(25):2954–63.
13. Takano M, Yamamoto M, Inami S, Murakami D, Ohba T, Seino Y, Mizuno K. Appearance of lipid-laden intima and neovascularization after implantation of bare-metal stents extended late-phase observation by intracoronary optical coherence tomography. J Am Coll Cardiol. 2009;55(1):26–32.
14. Mehran R, Dangas G, Abizaid AS, Mintz GS, Lansky AJ, Satler LF, Pichard AD, Kent KM, Stone GW, Leon MB. Angiographic patterns of in-stent restenosis: classification and implications for long-term outcome. Circulation. 1999; 100(18):1872–8.
15. Tearney GJ, Yabushita H, Houser SL, Aretz HT, Jang IK, Schlendorf KH, Kauffman CR, Shishkov M, Halpern EF, Bouma BE. Quantification of macrophage content in atherosclerotic plaques by optical coherence tomography. Circulation. 2003;107(1):113–9.
16. Cutlip DE, Windecker S, Mehran R, Boam A, Cohen DJ, van Es GA, Steg PG, Morel MA, Mauri L, Vranckx P, et al. Clinical end points in coronary stent trials: a case for standardized definitions. Circulation. 2007;115(17):2344–51.
17. Farb A, Sangiorgi G, Carter AJ, Walley VM, Edwards WD, Schwartz RS, Virmani R. Pathology of acute and chronic coronary stenting in humans. Circulation. 1999;99(1):44–52.
18. Hoffmann R, Mintz GS, Dussaillant GR, Popma JJ, Pichard AD, Satler LF, Kent KM, Griffin J, Leon MB. Patterns and mechanisms of in-stent restenosis. A serial intravascular ultrasound study. Circulation. 1996;94(6):1247–54.
19. Nakatani M, Takeyama Y, Shibata M, Yorozuya M, Suzuki H, Koba S, Katagiri T. Mechanisms of restenosis after coronary intervention: difference between plain old balloon angioplasty and stenting. Cardiovasc Pathol. 2003;12(1):40–8.
20. van Beusekom HM, Saia F, Zindler JD, Lemos PA, Swager-ten Hoor SL, van Leeuwen MA, de Feijter PJ, Serruys PW, van der Giessen WJ. drug-eluting stents show delayed healing: paclitaxel more pronounced than sirolimus. Eur Heart J. 2007;28(8):974–9.
21. Peters S. Inhibition of atherosclerosis by angiotensin II type 1 receptor antagonists. American journal of cardiovascular drugs: drugs, devices, and other interventions. 2013;13(4):221–4.
22. van Beusekom HM, van der Giessen WJ, van Suylen R, Bos E, Bosman FT, Serruys PW. Histology after stenting of human saphenous vein bypass grafts: observations from surgically excised grafts 3 to 320 days after stent implantation. J Am Coll Cardiol. 1993;21(1):45–54.
23. Hotchi J, Hoshiga M, Takeda Y, Yuki T, Fujisaka T, Ishihara T, Hanafusa T. Plaque-stabilizing effect of angiotensin-converting enzyme inhibitor and/or angiotensin receptor blocker in a rabbit plaque model. J Atheroscler Thromb. 2013;20(3):257–66.
24. Finn AV, Joner M, Nakazawa G, Kolodgie F, Newell J, John MC, Gold HK, Virmani R. Pathological correlates of late drug-eluting stent thrombosis: strut coverage as a marker of endothelialization. Circulation. 2007;115(18):2435–41.
25. Joner M, Nakazawa G, Finn AV, Quee SC, Coleman L, Acampado E, Wilson PS, Skorija K, Cheng Q, Xu X, et al. Endothelial cell recovery between comparator polymer-based drug-eluting stents. J Am Coll Cardiol. 2008;52(5):333–42.
26. Ohtani K, Egashira K, Ihara Y, Nakano K, Funakoshi K, Zhao G, Sata M, Sunagawa K. Angiotensin II type 1 receptor blockade attenuates in-stent restenosis by inhibiting inflammation and progenitor cells. Hypertension (Dallas, Tex: 1979). 2006;48(4):664–70.
27. Voors AA. Vascular benefits of angiotensin receptor blockers. Expert Opin Investig Drugs. 2007;16(7):987–97.
28. Kim BK, Kim JS, Park J, Ko YG, Choi D, Jang Y, Hong MK. Comparison of optical coherence tomographic assessment between first- and second-generation drug-eluting stents. Yonsei Med J. 2012;53(3):524–9.
29. Iannaccone M, D'Ascenzo F, Templin C, Omedè P, Montefusco A, Guagliumi G, Serruys PW, Di Mario C, Kochman J, Quadri G, et al. Optical coherence tomography evaluation of intermediate-term healing of different stent types: systemic review and meta-analysis. European heart journal cardiovascular imaging. 2017;18(2):159–66.

12

Left ventricle remodeling predicts the recurrence of ventricular tachyarrhythmias in implantable cardioverter defibrillator recipients for secondary prevention

Wei-Chieh Lee[1], Huang-Chung Chen[1], Yung-Lung Chen[1], Tzu-Hsien Tsai[1], Kuo-Li Pan[2], Yu-Sheng Lin[2] and Mien-Cheng Chen[1*]

Abstract

Background: Implantable cardioverter defibrillator (ICD) is an effective treatment for secondary prevention of ventricular tachycardia/ventricular fibrillation (VT/VF). Left ventricular (LV) remodeling may develop before ICD implant and over time. However, it remains unclear how LV remodeling affects subsequent risk for recurrence VT/VF in ICD recipients under optimal medical therapy.

Methods: From May of 2004 to June of 2015, 144 patients received ICD implantation for secondary prevention were enrolled in this study. All information interrogated from ICD devices during follow-up or ICD therapy history (anti-tachycardia pacing and shock therapy) were reviewed and validated the occurrences of VT/VF.

Results: At a mean follow-up of 1110.5 ± 860.6 days, 53 patients (36.8%) had recurrence of VT/VF episodes and 91 patients had no recurrence of VT/VF episode after ICD implant. Left ventricular end-diastolic volume (LVEDV) > 163.5 mL had significant predictive value for VT/VF recurrence (area under the curve: 0.602, $p = 0.041$). Moreover, the percentage of patients with LVEDV >163.5 mL was significantly higher in patients with recurrent VT/VF than patients without recurrent VT/VF (62.3 vs 40.0%, $p = 0.010$). Left ventricular ejection fraction ≤ 30% ($p = 0.031$), LVEDV > 163.5 mL ($p = 0.012$) and QRS width > 125 msec ($p = 0.049$) were significant predictors for VT/VF recurrence by univariate Cox regression analysis. However, only LVEDV > 163.5 mL (hazard ratio: 2.549, 95% confidence interval: 1.249 ~ 5.201, $p = 0.010$) and QRS width > 125 msec (hazard ratio: 2.173, 95% confidence interval: 1.030 ~ 4.586, $p = 0.042$) were independent predictors for recurrence of VT/VF after multivariable adjustment.

Conclusion: LV remodeling and QRS width > 125 msec were independent predictors for VT/VF recurrence in secondary prevention ICD recipients under optimal medical therapy, independent of LV ejection fraction.

Keywords: Implantable cardioverter defibrillator, Ventricular remodeling, Ventricular tachycardia

Background

Implantable cardioverter defibrillator (ICD) has been confirmed to be an effective treatment for selected patients who are survivors of sustained ventricular tachycardia/ventricular fibrillation (VT/VF) unrelated to transient correctable causes or are at risk of sudden cardiac death [1]. Several studies have consistently confirmed the preponderance of ICD therapy over anti-arrhythmic therapy in terms of primary or secondary prevention of sudden cardiac death and mortality in patients with heart failure and reduced left ventricular (LV) function [2–7]. However, ICD therapy is an expensive therapy and is reimbursed only for secondary prevention in many developing countries. Additionally, some ICD recipients for primary or secondary prevention may never experience recurrence of VT/VF and shock therapy during follow-up under optimal medical therapy,

* Correspondence: chenmien@ms76.hinet.net
[1]Division of Cardiology, Department of Internal Medicine, Kaohsiung Chang Gung Memorial Hospital, Chang Gung University College of Medicine, 123 Ta Pei Road, Niao Sung District, Kaohsiung City 83301, Taiwan
Full list of author information is available at the end of the article

including ß–blockers and renin-angiotensin-aldosterone antagonists, and modification of risk factors. Therefore, clinical predictors for recurrent VT/VF as the guidance for ICD replacement are requisite for limited healthcare resources in many developing countries. The majority of studies of clinical predictors for recurrent VT/VF enrolled both primary and secondary prevention ICD recipients. Klein et al. reported that LV ejection fraction < 40%, permanent atrial fibrillation and QRS duration > 150 msec are independent predictors for VT/VF recurrence in ICD recipients for primary and secondary prevention [8]. However, there are limited reports regarding clinical predictors for recurrent VT/VF in patients received ICD only for secondary prevention. Interestingly, Freedberg et al. reported no predictor for subsequent ICD therapy in patients receiving ICD for symptomatic VT or cardiac arrest [9].

Left ventricular remodeling associated with underling heart disease may develop before ICD implant and over time after implant. Moreover, ß–blockers and renin-angiotensin-aldosterone antagonists have been shown to inhibit or reverse LV remodeling rather than changes in LV ejection fraction [10]. However, it remains unclear how LV remodeling affects subsequent risk for recurrence VT/VF in ICD recipients for secondary prevention. Accordingly, we conducted this study to investigate the role of LV remodeling as a predictor for the recurrence of VT/VF in ICD recipients for secondary prevention under optimal medical therapy.

Methods

Patient population

From May of 2004 to June of 2015, 144 patients received ICD implantation for secondary prevention were enrolled in this study. All information interrogated from ICD devices during follow-up or ICD therapy history (anti-tachycardia pacing and shock therapy) were reviewed and validated the occurrences of VT/VF and ICD therapy. Ninety-one patients who did not have any VT/VF episode or ICD therapy during follow-up after ICD implant were defined as the "no recurrent VT/VF group", whereas 53 patients who had experienced VT/VF episodes and appropriate ICD therapies during follow-up after implant were defined as the "recurrent VT/VF group".

Definitions

Left ventricular diastolic dysfunction was categorized into 3 stages: stage I (impaired relaxation), stage II (pseudonormalization) and stage III (restrictive filling pattern) according to the echocardiographic patterns of mitral inflow velocity, mitral Doppler tissue imaging of mitral annular motion and pulmonary venous flow. The LV end-diastolic volume (LVEDV) and LV end-systolic volume (LVESV) were quantified by M-mode echocardiography and were corrected by two-dimensional guided biplanar Simpson's method of discs for measurement [11, 12].

Atrial fibrillation was defined as paroxysmal if atrial fibrillation episode lasting for 7 days or less, persistent if continuous atrial fibrillation episode lasting for more than 7 days, and longstanding persistent if continuous atrial fibrillation episode lasting for more than 1 year.

Study endpoints

The primary study endpoints were the recurrence of VT/VF and ICD therapy. The secondary endpoints were cardiovascular death (death related to heart failure and cardiac arrhythmia) and all-cause mortality (including sepsis, hepatic failure and brain hemorrhage).

Statistical analysis

Data are presented as mean ± SD or percentage. The clinical characteristics (general demographics, underling heart diseases, comorbidities, functional class of heart failure, QRS duration, medications, LVEDV, LVESV, LV function, VT/VF detection zone and VT ablation) between the study groups were compared using *t*-test for continuous variables or chi-square test for categorical variables. Receiver operating characteristic curve analysis was used to calculate the area under the curve for the optimal volume of LVEDV, LVESV and QRS width in predicting the recurrence of VT/VF. Univariate and multivariate Cox regression analyses were performed to identify the significant predictors for the recurrence of VT/VF after implant. Each independent variable was based on previous studies and conventional risk factors, and was expressed as a hazard ratio with 95% confidence interval. The Kaplan-Meier method and log-rank test were used to compare the event-free survival of the recurrence of VT/VF during follow-up. Statistical analysis was performed using statistical software (SPSS for Windows, version 22). A two-sided p value of < 0.05 was considered statistically significant.

Results

Baseline characteristics of study patients

At a mean follow-up of 1110.5 ± 860.6 days, 53 patients (36.8%) had recurrence of VT/VF episodes and 91 patients had no recurrence of any VT/VF episode after ICD implant (Fig. 1). Table 1 lists the clinical characteristics of the study group. In this study, 71.5% of patients received renin-angiotensin-aldosterone antagonists and 60.4% of patients received ß–blocker therapy. The average age of patients in recurrent VT/VF group was 60 ± 13 years, and 77.4% of the patients were male. The average age of patients in no recurrent VT/VF group was 63 ± 14 years, and 80.2% of the patients were male. Patients with coronary artery disease in recurrent VT/VF group had higher prevalence of revascularization with coronary artery bypass graft surgery than patients with coronary artery

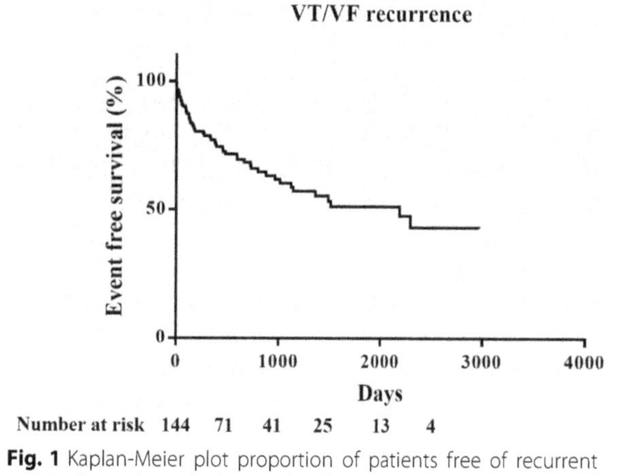

Fig. 1 Kaplan-Meier plot proportion of patients free of recurrent ventricular tachycardia/ventricular fibrillation (VT/VF) events after implant in the study cohort

disease in no recurrent VT/VF group. There was no significant difference in age, gender, body mass index, underling heart diseases, prevalence of comorbidities and atrial fibrillation, frequency of medications related to comorbidities and anti-arrhythmics, the average dosage of ß-blocker and anti-arrhythmics, QRS duration, the percentages of left bundle branch block and ventricular-dependent pacing, stage of LV diastolic dysfunction and heart failure status between the two groups. There was no significant difference in the prevalence of unstable VT ($p = 0.590$) and VT ablation plus medications (anti-arrhythmics and ß-blocker) ($p = 0.358$) between the two groups. Seventy nine patients received single chamber ICD and 65 patients received dual chamber ICD. There was no significant difference in the ICD type and the percentage of cardiac resynchronization therapy defibrillator recipients between the two groups. The lowest VT- and VF-detection rates were similar between two groups. Fifteen patients (10.4%) received catheter ablation and modification of arrhythmic substrates, including 6 patients (6.6%) in no recurrent VT/VF group, and 9 patients (17.0%) in recurrent VT/VF group ($p = 0.087$) (Table 1).

Determinants of recurrence of VT/VF during follow-up

Although there was no significant difference in LV ejection fraction between the two groups, LVEDV and LVESV were larger in patients with recurrent VT/VF than patients without recurrent VT/VF (Table 1). Receiver operating characteristic curve analysis was used to calculate the area under the curve for the optimal volume of LVEDV and LVESV in predicting the recurrence of VT/VF. Only LVEDV > 163.5 mL had significant predictive value for the recurrence of VT/VF (area under the curve: 0.602, $p = 0.041$). Moreover, the percentage of patients with LVEDV >163.5 mL was significantly higher in patients with recurrent VT/VF than patients without recurrent VT/VF ($p = 0.010$). Receiver operating characteristic curve analysis was also used to calculate the area under the curve for the optimal duration of QRS width in predicting the recurrence of VT/VF. QRS width over 125 msec had the best predictive value, although it did not reach statistical significance (area under the curve: 0.563, $p = 0.209$). Eighty-six patients (59.7%) had follow-up echocardiograms at a median follow-up period of 939.5 days. Notably, LVEDV at follow-up were significantly larger in patients with recurrent VT/VF than patients without recurrent VT/VF (191.00 ± 76.61 vs. 158.15 ± 57.82 mL, $p = 0.028$). Moreover, there was a trend, but not statistically significant that patients with no recurrent VT/VF were more likely to have reverse remodeling of LVEDV more prominently (-21.73 ± 54.49 vs. -0.74 ± 55.72 mL, $p = 0.083$) and more frequently (58.3% vs. 44.7%, $p = 0.266$) compared with patients with recurrent VT/VF (Fig. 2). The LV ejection fraction at follow-up remained similar between patients with recurrent VT/VF and patients without recurrent VT/VF (47.2 ± 16.3 vs. 46.7 ± 16.2%, $p = 0.885$).

By univariate Cox regression analyses, LV ejection fraction ≤ 30% ($p = 0.031$), larger LVEDV ($p = 0.028$), LVEDV > 163.5 mL ($p = 0.012$), and larger LVESV ($p = 0.025$) were significant predictors for VT/VF recurrence during follow-up (Table 2). QRS width > 125 msec was also a significant predictor for VT/VF recurrence during follow-up ($p = 0.049$). There was a trend, but not statistically significant that anti-arrhythmics had a protective role for VT/VF recurrence (hazard ratio: 0.611, 95% confidence interval: 0.298 ~ 1.252, $p = 0.178$) (Table 2). However, only LVEDV > 163.5 mL (hazard ratio: 2.549, 95% confidence interval: 1.249 ~ 5.201, $p = 0.010$) and QRS width > 125 msec (hazard ratio: 2.173, 95% confidence interval: 1.030 ~ 4.586, $p = 0.042$) were independent predictors for recurrence of VT/VF during follow-up after multivariate adjustment (Table 2) (Fig. 3).

Cardiovascular death and all-cause mortality during follow-up

The average follow-up periods in the no VT/VF recurrence group and the recurrent VT/VF group were 1019.5 ± 791.4 days and 1266.7 ± 1028.5 days, respectively ($p = 0.108$). The 1-year cardiovascular mortality was significant higher in the recurrent VT/VF group than the no recurrence VT/VF group (9.4% vs. 1.1%, $p = 0.028$) (Table 1). However, there was no significant difference in the 1-year all-cause mortality between the two groups (9.4% vs. 5.5%, $p = 0.499$).

Discussion

This study identifies and reports 36.8% of ICD recipients for secondary prevention having recurrent VT/VF at a mean follow-up of 1110.5 ± 860.6 days. LVEDV > 163.5 mL

Table 1 Baseline characteristics of study patients

	No VT/VF group ($N = 91$)	Recurrent VT/VF group ($N = 53$)	*p* value
General demographics			
Age (year)	63 ± 14	60 ± 13	0.166
Male gender	73 (80.2)	41 (77.4)	0.419
BMI	25.5 ± 4.7	25.1 ± 3.8	0.686
Heart disease			
Congenital heart	4 (4.4)	0 (0)	0.297
CAD	51 (56.0)	29 (54.7)	0.979
Treatment in CAD patients			0.020
CABG	5 (9.8)	10 (34.5)	
PCI	41 (80.4)	18 (62.1)	
Medical treatment	5 (9.8)	1 (3.4)	
DCM	16 (17.6)	11 (20.8)	0.397
HOCM	4 (4.4)	2 (1.9)	0.391
Idiopathic VF	8 (8.8)	3 (5.7)	0.370
Brugada syndrome	3 (3.3)	3 (5.7)	0.388
Long QT syndrome	4 (4.4)	3 (3.8)	0.391
Valvular heart disease	8 (8.8)	8 (15.1)	0.187
Comorbidity			
Hypertension	52 (57.1)	26 (49.1)	0.222
Diabetes	24 (26.4)	20 (37.7)	0.108
Prior stroke	10 (11.0)	7 (13.2)	0.441
Hyperlipidemia	28 (30.8)	14 (26.4)	0.360
ESRD	6 (6.6)	5 (9.4)	0.377
Atrial fibrillation (%)			0.634
No	67 (73.6)	40 (75.5)	
Paroxysmal	17 (18.7)	11 (20.8)	
Persistent	7 (7.7)	2 (3.8)	
Heart failure			0.865
Without heart failure	29 (31.9)	16 (30.2)	
NYHA functional class I	16 (17.6)	11 (20.8)	
NYHA functional class II	27 (29.7)	13 (24.5)	
NYHA functional class III	14 (15.4)	8 (15.1)	
NYHA functional class IV	5 (5.5)	5 (9.4)	
Diastolic function (%)			0.322
Normal	11 (12.9)	11 (22.9)	
Stage I	40 (47.1)	24 (50.0)	
Stage II	14 (31.8)	8 (22.9)	
Stage III	5 (8.2)	5 (4.2)	
QRS length (msec)	115.3 ± 30.7	121.8 ± 32.3	0.231
LBBB	2 (2.2)	4 (7.5)	0.121
Medications			
ACEI/ARB	63 (69.2)	32 (60.4)	0.184
ß-blocker	59 (64.8)	28 (52.8)	0.107

Table 1 Baseline characteristics of study patients *(Continued)*

Bisoprolol (the average dose) (mg)	3.5 ± 2.2	3.2 ± 1.5	0.530
Carvedilol (the average dose) (mg)	17.2 ± 10.0	9.1 ± 13.1	0.651
Diuretic	30 (33.0)	15 (28.3)	0.348
Statin	29 (31.9)	20 (37.7)	0.473
Spironolactone	11 (12.1)	11 (20.8)	0.125
Anti-platelet agent	54 (59.3)	29 (54.7)	0.604
Warfarin	12 (13.2)	9 (17.0)	0.626
NOAC	3 (3.3)	0 (0)	0.297
Anti-arrhythmic medications			
Amiodarone	62 (68.1)	33 (62.3)	0.295
The average dose (mg)	196.8 ± 85.4	214.3 ± 103.3	0.371
Dronedarone	2 (2.2)	0 (0)	0.532
The average dose (mg)	800		
Quinidine	2 (2.2)	0 (0)	0.532
The average dose (mg)	600		
Mexiletine	2 (2.2)	0 (0)	0.532
The average dose (mg)	300		
Sotalol	1 (1.1)	0 (0)	1.000
The average dose (mg)	160		
CRT-D	1 (1.1)	3 (5.7)	0.108
ICD chamber			0.731
Single	51 (56.0)	28 (52.8)	
Dual	40 (44.0)	25 (47.2)	
Ventricular-dependent pacing	4 (4.4)	1 (1.9)	0.428
Hemodynamic condition			0.590
Stable	60 (65.9)	32 (60.4)	
Unstable	31 (34.1)	21 (39.6)	
Lowest VT-detection zone (bpm)	165.9 ± 13.2	165.4 ± 10.5	0.865
Lowest VF-detection zone (bpm)	209.2 ± 13.5	208.2 ± 15.8	0.773
Post VT ablation (%)	6 (6.6)	9 (17.0)	0.087
Success	3 (50)	3 (33.3)	0.518
Failure	3 (50)	6 (66.7)	
Combination of VT ablation plus medications (anti-arrhythmics and ß-blocker)	6 (6.6)	6 (11.3)	0.358
LV systolic function			
LVEF (%)	49.5 ± 16.7	44.6 ± 18.5	0.105
LVEDV (mL)	162.0 ± 68.1	186.4 ± 84.5	0.060
LVEDV > 163.5 mL	36 (40.0)	33 (62.3)	0.010
LVESV (mL)	88.2 ± 61.3	111.4 ± 81.6	0.055
1-year CV mortality	1 (1.1)	5 (9.4)	0.028
1-year all-cause mortality	5 (5.5)	5 (9.4)	0.499
Follow-up time (days)	1019.5 ± 791.4	1266.7 ± 1028.5	0.108

Data are expressed as mean ± SD or as number (percentage)

**Abbreviations: VT* ventricular tachycardia, *VF* ventricular fibrillation, *BMI* body mass index, *CAD* coronary artery disease, *CABG* coronary artery bypass graft surgery, *PCI* percutaneous coronary intervention, *DCM* dilated cardiomyopathy, *HOCM* hypertrophic obstructive cardiomyopathy, *RVOT* right ventricular outflow tract, *ESRD* end stage renal disease, *LVEF* left ventricular ejection fraction, *LVEDV* left ventricular end diastolic volume, *LVESV* left ventricular end systolic volume, *NYHA* New York Heart Association, *LBBB* left bundle branch block, *NOAC* non-vitamin K oral anticoagulants, CRT-D, cardiac resynchronization therapy-defibrillator, *ACEI* angiotensin-converting-enzyme inhibitor, *ARB* angiotensin receptor blocker, *CV* cardiovascular

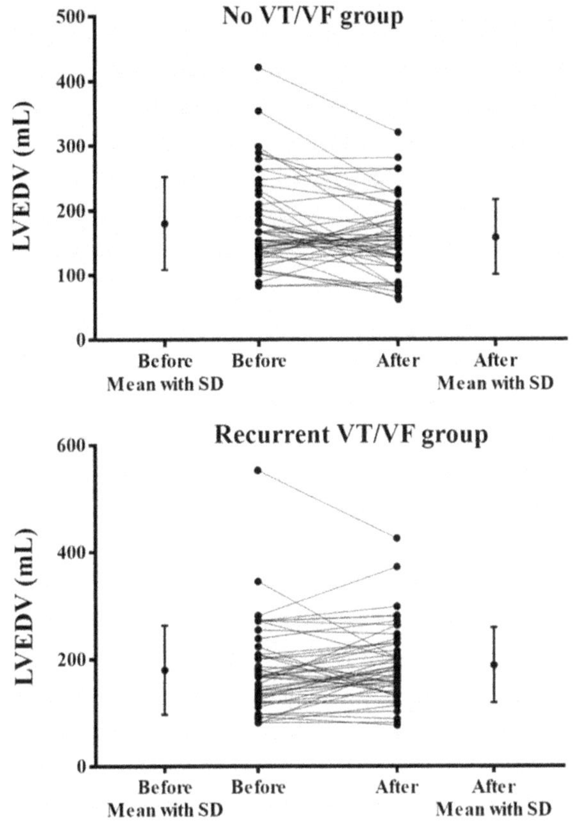

Fig. 2 Changes in follow-up left ventricular end-diastolic volume (LVEDV) in the no ventricular tachycardia/ventricular fibrillation (VT/VF) recurrence group (*upper panel*) and the recurrent VT/VF group (*lower panel*). SD: standard deviation

and QRS width > 125 msec were independent predictors for recurrence of VT/VF during follow-up after multivariable adjustment.

In the multicentre COMFORT trial, Zaman et al. reported that secondary prevention ICD recipients had more recurrent VT/VF than primary prevention ICD recipients (37.1% vs. 19.9% at 2-year follow-up) [13]. In our study, 36.8% of ICD recipients for secondary prevention had recurrent VT/VF, which was comparable to the recurrent rate reported in the COMFORT trial.

Ventricular tachyarrhythmia is an important cause of cardiovascular mortality, morbidity and heart failure hospitalization in a wide variety of heart diseases [14]. Implantable cardioverter defibrillator is now widely used in patients who survive sustained VT or VF, or who are at high risk for sudden cardiac death [1, 15]. Although ICDs can decrease risk of arrhythmic death, long-term total mortality still depends on the severity of the underlying heart diseases and associated comorbidities with the increase in nonarrhythmic deaths completely offsetting the decrease in arrhythmic deaths [14]. In our study, cardiovascular mortality was significant higher in the recurrent VT/VF group than the no recurrence VT/VF group, whereas there was no difference in the all-cause mortality (including nonarrhythmic deaths) between the two groups.

According to current guideline, LV ejection fraction has been selected as the most important criteria for ICD implantation in primary and secondary prevention settings [1]. However, several studies have shown improvement of LV ejection fraction during follow-up in primary prevention ICD recipients [16, 17]. Notably, Kini et al. reported that approximately 25% of primary prevention ICD recipients may no longer meet guideline indications for ICD use at

Table 2 Univariate and multivariate Cox regression analyses in terms of VT/VF recurrence

	Univariate analysis			Multivariate analysis		
Variables	Hazard ratio	95% CI	*p*-value	Hazard ratio	95% CI	*p*-value
Atrial fibrillation (paroxysmal and persistent)	1.095	0.584 ~ 2.052	0.777			
LVEF (%)	0.986	0.970 ~ 1.001	0.074			
LVEF ≦ 30%	1.995	1.064 ~ 3.740	0.031			
LVEDV (mL)	1.004	1.000 ~ 1.007	0.028			
LVEDV > 163.5 mL	2.042	1.170 ~ 3.562	0.012	2.549	1.249 ~ 5.201	0.010
LVESV (mL)	1.004	1.001 ~ 1.008	0.025			
Heart failure NYHA functional class ≧ 3	1.293	0.688 ~ 2.430	0.425			
QRS width (msec)	1.008	1.000 ~ 1.016	0.059			
QRS width > 125 msec	2.067	1.003 ~ 4.260	0.049	2.173	1.030 ~ 4.586	0.042
Ischemic cardiomyopathy	0.998	0.580 ~ 1.717	0.995			
Dilated cardiomyopathy	0.851	0.437 ~ 1.655	0.634			
Anti-arrhythmic drugs	0.611	0.298 ~ 1.252	0.178			
Post VT ablation	0.844	0.272 ~ 2.615	0.768			

*Abbreviations: *VT* ventricular tachycardia, *VF* ventricular fibrillation, *CI* confidence interval, *LVEF* left ventricular ejection fraction, *LVEDV* left ventricular end diastolic volume, *LVESV* left ventricular end systolic volume, *NYHA* New York Heart Association

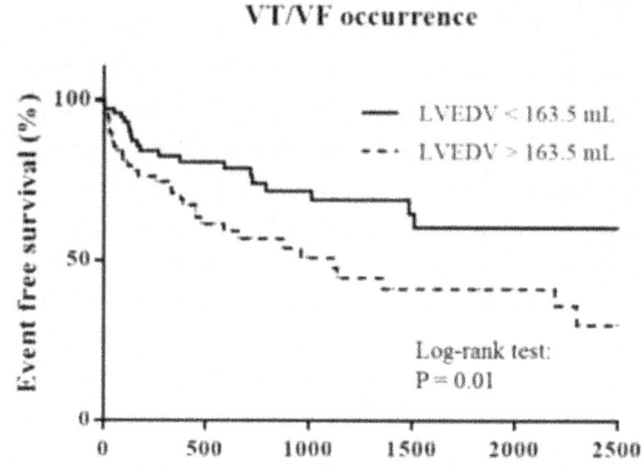

Number at risk						
LVEDV < 163.5 mL	74	43	26	15	6	2
LVEDV > 163.5 mL	70	28	15	10	7	2

Fig. 3 Kaplan-Meier plot proportion of patients free of recurrent ventricular tachycardia/ventricular fibrillation (VT/VF) events after implant stratified by left ventricular end-diastolic volume (LVEDV) of 163.5 mL

the time of generator replacement due to improvement of LV ejection fraction, and these ICD recipients received subsequent ICD therapies at a significantly lower rate [16]. Additionally, in MADIT-CRT trial, patients who achieve LV ejection fraction normalization (>50%) during follow-up have very low absolute and relative risk of ventricular tachyarrhythmias and a favorable clinical course within 2.2 years of follow-up, and downgrade from cardiac resynchronization therapy-defibrillator to cardiac resynchronization therapy-pacemaker at the time of battery depletion for cost savings could be considered in these patients if no ventricular tachyarrhythmias have recurred [17]. However, ICD therapy is reimbursed only for secondary prevention in many countries, and limited data regarding LV remodeling as predictor for recurrent VT/VF are available for secondary prevention ICD recipients. Klein et al. reported that LV ejection fraction < 40%, permanent atrial fibrillation and QRS duration > 150 msec are independent predictors for VT/VF recurrence in ICD recipients predominantly for secondary prevention [8]. However, Freedberg et al. reported that LV ejection fraction was not a predictor for subsequent ICD therapy in secondary prevention ICD recipients [9]. In our study for secondary prevention ICD recipients, LVEDV > 163.5 mL and QRS width > 125 msec were independent predictors for recurrence of VT/VF during follow-up after multivariable adjustment (including LV ejection fraction, atrial fibrillation and heart failure status), and LVEF ≤ 30% was no longer a predictor after multivariable adjustment (Table 2).

Study limitations

There are several limitations in this study. Firstly, this retrospective analysis bears the inherent limitations of these types of studies. Secondly, LVEDVs were estimated by M-mode echocardiography and were corrected by two-dimensional guided biplanar Simpson's method of discs for measurement and this quantified method has been proven to be an acceptable method to evaluate LV volume. Moreover, there was a trend that patients with no recurrent VT/VF were more likely to have reverse remodeling of LVEDV during follow-up compared with patients with recurrent VT/VF (Fig. 2).

Conclusions

LV remodeling and QRS width > 125 msec were independent predictors for recurrence of VT/VF during follow-up in secondary prevention ICD recipients under optimal medical therapy, independent of LV ejection fraction.

Abbreviations

ICD: Implantable cardioverter defibrillator; LV: Left ventricular; LVEDV: LV end-diastolic volume; LVESV: LV end-systolic volume; VT/VF: Ventricular tachycardia/Ventricular fibrillation

Acknowledgements

Not applicable.

Funding

None.

Author's contributions

WCL, HCC, YLC, THT, KLP, YSL and MCC designed the research; WCL, HCC and MCC performed the research; WCL, HCC, YLC and MCC analyzed the data; WCL and MCC wrote the paper. All authors read and approved the final manuscript.

Competing interests

The authors declare that they have no competing interests.

Author details
[1]Division of Cardiology, Department of Internal Medicine, Kaohsiung Chang Gung Memorial Hospital, Chang Gung University College of Medicine, 123 Ta Pei Road, Niao Sung District, Kaohsiung City 83301, Taiwan. [2]Division of Cardiology, Chang Gung Memorial Hospital, Chiayi, Taiwan.

References

1. Russo AM, Stainback RF, Bailey SR, Epstein AE, Heidenreich PA, Jessup M, Kapa S, Kremers MS, Lindsay BD, Stevenson LW. ACCF/HRS/AHA/ASE/HFSA/SCAI/SCCT/SCMR 2013 appropriate use criteria for implantable cardioverter-defibrillators and cardiac resynchronization therapy: a report of the American College of Cardiology Foundation appropriate use criteria task force, Heart Rhythm Society, American Heart Association, American Society of Echocardiography, Heart Failure Society of America, Society for Cardiovascular Angiography and Interventions, Society of Cardiovascular Computed Tomography, and Society for Cardiovascular Magnetic Resonance. J Am Coll Cardiol. 2013;61:1318–68.
2. Bardy GH, Lee KL, Mark DB, Poole JE, Packer DL, Boineau R, Domanski M, Troutman C, Anderson J, Johnson G, McNulty SE, Clapp-Channing N, Davidson-Ray LD, Fraulo ES, Fishbein DP, Luceri RM, Ip JH. Sudden Cardiac Death in Heart Failure Trial (SCD-HeFT) investigators. Amiodarone or an implantable cardioverter-defibrillator for congestive heart failure. N Engl J Med. 2005;352:225–37.
3. Buxton AE, Lee KL, Fisher JD, Josephson ME, Prystowsky EN, Hafley G. A randomized study of the prevention of sudden death in patients with coronary artery disease. Multicenter Unsustained Tachycardia Trial Investigators. N Engl J Med. 1999;341:1882–90.
4. Kadish A, Dyer A, Daubert JP, Quigg R, Estes NA, Anderson KP, Calkins H, Hoch D, Goldberger J, Shalaby A, Sanders WE, Schaechter A, Levine JH. Defibrillators in Non-Ischemic Cardiomyopathy Treatment Evaluation (DEFINITE) Investigators. Prophylactic defibrillator implantation in patients with nonischemic dilated cardiomyopathy. N Engl J Med. 2004;350:2151–8.
5. Moss AJ, Zareba W, Hall WJ, Klein H, Wilber DJ, Cannom DS, Daubert JP, Higgins SL, Brown MW, Andrews ML. Multicenter Automatic Defibrillator Implantation Trial II Investigators. Prophylactic implantation of a defibrillator in patients with myocardial infarction and reduced ejection fraction. N Engl J Med. 2002;346:877–83.
6. Bristow MR, Saxon LA, Boehmer J, Krueger S, Kass DA, De Marco T, Carson P, DiCarlo L, DeMets D, White BG, DeVries DW, Feldman AM. Comparison of Medical Therapy, Pacing, and Defibrillation in Heart Failure (COMPANION) Investigators. Cardiac-resynchronization therapy with or without an implantable defibrillator in advanced chronic heart failure. N Engl J Med. 2004;350:2140–50.
7. Moss AJ, Hall WJ, Cannom DS, Daubert JP, Higgins SL, Klein H, Levine JH, Saksena S, Waldo AL, Wilber D, Brown MW, Heo M. Improved survival with an implanted defibrillator in patients with coronary disease at high risk for ventricular arrhythmia. Multicenter Automatic Defibrillator Implantation Trial Investigators. N Engl J Med. 1996;335:1933–40.
8. Klein G, Lissel C, Fuchs AC, Gardiwal A, Oswald H, Desousa M, Pichlmaier AM, Lichtinghagen R, Geerlings H, Lippolt P, Niehaus M, Drexler H, Korte T. Predictors of VT/VF-occurrence in ICD patients: results from the PROFIT-Study. Europace. 2006;8:618–24.
9. Freedberg NA, Hill JN, Fogel RI, Prystowsky EN, CARE Group. Recurrence of symptomatic ventricular arrhythmias in patients with implantable cardioverter defibrillator after the first device therapy: implications for antiarrhythmic therapy and driving restrictions. J Am Coll Cardiol. 2001;37:1910–5.
10. Frigerio M, Roubina E. Drugs for left ventricular remodeling in heart failure. Am J Cardiol. 2005;96:10L–8L.
11. Crawford MH, Grant D, O'Rourke RA, Starling MR, Groves BM. Accuracy and reproducibility of new M-mode echocardiographic recommendations for measuring left ventricular dimensions. Circulation. 1980;61:137–43.
12. Lang RM, Bierig M, Devereux RB, Flachskampf FA, Foster E, Pellikka PA, Picard MH, Roman MJ, Seward J, Shanewise JS, Solomon SD, Spencer KT, Sutton MS, Stewart WJ. Recommendations for chamber quantification: A report from the American Society of Echocardiography's Guidelines and Standards Committee and the Chamber Quantification Writing Group, developed in conjunction with the European Association of Echocardiography, a branch of the European Society of Cardiology. J Am Soc Echocardiogr. 2005;18:1440–63.
13. Zaman S, Sivagangabalan G, Chik W, Stafford W, Hayes J, Denman R, Young G, Sanders P, Kovoor P. Ventricular tachyarrhythmia recurrence in primary versus secondary implantable cardioverter-defibrillator patients and role of electrophysiology study. J Interv Card Electrophysiol. 2014;41:195–202.
14. Dorian P, Hohnloser SH, Thorpe KE, Roberts RS, Kuck KH, Gent M, Connolly SJ. Mechanisms underlying the lack of effect of implantable cardioverter-defibrillator therapy on mortality in high-risk patients with recent myocardial infarction: insights from the Defibrillation in Acute Myocardial Infarction Trial (DINAMIT). Circulation. 2010;122:2645–52.
15. Goldenberg I, Gillespie J, Moss AJ, Hall WJ, Klein H, McNitt S, Brown MW, Cygankiewicz I, Zareba W. Long-term benefit of primary prevention with an implantable cardioverter-defibrillator: an extended 8-year follow-up study of the Multicenter Automatic Defibrillator Implantation Trial II. Circulation. 2010;122:1265–71.
16. Kini V, Soufi MK, Deo R, Epstein AE, Bala R, Riley M, Groeneveld PW, Shalaby A, Dixit S. Appropriateness of primary prevention implantable cardioverter-defibrillators at the time of generator replacement: are indications still met? J Am Coll Cardiol. 2014;63:2388–94.
17. Ruwald MH, Solomon SD, Foster E, Kutyifa V, Ruwald AC, Sherazi S, McNitt S, Jons C, Moss AJ, Zareba W. Left ventricular ejection fraction normalization in cardiac resynchronization therapy and risk of ventricular arrhythmias and clinical outcomes: results from the Multicenter Automatic Defibrillator Implantation Trial With Cardiac Resynchronization Therapy (MADIT-CRT) trial. Circulation. 2014;130:2278–86.

13

Comparing the effectiveness and safety between triple antiplatelet therapy and dual antiplatelet therapy in type 2 diabetes mellitus patients after coronary stents implantation

Pravesh Kumar Bundhun, Tao Qin and Meng-Hua Chen*

Abstract

Background: Since antiplatelet therapy in type 2 diabetes mellitus (T2DM) patients is very important after intracoronary stenting, and because the most commonly used therapies have been the dual antiplatelet therapy (DAPT) consisting of aspirin and clopidogrel and the triple antiplatelet therapy (TAPT) consisting of aspirin, clopidogrel and cilostazol, we aim to compare the effectiveness and safety between triple antiplatelet therapy and dual antiplatelet therapy in T2DM patients.

Methods: Systematic literature search was done from the databases of PubMed, Cochrane, Embase, China National Knowledge Infrastructure (CNKI) and WanFang. Randomized controlled trials (RCTs) comparing the effectiveness and safety between triple therapy and dual therapy in T2DM patients after coronary stents placement were included. Endpoints included major adverse cardiac effects (MACEs), target lesion revascularization (TLR), target vessel revascularization (TVR), death, stent thrombosis, bleeding and adverse drug reactions during a 9–12 months period, as well as platelet activities.

Results: Four studies including 1005 patients reporting the adverse clinical outcomes and six studies including 519 patients reporting the platelet activities, with a total of 1524 patients have been analyzed in this meta-analysis. The pooling analysis shows that TAPT has significantly decreased the occurrence of MACEs (RR: 0.55; 95 % CI: 0.36–0.86, $P = 0.009$), TLR (RR 0.41; 95 % CI: 0.21–0.80, $P = 0.008$), TVR (RR 0.55; 95 % CI: 0.34–0.88, $P = 0.01$) and the overall incidence of Death/ Myocardial Infarction (MI)/TVR (RR 0.54; 95 % CI: 0.31–0.94, $P = 0.03$) during this 9 to 12 months follow up period after stents implantation. Stent thrombosis was almost similar in both groups. Bleeding seemed to favor DAPT but the result was not statistically significant. Platelet aggregation, platelet reactivity index (PRI) and platelet reactivity unit (PRU) were also reduced with Weight Mean Difference (WMD) of (−13.80; 95 % CI: −17.03 to −10.56, $P < 0.00001$), (−22.87; 95 % CI: −23.66 to −22.07, $P < 0.00001$) and (−44.17; 95 % CI: −58.56 to −29.77, $P < 0.00001$) respectively.

Conclusion: Since MACEs have been significantly decreased in the triple group, TAPT appears to be more effective than DAPT in T2DM patients after intracoronary stenting. No significant difference in stent thrombosis and bleeding risks between these 2 groups shows TAPT to be almost as safe as DAPT in these diabetic patients.

Keywords: Antiplatelet therapy, Cilostazol, Type 2 diabetes mellitus, Coronary stents implantation

* Correspondence: cmhnn@sina.com
Institute of Cardiovascular Diseases, the First Affiliated Hospital of Guangxi Medical University, Nanning, Guangxi 530027, P. R. China

Background

Nowadays percutaneous coronary intervention (PCI) is becoming the preferred invasive procedure in patients suffering from coronary artery disease (CAD) and acute coronary syndrome (ACS) which are chronic macrovascular complications in type 2 diabetes mellitus (T2DM) patients. Several studies have shown that T2DM patients are more exposed to many adverse clinical outcomes such as major adverse cardiac effects (MACEs), target lesion revascularization (TLR), target vessel revascularization (TVR) and stent thrombosis after intracoronary stenting [1]. Platelet dysfunction is among one of the reasons T2DM patients have an increased risk of atherothrombotic events [2, 3]. In particular, T2DM patients have increased platelet reactivity warranting the use of platelet-inhibiting strategies in order to reduce their ischemic risk after stents implantation. Since cardiovascular disease is the leading cause of morbidity and mortality in patients with T2DM and because the latter usually present with atypical symptoms in these patients, antiplatelet therapies in these high risk patients after coronary stents placement are extremely important. Although currently approved antiplatelet treatment strategies have proven useful in improving outcomes, T2DM patients continue to have a higher risk of adverse cardiovascular events especially after stents implantation. Several antiplatelet therapies have been tried but the most commonly used have been the dual antiplatelet therapy (DAPT) consisting of aspirin and clopidogrel, as mentioned in Emmanouil's study [4], and the triple antiplatelet therapy (TAPT) consisting of aspirin, clopidogrel and cilostazol [5–9]. Studies show that TAPT has been a better option in T2DM patients compared to DAPT [10] but the treatments have not yet been well established systematically. Therefore, by performing a meta-analysis, we sought to evaluate systematically whether TAPT is more effective and safe to use compared to DAPT in T2DM patients after coronary stents implantation.

The abbreviations and acronyms used in this meta-analysis have been represented in Table 1.

Table 1 Abbreviations and acronyms

T2DM	Type 2 diabetes mellitus
PCI	Percutaneous coronary intervention
DAPT	Dual antiplatelet therapy
TAPT	Triple antiplatelet therapy
TVR	Target vessel revascularization
TLR	Target lumen revascularization
MACEs	Major adverse cardiac effects
PRI	Platelet reactivity index
WMD	Weight mean difference

Methods

Eligibility and search strategy

Relevant randomized controlled trials (RCTs) were identified through a computerized literature search from PubMed, Cochrane, Embase/Science Direct, China National Knowledge Infrastructure (CNKI) and WanFang databases using the search terms "Diabetes + Coronary Stents + Dual and/or Triple Anti platelet therapy". Different wordings of the same meanings have also been used such as "PTCA/PCI, DAPT, TAPT, T2DM, coronary angioplasty and anti-platelets". No language restrictions were used. All data were independently extracted by two investigators and then the results were compared, and disagreements were resolved by discussing with a third investigator before December 2014.

Inclusion and exclusion criteria

Studies included in our meta-analysis were trials that: (a) randomly assigned patients for RCTs (b) included T2DM patients (wherever possible, selecting only T2DM patients in studies consisting of both T2DM and non-T2DM or retrieving the number of diabetic patients among other disease conditions such as acute coronary syndrome or long coronary lesion) (c) compared TAPT (aspirin, clopidogrel and cilostazol) with DAPT (aspirin and clopidogrel) (d) reported any of the corresponding endpoints including MACEs, TLR, TVR, stent thrombosis, bleeding and adverse drug reactions as well as platelet aggregation, PRI and PRU.

Exclusion criteria were trials (a) of retrospective non-randomized studies (b) including only non-diabetic patients (c) including another drug instead of cilostazol in the TAPT group (d) considering only DAPT or TAPT separately without comparison (e) with duplicate reports.

Data extraction and quality assessment

Two authors (P.K.B. and T.Q.) independently reviewed the data and assessed the eligibility and methodological quality of each eligible trial. Information regarding study and patient characteristics, intervention strategies, and the pre-specified clinical outcomes was systematically extracted. Disagreements were discussed between the authors, and if the authors could not reach a consensus, disagreements were resolved by the third author (M.H.C.). The bias risk of trials was assessed with the components recommended by the Cochrane Collaboration, including sequence generation of the allocation, allocation concealment, blinding of participants, personnel, and outcome assessors, incomplete outcome data, selective outcome reporting, and other sources of bias. Quality scale was used to assess the trials: (A) true randomization and allocation concealed, and (B) process of randomization not given and concealment of allocation unclear. This approach was recommended by Cochrane Collaboration.

Definitions, outcomes and follow-up

Major adverse cardiac effects: MACEs were defined as death of cardiac or procedure-related origin, MI, and repeat target lesion revascularization after stents implantation. Major adverse cardiovascular and cerebrovascular events (MACCEs) have also been considered together in this section.

Revascularization: included TLR and TVR. Revascularization was clinically indicated if there was >70 % diameter stenosis on angiography or >50 % stenosis together with a positive stress test or ischemic symptoms. TLR was defined as clinically indicated percutaneous or surgical revascularization of the index lesion during follow-up.

Stent thrombosis: which could occur acutely (within 24 h), sub-acutely (within 30 days), or as late as 1 year (late) after stent placement throughout the whole follow up period.

Bleeding: was defined as any hemorrhagic event which could occur with the use of the anti-platelets after stents implantation and included minor, major or minimal bleeding in this study.

Adverse drug reactions: included the adverse effects associated with the use of these anti-platelets. For example, rashes, gastrointestinal troubles, thrombocytopenia, liver dysfunction and finally drug discontinuation due to these adverse effects.

Platelet aggregation: defined as the clumping together of platelets in the blood.

PRI and PRU: dealt with the reactivity and activation of platelets after antiplatelet use.

The follow-up for these adverse clinical outcomes as well as the adverse drug reactions was for a period of 9 months in two studies and 12 months in the other two studies. For the platelet aggregation, PRI and PRU, the follow up period was randomly assumed to be during any given time after stents implantation.

Statistical analysis

Risk ratio (RR) with 95 % confidence interval (CI) was used to express the pooled effect on discontinuous variables. For continuous variables, standard deviation for each group was calculated using the formula $s=\sqrt{\frac{1}{N-1}\sum_{i=1}^{N}(x_i-\bar{x})^2}$ and data were evaluated by means of weighted mean differences (WMDs) and 95 % confidence intervals (CIs). Heterogeneity across the trials was assessed using the Cochrane Q-statistic ($p \leq 0.05$ was considered significant) and I^2-statistic. I^2 describes the percentage of total variation across studies that is due to heterogeneity rather than chance. A value of 0 % indicates no heterogeneity, and larger values indicate increased heterogeneity. If I^2 was <50 %, fixed effect model was used. However, if I^2 was >50 %, a random effect model was used [11]. Publication bias was visually estimated by assessing funnel plots. The pooled analyses were performed with RevMan 5.3.

Results

Selected studies and baseline characteristics

From the initial literature search, 211 items in PubMed, 597 in Embase, 341 in CNKI, 416 in WanFang databases and 19 in the Cochrane database were identified. After an elaborative screening, 15 RCTs satisfied our inclusion criteria studies. However, after eliminating the duplicate studies, 10 RCTs have been finally selected for our meta-analysis.

Among these ten studies, four studies including 1005 patients (487 in the DAPT, 518 in the TAPT group) reported the adverse clinical outcomes in these T2DM patients whereas the remaining six studies with 519 patients (287 in the DAPT group, 232 in the TAPT group) reported the platelet activities. A total of 1524 patients (774 and 750 patients following TAPT and DAPT respectively) fulfilled the inclusion criteria and have been finally included in our meta-analysis. Figure 1 shows the flow of the process for identifying potentially eligible trials and the reasons for exclusion.

Trials included in this meta-analysis with their total number of patients (including DAPT and TAPT) and their corresponding endpoints have been represented in Table 2.

According to Table 2, four studies reported adverse cardiovascular outcomes as their endpoints. The other remaining trials dealt with platelet activities.

Table 3 summarizes the baseline characteristics for each of the included trials. No significant differences have been found in the baseline characteristics between the 2 groups.

Patients in most of the studies used beta-blockers and ACEI/ARB routinely. Moreover, patients in few of the studies also use statins as part of their routine medications. The use of glycoprotein IIb/IIIa was dependent on the physician's decision during the procedure.

For the studies related to platelet activities, such as platelet aggregation, PRI and PRU; the mean has been calculated first as well as the standard deviation. In a few of the studies, since there was a period of crossover adding cilostazol to the DAPT or removing cilostazol from the TAPT after complete washout; the participants have been considered as different individuals before and after the crossover period despite of being the same patients. For example, in Angiolillo's study there were 20 participants. These 20 participants were treated first with DAPT for 2 weeks and then after a washout period, the same 20 participants were treated with TAPT. In such a case, we have considered the number of patients undergoing DAPT to

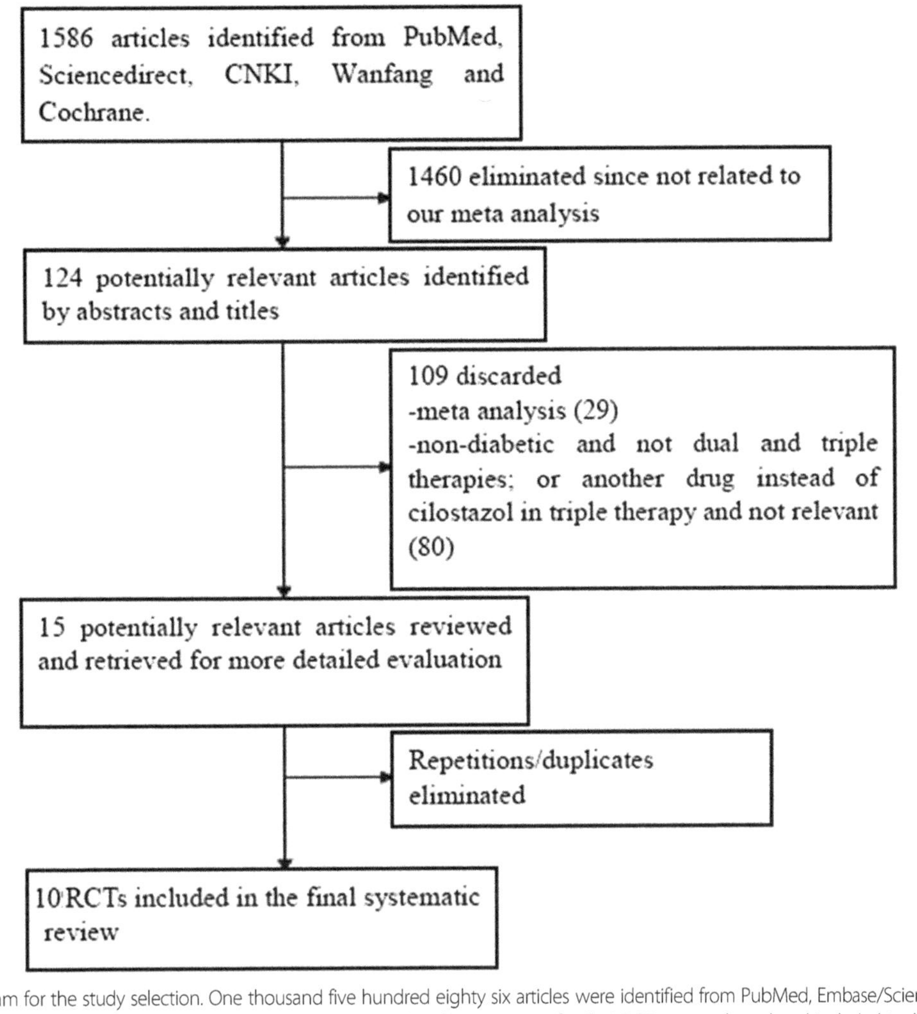

Fig. 1 Flow diagram for the study selection. One thousand five hundred eighty six articles were identified from PubMed, Embase/Science Direct, CNKI, Wanfang and Cochrane databases. After considering the inclusion and exclusion criteria, finally 8 RCTs were selected and included in this meta-analysis. Showing the detailed flow chart of study selection

Table 2 Shows the endpoints reported by each of the included trials

Trials	No of patients (DAPT + TAPT)	Follow up period (month)	Reported endpoints/outcomes
Han 2009 [6]	263	12	MACEs, TVR, and ADR.
Lee 2011 [33]	176	12	MACEs, TVR, TLR, ST, D/MI/TVR, BL and ADR.
Lee 2008 [5]	400	9	MACEs, TVR, TLR, ST, D/MI/TVR, BL and ADR.
Lee 2007 [34]	166	9	MACEs, TVR, TLR, ST, D/MI/TVR, BL and ADR.
Yang 2011 [35]	154	–	PRU and PA
Yang 2007 [36]	55	7	PA
Capranzano 2012 [37]	80	1	PRU and PRI
Angiolillo 2008 [38]	40	1	PRI and PA
Angiolillo 2011 [39]	106	1	PRI
Ha 2013 [40]	84	2	PRU and PA

Abbreviations: *MACEs* major adverse cardiac effects, *TVR* target vessel revascularization, *TLR* target lesion revascularization, *BL* bleeding, *ST* stent thrombosis, *ADR* adverse drug reactions, *D* death, *MI* myocardial infarction, *PA* platelet aggregation, *PRI* platelet reactivity index, *PRU* platelet reactivity unit

Table 3 Baseline characteristics of patients from the included studies

Study/Year	Age (yrs)	Male (%)	Ht (%)	Hc (%)	Cs (%)	Q[a]
	T/D	T/D	T/D	T/D	T/D	
Lee 2007 [34]	60.9/61.2	64.8/63.6	54.8/55.2	30.0/28.4	37.6/37.2	B
Lee 2008 [5]	61.0/60.7	59.0/57.0	59.5/59.5	30.5/28.5	24.0/31.5	B
Yang 2011 [35]	63.5/63.5	62.3/62.3	55.8/55.8	37.7/37.7	28.6/28.6	B
Yang 2009 [36]	63.4/63.8	40.0/60.0	61.9/57.1	28.6/41.2	14.3/20.6	B
Capranzano 2012 [37]	60.4/60.4	60.2/60.2	91.2/91.2	97.0/97.0	37.1/37.1	B
Angiolillo 2008 [38]	64.0/64.0	60.0/60.0	96.0/96.0	92.0/92.0	24.0/24.0	B
Angiolillo 2011 [39]	60.5/60.5	63.0/63.0	95.0/95.0	100.0/100.0	28.0/28.0	B
Ha 2013 [40]	64.9/62.3	67.7/76.1	71.4/76.1	33.3/42.5	23.8/23.8	B
Lee 2011 [33]	60.9/62.1	70.0/71.5	58.4/64.7	42.4/45.0	30.4/30.1	B
Han 2009 [6]	59.6/60.2	73.8/72.9	57.9/56.1	45.5/45.4	–	B

Abbreviations:NM not mentioned, *Ht* hypertension, *Hc* hypercholesterolemia; *Cs* current smoker, *T* triple therapy, *D* dual therapy
[a]Quality scale: A:true randomization and allocation concealed; B:process of randomization not given and concealment of allocation unclear

be 20 and the number of patients undergoing TAPT to be 20. And finally we have considered the total number of patients to be 40. These values have been used in the results.

All the patients were above 60 years old of age and most of them were males. In three studies, the percentage of patients suffering from hypertension was above 90 % while in the remaining studies, 50–70 % suffered from high blood pressure. Three studies reported a hyperlipidemia level of more than 90 % whereas the amount of participants who were smokers did not exceed 40 %.

The mean Quantitative Angiographic Measurement of the included studies showing the lesion length, stented length, minimal lumen diameter before and after the procedure and the diameter of the stenosis before and after the procedure have been illustrated in Table 4.

There were no differences in angiographic measurements between the 2 groups in those included studies.

Result of the meta-analysis

The pooling analysis shows that TAPT significantly decreased the occurrence of overall MACEs among the 1005 patients reporting this outcome with (RR: 0.55, 95 % CI: 0.36–0.86; $P = 0.009$), TLR (RR 0.41; 95 % CI: 0.21–0.80; $P = 0.008$) and TVR (RR 0.55; 95 % CI: 0.34–0.88; $P = 0.01$) in these T2DM patients after coronary stents implantation. TAPT treatment showed superiority in reducing the overall Death/MI/TVR (RR 0.54; 95 % CI: 0.31–0.94; $P = 0.03$) compared to DAPT. Stent thrombosis (RR 0.95; 95 % CI: 0.19–4.76, $P = 0.95$) was similar in both groups and the result for bleeding (RR 0.80; 95 % CI: 0.40–1.59, $P = 0.52$) was not statistically significant. TAPT showed to be more beneficial in these T2DM patients by significantly reducing the platelet aggregation WMD: (−13.80; 95 % CI: −17.03 to −10.56, $P < 0.00001$), PRI WMD: (−22.87; 95 % CI: −23.66 to −22.07, $P < 0.00001$) and PRU WMD: (−44.17; 95 % CI: −58.56 to −29.77, $P < 0.00001$) respectively.

Results for the associated adverse effects between these 2 groups were as follow: (RR 2.67; 95 % CI: 1.26–5.65; $P = 0.01$) for rashes being higher in the TAPT group; (RR 1.76; 95 % CI: 0.77–4.01; $P = 0.18$) for gastrointestinal troubles; (RR 0.33; 95 % CI: 0.01–8.13; $P = 0.50$) for thrombocytopenia; (RR 0.72; 95 % CI: 0.16–3.18; $P = 0.67$) for hepatic dysfunction; (RR 6.18;

Table 4 Shows the mean Quantitative Angiographic Measurement of the included studies[a]

Variables (mm)	TAPT group ($n = 377$)	DAPT group ($n = 365$)
Reference diameter	2.81	2.79
Lesion length	31.5	31.7
Stented length	37.45	36.05
Minimal lumen diameter in segment before procedure	0.81	0.79
Minimal lumen diameter in segment after procedure	2.25	2.24
Minimal lumen diameter in stent after procedure	2.57	2.58
Stenosis diameter in segment before procedure (%)	70.3	70.4
Stenosis diameter in segment after procedure (%)	17.7	17.2
Stenosis diameter in stent after procedure (%)	8.45	7.57
Acute gain in segment	1.44	1.46
Acute gain in stent	1.76	1.79

[a]Data from trials Lee 2007 [34], Lee 2008 [5] and Lee 2011 [33] have been included in this table. Quantitative Angiographic Measurement data for study Han 2009 [6] was not available and therefore have been omitted

95 % CI: 0.76–50.20; $P = 0.09$) for palpitation and (RR 3.56; 95 % CI: 0.76–16.54; $P = 0.11$) for headache. Moreover, the risk ratio for patients to discontinue TAPT due to these adverse effects was (RR 3.75; 95 % CI: 2.18–6.46; $P < 0.00001$). The detailed results have been illustrated in Figs. 2, 3 and 4.

The funnel plots assessing publication bias in the included studies have been illustrated in Fig. 5a and b.

For all of the above analyses, sensitivity analyses yielded consistent results. Based on a visual inspection of the funnel plots, there has been no evidence of publication bias for the included studies that assessed all clinical endpoints.

Discussion

Aim and results of this study

The aim of the current study was to perform a comprehensive meta-analysis of several RCTs comparing and analyzing the effectiveness and safety between TAPT (aspirin, clopidogrel and cilostazol) and DAPT (aspirin and clopidogrel) in T2DM patients after coronary stents implantation.

Results from this study including 1005 patients reporting adverse clinical outcomes as their endpoints show that TAPT is more effective than DAPT in several aspects in T2DM patients. TAPT has significantly decreased platelet aggregation, PRI and PRU among the 519 patients analyzed. MACEs, TLR and TVR which are more prominent among diabetic patients, have also decreased significantly with the use of this cilostazol based TAPT. Stent thrombosis was similar in both groups. However, TAPT did not significantly increase the bleeding in these T2DM patients.

Mechanisms of cilostazol in this TAPT

Several reasons are associated with these benefits and effectiveness of this TAPT. First of all, cilostazol has a different mechanism of action compared to aspirin and clopidogrel. It is a phosphodiesterase III (PDE3) inhibitor that plays the role of increasing cyclic adenosine monophosphate within platelets and thus leads to reduced aggregation of platelets [12]. Cilostazol can also inhibit expression of stent-induced P-selectin and the subsequent Mac-1–mediated leukocyte activation that is the trigger of restenosis after PCI [13]. To further explain this mechanism is thought to be the inhibition of neo-intimal proliferation, considered to be a major mechanism of restenosis after PCI caused by smooth muscle cells (SMC) migration, proliferation, and matrix synthesis. SMC migration and proliferation are induced by growth factors released from activated platelets. As an antiplatelet medication, cilostazol controls the induction by platelet-derived growth factors. More importantly, cilostazol is thought to directly inhibit SMC growth. In addition, there is much evidence that Mac-1 is one of the key proteins in the mechanism of restenosis. Studies have demonstrated clinically that PCI induced activation and upregulation of Mac-1 on the surface of neutrophils and that Mac-1 kinetics were linked to angiographic late lumen loss—known as neo-intimal thickening. Cilostazol may inhibit Mac-1–mediated leukocyte activation (act as a Mac-1 blocker) directly or through P-selectin–mediated platelet activation, which may lead to a reduction in the rate of restenosis after coronary stent implantation. This unique property of cilostazol makes it different from all the other anti-platelet agents.

Moreover, since T2DM have platelets hyperactivity, and are usually victims of aspirin and clopidogrel hyporesponsiveness, this adjunctive cilostazol can help to inhibit platelet aggregations and activation which might not be completely possible with the use of DAPT [14]. These mechanisms could be used to explain the better effect of this cilostazol-based TAPT compared to DAPT especially in these T2DM patients who are more at risk of these serious adverse cardiac events after coronary stenting.

TAPT and DAPT in other studies

Similar to our results which showed that TAPT decreased MACEs, TLR as well as TVR, Mohammad's study published in 2010 also indicated that TAPT was more effective after drug eluting stents (DES) placement since it was associated with decreased TLR and MACEs in high risk patients [15]. Another example is Bangalore's meta-analysis consisting of 41 trials conducted in 2014 [16]. This meta-analysis was also in favor of using cilostazol associated TAPT due to a significant reduction in both stent thrombosis and restenosis but, however, his study was not restricted to T2DM patients. Min's study published in 2007 (including 23 % of the population with T2DM using TAPT and 29 % using DAPT) also concluded that the cilostazol based TAPT seemed to be more effective at preventing in-stent neointimal hyperplasia than a dual antiplatelet regimen [17]. Moreover, the results from the DECREASED registry showed that TAPT significantly reduced 12-month risks of stent thrombosis and MI after DES implantation compared with DAPT without any increase risk of bleeding complications [18]. In another meta-analysis, this time conducted by Sakurai, in 2013, TAPT was associated with significantly effective outcomes for TLR and TVR without any increase in MACEs [19]. A study by Kim published in 2011 including almost 30 % T2DM using TAPT, also supports our results showing that compared with high-dose clopidogrel in DAPT, adjunctive cilostazol significantly enhanced platelet inhibition and reduced the rate of high platelet reactivity showing that TAPT is apparently more effective than DAPT [20]. Moreover, the study by Douglas et al. which included 23 % of diabetic patients treated with TAPT and 28 %

Study or Subgroup	TAPT Events	TAPT Total	DAPT Events	DAPT Total	Weight	Risk Ratio M-H, Fixed, 95% CI
1.1.1 Target Lesion Revascularization (TLR)						
Lee2007	2	85	6	81	3.5%	0.32 [0.07, 1.53]
Lee2008	5	200	14	200	8.0%	0.36 [0.13, 0.97]
Lee2011	5	92	8	84	4.8%	0.57 [0.19, 1.68]
Subtotal (95% CI)		**377**		**365**	**16.3%**	**0.41 [0.21, 0.80]**
Total events	12		28			
Heterogeneity: Chi^2 = 0.53, df = 2 (P = 0.77); I^2 = 0%						
Test for overall effect: Z = 2.63 (P = 0.008)						
1.1.2 Target Vessel Revascularization (TVR)						
Han2009	11	141	13	122	8.0%	0.73 [0.34, 1.57]
Lee2007	3	85	6	81	3.5%	0.48 [0.12, 1.84]
Lee2008	7	200	16	200	9.2%	0.44 [0.18, 1.04]
Lee2011	5	92	9	84	5.4%	0.51 [0.18, 1.45]
Subtotal (95% CI)		**518**		**487**	**26.1%**	**0.55 [0.34, 0.88]**
Total events	26		44			
Heterogeneity: Chi^2 = 0.87, df = 3 (P = 0.83); I^2 = 0%						
Test for overall effect: Z = 2.51 (P = 0.01)						
1.1.3 Death/MI/TVR						
Lee2007	3	85	6	81	3.5%	0.48 [0.12, 1.84]
Lee2008	8	200	16	200	9.2%	0.50 [0.22, 1.14]
Lee2011	7	92	10	84	6.0%	0.64 [0.25, 1.60]
Subtotal (95% CI)		**377**		**365**	**18.7%**	**0.54 [0.31, 0.94]**
Total events	18		32			
Heterogeneity: Chi^2 = 0.20, df = 2 (P = 0.91); I^2 = 0%						
Test for overall effect: Z = 2.16 (P = 0.03)						
1.1.4 Stent thrombosis						
Lee2007	1	85	1	81	0.6%	0.95 [0.06, 14.98]
Lee2008	0	200	1	200	0.9%	0.33 [0.01, 8.13]
Lee2011	1	92	0	84	0.3%	2.74 [0.11, 66.40]
Subtotal (95% CI)		**377**		**365**	**1.7%**	**0.95 [0.19, 4.76]**
Total events	2		2			
Heterogeneity: Chi^2 = 0.84, df = 2 (P = 0.66); I^2 = 0%						
Test for overall effect: Z = 0.06 (P = 0.95)						
1.1.5 Bleeding						
Han2009	4	141	2	122	1.2%	1.73 [0.32, 9.28]
Lee2007	1	85	1	81	0.6%	0.95 [0.06, 14.98]
Lee2008	3	200	3	20	3.1%	0.10 [0.02, 0.46]
Lee2011	7	92	6	84	3.6%	1.07 [0.37, 3.04]
Subtotal (95% CI)		**518**		**307**	**8.5%**	**0.80 [0.40, 1.59]**
Total events	15		12			
Heterogeneity: Chi^2 = 8.18, df = 3 (P = 0.04); I^2 = 63%						
Test for overall effect: Z = 0.64 (P = 0.52)						
1.1.6 Major Adverse Cardiac Effects (MACEs)						
Han2009	14	141	18	122	11.1%	0.67 [0.35, 1.30]
Lee2007	2	85	6	81	3.5%	0.32 [0.07, 1.53]
Lee2008	6	200	14	200	8.0%	0.43 [0.17, 1.09]
Lee2011	7	92	10	84	6.0%	0.64 [0.25, 1.60]
Subtotal (95% CI)		**518**		**487**	**28.6%**	**0.55 [0.36, 0.86]**
Total events	29		48			
Heterogeneity: Chi^2 = 1.20, df = 3 (P = 0.75); I^2 = 0%						
Test for overall effect: Z = 2.62 (P = 0.009)						
Total (95% CI)		**2685**		**2376**	**100.0%**	**0.55 [0.44, 0.70]**
Total events	102		166			
Heterogeneity: Chi^2 = 12.90, df = 20 (P = 0.88); I^2 = 0%						
Test for overall effect: Z = 4.87 (P < 0.00001)						
Test for subgroup differences: Chi^2 = 2.33, df = 5 (P = 0.80), I^2 = 0%						

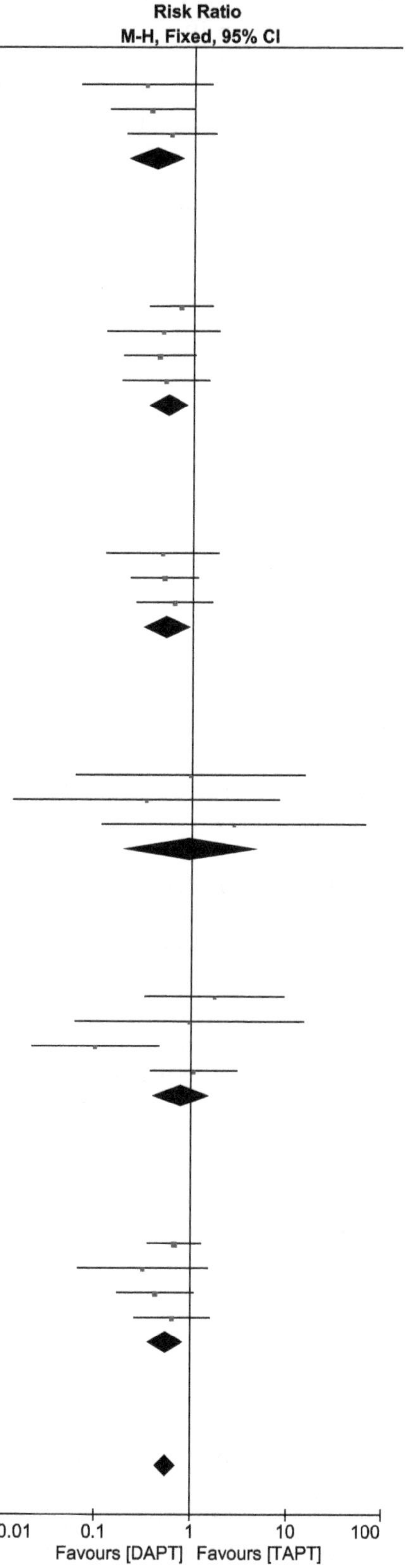

Fig. 2 Forest plot comparing the adverse clinical outcomes between TAPT and DAPT in T2DM patients after intracoronary stenting. Adverse clinical outcomes have decreased with the use of this TAPT during a follow up period of 9 to 12 months after coronary stenting

Study or Subgroup	TAPT Mean	TAPT SD	TAPT Total	DAPT Mean	DAPT SD	DAPT Total	Weight	Mean Difference IV, Random, 95% CI
1.2.1 Platelet aggregation								
Angiolillo2008	32	3.23	20	54.5	1.24	20	9.9%	-22.50 [-24.02, -20.98]
Ha2013	44.5	0.31	42	56.8	0.5	42	10.1%	-12.30 [-12.48, -12.12]
Yang2009	38.7	1.65	21	50.1	1.71	34	10.0%	-11.40 [-12.31, -10.49]
Yang2011	69	3.21	52	78.3	1.83	102	10.0%	-9.30 [-10.24, -8.36]
Subtotal (95% CI)			**135**			**198**	**40.1%**	**-13.80 [-17.03, -10.56]**
Heterogeneity: Tau² = 10.63; Chi² = 216.55, df = 3 (P < 0.00001); I² = 99%								
Test for overall effect: Z = 8.36 (P < 0.00001)								
1.2.2 Platelet Reactivity Index (PRI)								
Angiolillo2008	36.3	0.76	20	59.9	0.92	20	10.1%	-23.60 [-24.12, -23.08]
Angiolillo2011	29.6	0.45	57	52.6	0.48	49	10.1%	-23.00 [-23.18, -22.82]
Capranzano2012	33	0.005	40	55.1	0.13	40	10.1%	-22.10 [-22.14, -22.06]
Subtotal (95% CI)			**117**			**109**	**30.3%**	**-22.87 [-23.66, -22.07]**
Heterogeneity: Tau² = 0.47; Chi² = 122.95, df = 2 (P < 0.00001); I² = 98%								
Test for overall effect: Z = 56.29 (P < 0.00001)								
1.2.3 Platelet Reactivity Unit (PRU)								
Capranzano2012	160.8	1.95	40	204.7	1.99	40	10.0%	-43.90 [-44.76, -43.04]
Ha2013	138.7	5.36	42	198.8	2.86	42	9.8%	-60.10 [-61.94, -58.26]
Yang2011	219.4	6.5	52	247.9	3.06	102	9.8%	-28.50 [-30.36, -26.64]
Subtotal (95% CI)			**134**			**184**	**29.7%**	**-44.17 [-58.56, -29.77]**
Heterogeneity: Tau² = 161.15; Chi² = 560.63, df = 2 (P < 0.00001); I² = 100%								
Test for overall effect: Z = 6.01 (P < 0.00001)								
Total (95% CI)			**386**			**491**	**100.0%**	**-25.59 [-29.16, -22.02]**
Heterogeneity: Tau² = 32.93; Chi² = 16782.47, df = 9 (P < 0.00001); I² = 100%								
Test for overall effect: Z = 14.04 (P < 0.00001)								
Test for subgroup differences: Chi² = 37.31, df = 2 (P < 0.00001), I² = 94.6%								

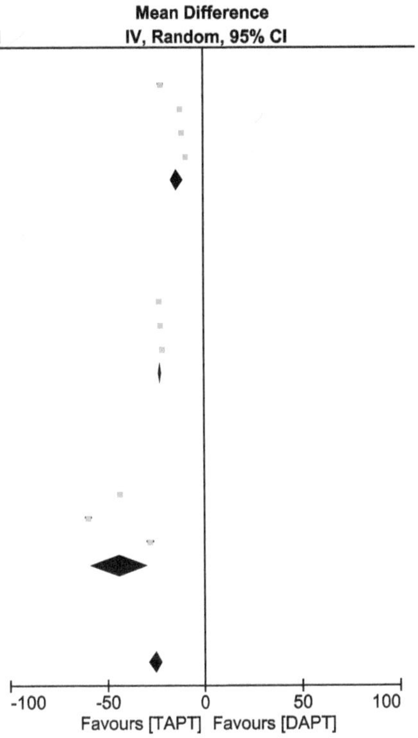

Fig. 3 Forest plot comparing the platelet activities between TAPT and DAPT in T2DM after intracoronary stenting. A lower platelet aggregation, platelet reactivity index and platelet reactivity unit in the TAPT group shows that TAPT seems to be more effective in these T2DM patients

treated with DAPT showed that cilostazol-treated patients with oral hypoglycemic medications experienced a highly significant 63 % reduction in the risk of restenosis ($P < 0.006$) [21]. The study by Jeong et al. demonstrated that among his 30 % T2DM patients using TAPT and 13.3 % using the standard DAPT, the use of TAPT may achieve adequate inhibition of ADP-induced platelet aggregation to suppress the occurrence of major adverse cardiovascular events [22]. Finally, the CIDES trial which dealt with only T2DM patients showed that cilostazol was better than clopidogrel after drug eluting stents implantation in these patients. However, this study did not compare TAPT with DAPT; but instead, compared the clinical outcomes with the use of cilostazol and clopidogrel separately [23]. All of these studies show that TAPT is more effective and could safely be used as it is expected not to cause any increase in bleeding. In other words, apart from being more effective, TAPT is expected to be at least as safe as DAPT in T2DM patients.

However, even if many studies support our results, there are still a few studies whose results were completely different from our study. For example, the multicenter randomized trial conducted by Suh criticized the use of cilostazol as a component of the TAPT after stents implantation. But, the author accepted that his CILON-T trial had a different composition of patients and primary endpoints. The trial did not assess the beneficial role of cilostazol during PCI and included relatively low-risk patients. The author also precised that DECLARE DIABETES and DECLARE LONG studies which we have used in our meta-analysis had enrolled only high risk patients such as diabetes mellitus or long lesions. He also mentioned that his study was not designed to evaluate the post-treatment platelet reactivity [24]. Similarly, Jeon's study conducted in 2010 demonstrated that there was no significant difference in the prevention of stent thrombosis between TAPT and DAPT groups but however, his study had a mixture of low and high risk patients [25]. Moreover, results from the HOST-ASSURE trial published in 2013 showed that the outcomes of both DAPT and TAPT were almost the same. TAPT was non inferior to double dose clopidogrel DAPT. However, the short follow-up period of 1 month could be a reason for this completely different result [26].

Other anti-platelet agents

Apart from this cilostazol based TAPT, there are other anti-platelet agents which can be used after intracoronary stenting. For example, the early use of glycoprotein IIb/IIIa inhibitors can reduce the occurrence of death or myocardial infarction in patients with acute coronary

Study or Subgroup	TAPT Events	TAPT Total	DAPT Events	DAPT Total	Weight	Risk Ratio M-H, Fixed, 95% CI
1.2.1 Rashes						
Han2009	3	141	1	122	2.5%	2.60 [0.27, 24.63]
Lee2007	4	85	1	81	2.4%	3.81 [0.44, 33.39]
Lee2008	15	200	5	200	11.9%	3.00 [1.11, 8.10]
Lee2011	3	92	2	84	5.0%	1.37 [0.23, 8.00]
Subtotal (95% CI)		**518**		**487**	**21.8%**	**2.67 [1.26, 5.65]**
Total events	25		9			
Heterogeneity: Chi² = 0.71, df = 3 (P = 0.87); I² = 0%						
Test for overall effect: Z = 2.57 (P = 0.01)						
1.2.2 GI troubles						
Han2009	0	141	1	122	3.8%	0.29 [0.01, 7.02]
Lee2007	4	85	1	81	2.4%	3.81 [0.44, 33.39]
Lee2008	9	200	5	200	11.9%	1.80 [0.61, 5.28]
Lee2011	2	92	1	84	2.5%	1.83 [0.17, 19.77]
Subtotal (95% CI)		**518**		**487**	**20.6%**	**1.76 [0.77, 4.01]**
Total events	15		8			
Heterogeneity: Chi² = 1.72, df = 3 (P = 0.63); I² = 0%						
Test for overall effect: Z = 1.35 (P = 0.18)						
1.2.3 Thrombocytopenia						
Lee2007	0	85	0	81		Not estimable
Lee2008	0	200	1	200	3.6%	0.33 [0.01, 8.13]
Lee2011	0	92	0	84		Not estimable
Subtotal (95% CI)		**377**		**365**	**3.6%**	**0.33 [0.01, 8.13]**
Total events	0		1			
Heterogeneity: Not applicable						
Test for overall effect: Z = 0.67 (P = 0.50)						
1.2.4 Hepatic Dysfunction						
Lee2007	0	85	1	81	3.6%	0.32 [0.01, 7.69]
Lee2008	2	200	1	200	2.4%	2.00 [0.18, 21.88]
Lee2011	0	92	1	84	3.7%	0.30 [0.01, 7.38]
Subtotal (95% CI)		**377**		**365**	**9.8%**	**0.72 [0.16, 3.18]**
Total events	2		3			
Heterogeneity: Chi² = 1.23, df = 2 (P = 0.54); I² = 0%						
Test for overall effect: Z = 0.43 (P = 0.67)						
1.2.5 Drug discontinuation						
Lee2007	13	85	1	81	2.4%	12.39 [1.66, 92.55]
Lee2008	29	200	5	200	11.9%	5.80 [2.29, 14.68]
Lee2011	17	92	9	84	22.4%	1.72 [0.81, 3.66]
Subtotal (95% CI)		**377**		**365**	**36.7%**	**3.75 [2.18, 6.46]**
Total events	59		15			
Heterogeneity: Chi² = 6.31, df = 2 (P = 0.04); I² = 68%						
Test for overall effect: Z = 4.77 (P < 0.00001)						
1.2.6 Headache						
Han2009	4	141	1	122	2.5%	3.46 [0.39, 30.55]
Lee2011	4	92	1	84	2.5%	3.65 [0.42, 32.03]
Subtotal (95% CI)		**233**		**206**	**5.0%**	**3.56 [0.76, 16.54]**
Total events	8		2			
Heterogeneity: Chi² = 0.00, df = 1 (P = 0.97); I² = 0%						
Test for overall effect: Z = 1.62 (P = 0.11)						
1.2.7 Palpitation						
Han2009	5	141	0	122	1.3%	9.53 [0.53, 170.58]
Lee2011	1	92	0	84	1.2%	2.74 [0.11, 66.40]
Subtotal (95% CI)		**233**		**206**	**2.5%**	**6.18 [0.76, 50.20]**
Total events	6		0			
Heterogeneity: Chi² = 0.34, df = 1 (P = 0.56); I² = 0%						
Test for overall effect: Z = 1.70 (P = 0.09)						
Total (95% CI)		**2633**		**2481**	**100.0%**	**2.74 [1.94, 3.87]**
Total events	115		38			
Heterogeneity: Chi² = 15.68, df = 18 (P = 0.61); I² = 0%						
Test for overall effect: Z = 5.70 (P < 0.00001)						
Test for subgroup differences: Chi² = 7.86, df = 6 (P = 0.25), I² = 23.7%						

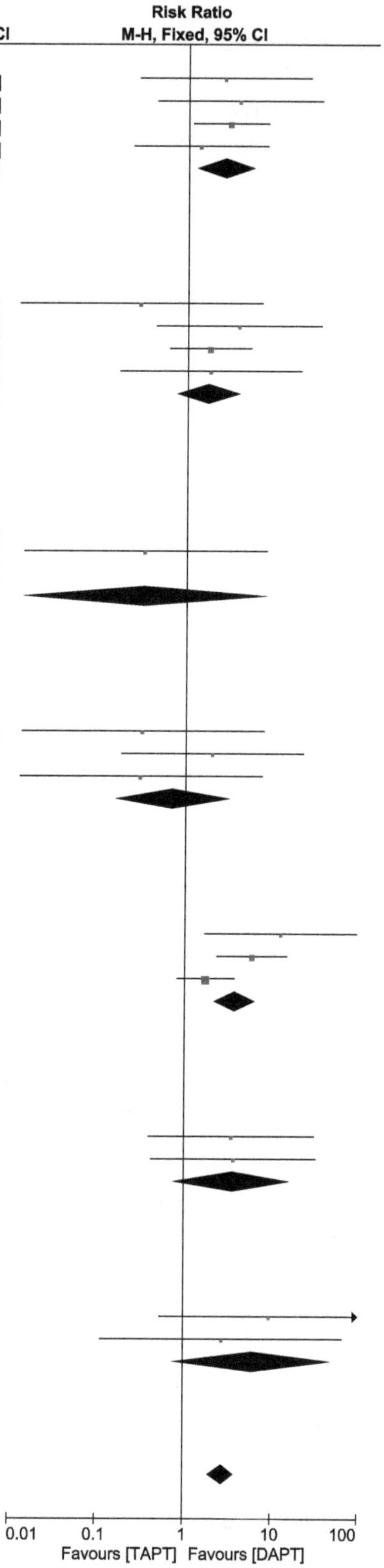

Fig. 4 Forest plot comparing the adverse drug reactions between TAPT and DAPT in T2DM patients after intracoronary stenting. More adverse effects are associated with cilostazol use in this TAPT compared to DAPT in these T2DM patients

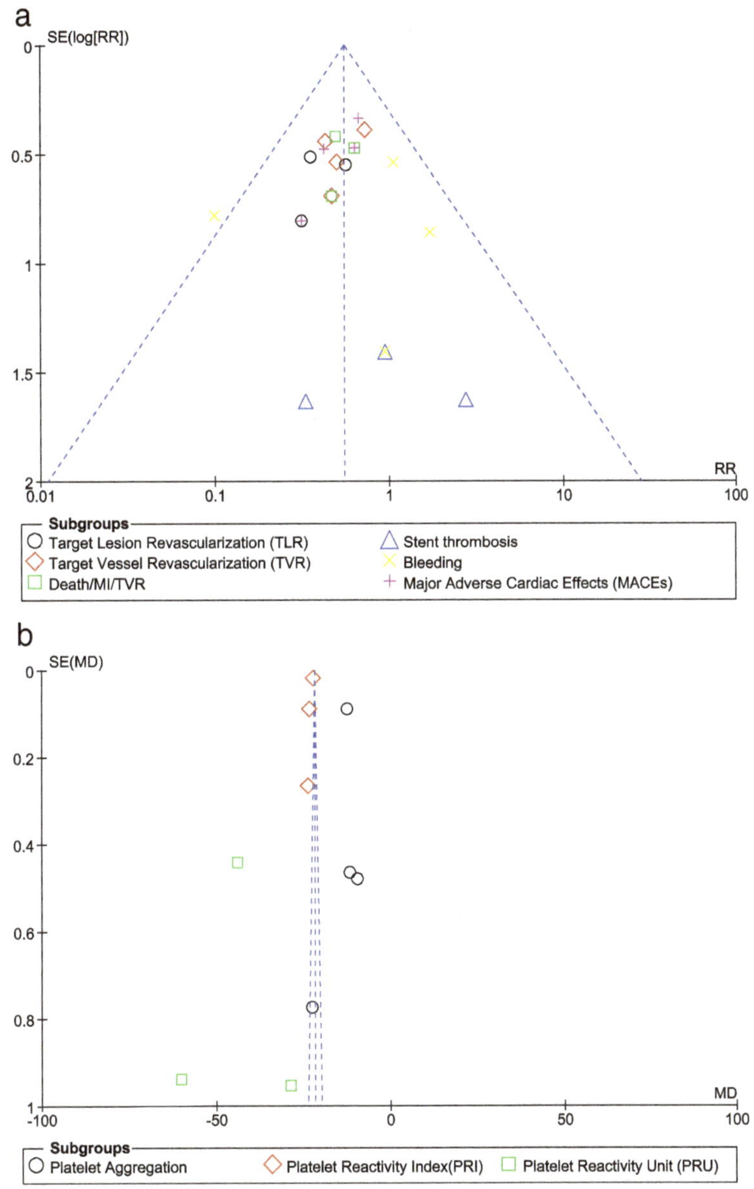

Fig. 5 a and **b** Funnel plots assessing publication bias in the included studies. For all of the above analyses, sensitivity analyses yielded consistent results. Based on a visual inspection of the funnel plots, there has been no evidence of publication bias for the included studies that assessed all clinical end points

syndromes who are not routinely scheduled for early revascularization. The event reduction is clinically most meaningful in patients at high risk of intracoronary thrombotic complications [27]. However, this drug can only be used for the short term in-hospital follow up. Moreover, the study by Geeganage's showed that TAPT based on i.v GPIIb/IIIa inhibitors was associated with a higher bleeding complication than that of the standard DAPT; however, the diabetic status of these patients was unknown [28].

New drugs such as prasugrel and ticagrelor are gradually becoming known among the antiplatelet agents. However, these drugs are associated with a higher bleeding tendency and they lack the anti-restenosis property which is only possible with the use of cilostazol and hence, rendering this cilostazol based TAPT to be a better option for T2DM patients.

Other potential benefits of cilostazol

Apart from being a part of TAPT, cilostazol alone has other potential indications. Studies have shown that cilostazol could reduce the symptoms of intermittent claudication [29, 30]. Cilostazol could also be used for the prevention of stroke in patients with non-cardio-embolic stroke [31]. Surprisingly, cilostazol has also shown to be beneficial to the heart. It can: increase the heart rate in patients with bradycardia, preventing ventricular fibrillation in patients suffering from Brugada syndrome, benefit patients with third degree atrio-ventricular block and could possibly act as a cardio-protective drug in patients with heart failure [32].

Novelty in this study

Contrary to other studies, this meta-analysis has strictly been conducted on T2DM patients and has combined the adverse cardiovascular outcomes such as MACEs, TLR, TVR and stent thrombosis with platelet reactivity such as PRI and PRU; and has included all of them into one study. It can be said that TAPT could be a more promising drug therapy than the standard DAPT in T2DM patients after intracoronary stenting both in terms of effectiveness and safety.

Limitations

Few limitations were as follow: First of all, because of the short follow up period and due to the limited study number and population size, the power of the analysis might be restricted to some extent. One study had a follow up of up to 2 years but this could not be considered for comparison because other studies did not have such long follow up periods. Secondly, due to the small population size, the results of this study may be affected to an extent. Also, the availability of new anti-platelet therapies such as prasugrel and ticagrelor could render TAPT useless in clinical practice. Unfortunately another limitation which restricts the use of this TAPT is that cilostazol is associated with a few adverse drug reactions such as rashes (RR 2.67; $P = 0.01$); gastrointestinal troubles (RR 1.76; $P = 0.18$); thrombocytopenia (RR 0.33; $P = 0.50$), hepatic dysfunction (RR 0.72; $P = 0.67$); palpitation (RR 6.18; $P = 0.09$) and headache (RR 3.56; $P = 0.11$). However, despite most of these adverse drug reactions being statistically insignificant in our study, drug discontinuation was significantly higher in the triple group (RR 3.75; $P < 0.00001$).

Conclusion

Since MACEs have been significantly decreased in the triple group, TAPT appears to be more effective than DAPT in T2DM patients after intracoronary stenting. The insignificant differences in stent thrombosis, bleeding and most adverse drug reactions between these 2 groups result in TAPT to be almost as safe as DAPT in these diabetic patients.

Competing interests

The authors declare that they have no competing interests.

Authors' contributions

PKB was responsible for the conception and design, acquisition of data, analysis and interpretation of data, drafting the initial manuscript and revising it critically for important intellectual content. TQ was responsible for acquisition of data, interpretation of data and for revising the manuscript critically for important intellectual content. MHC was responsible for the conception and design, acquisition of data, interpretation of data, and for revising the manuscript critically for important intellectual content. All authors read and approved the final manuscript.

Acknowledgements

There was no external funding source for this research.

References

1. De Luca G, Dirksen MT, Spaulding C, Kelbæk H, Schalij M, Thuesen L, et al. Impact of diabetes on long-term outcome after primary Angioplasty: insights from the DESERT cooperation. Diabetes Care. 2013;36(4):1020–5.
2. Colwell JA, Nesto RW. The platelet in diabetes: focus on prevention of ischemic events. Diabetes Care. 2003;26:2181–8.
3. Geisler T, Anders N, Paterok M, Langer H, Stellos K, Lindemann S, et al. Platelet response to clopidogrel is attenuated in diabetic patients undergoing coronary stent implantation. Diabetes Care. 2007;30:372–4.
4. Brilakis ES, Patel VG, Banerjee S. Medical management after coronary stent implantation: a review. JAMA. 2013;310(2):189–98.
5. Lee SW, Park SW, Kim YH, Yun SC, Park DW, Lee CW, et al. Drug-eluting stenting followed by cilostazol treatment reduces late restenosis in patients with diabetes mellitus the DECLARE-DIABETES Trial (a randomized comparison of triple antiplatelet therapy with dual antiplatelet therapy after drug-eluting stent implantation in diabetic patients). J Am Coll Cardiol. 2008;51:1181–7.
6. Han Y, Li Y, Wang S, Jing Q, Wang Z, Wang D, et al. Cilostazol in addition to aspirin and clopidogrel improves long-term outcomes after percutaneous coronary interve ntion in patients with acute coronary syndromes: a randomized, controlled study. Am Heart J. 2009;157(4):733–9.
7. Bertrand ME, Rupprecht HJ, Urban P, Gershlick AH, CLASSICS Investigators. Double-blind study of the safety of clopidogrel with and without a loading dose in combination with aspirin compared with ticlopidine in combination with aspirin after coronary stenting: the clopidogrel aspirin stent international cooperative study (CLASSICS). Circulation. 2000;102:624–9.
8. Wallentin L, Becker RC, Budaj A, Cannon CP, Emanuelsson H, Held C, et al. Ticagrelor versus clopidogrel in patients with acute coronary syndromes. N Engl J Med. 2009;361:1045–57.
9. Wiviott SD, Braunwald E, McCabe CH, Montalescot G, Ruzyllo W, Gottlieb S, et al. Prasugrel versus clopidogrel in patients with acute coronary syndromes. N Engl J Med. 2007;357:2001–15.
10. Angiolillo DJ, Fernandez-Ortiz A, Bernardo E, Ramírez C, Sabaté M, Jimenez-Quevedo P, et al. Platelet function profiles in patients with type 2 diabetes and coronary artery disease on combined aspirin and clopidogrel treatment. Diabetes. 2005;54:2430–5.
11. Higgins JP, Thompson SG, Deeks JJ, Altman DG. Measuring inconsistency in meta-analyses. BMJ. 2003;327:557–60.
12. Savi P, Zachayus JL, Delesque-Touchard N, Labouret C, Herve C, Uzabiaga MF, et al. The active metabolite of clopidogrel disrupts P2Y12 receptor oligomers and partitions them out of lipid rafts. Proc Natl Acad Sci U S A. 2006;103:11069–74.
13. Sumpio BE, Aruny J. Cilostazol inhibits leukocyte integrin Mac-1, leading to a potential reduction in restenosis after coronary stent implantation. Perspect Vasc Surg Endovasc Ther. 2005;17:265–7.
14. Angiolillo DJ. Antiplatelet therapy in diabetes: efficacy and limitations of current treatment strategies and future directions. Diabetes Care. 2009;32(4):531–40.
15. Mohammad RA, Goldberg T, Dorsch MP, Cheng JW. Antiplatelet therapy after placement of a drug-eluting stent: a review of efficacy and safety studies. Clin Ther. 2010;32(14):2265–81.
16. Bangalore S, Singh A, Toklu B, DiNicolantonio JJ, Croce K, Feit F, et al. Efficacy of cilostazol on platelet reactivity and cardiovascular outcomes in patients undergoing percutaneous coronary intervention: insights from a meta-analysis of randomised trials. Open Heart. 2014;1(1), e000068.

17. Min P-K, Jung J, Ko YG, Choi D, Jang Y, Shim WH. Effect of cilostazol on in-stent neointimal hyperplasia after coronary artery stenting. Circ J. 2007;71:1685–90.
18. Lee S-W, Park S, Yun S, Kim YH, Park DW, Kim WJ, et al. Triple antiplatelet therapy reduces ischemic events after drug-eluting stent implantation: Drug-eluting stenting followed by cilostazol treatment reduces adverse serious cardiac events (DECREASE registry). Am Heart J. 2010;284–91.
19. Sakurai R, Koo BK, Kaneda H, Bonneau HN, Nagai R. Cilostazol added to aspirin and clopidogrel reduces revascularization without increases in major adverse events in patients with drug-eluting stents: a meta-analysis of randomized controlled trials. Int J Cardiol. 2013;167:2250–8.
20. Kim IS, Jeong YH, Park Y, Park KS, Yun SE, Park JR, et al. Platelet inhibition by adjunctive cilostazol versus high maintenance-dose clopidogrel in patients with acute myocardial infarction according to cytochrome P450 2C19 genotype. JACC Cardiovasc Interv. 2011;4:381–91.
21. Douglas Jr JS, Holmes Jr DR, Kereiakes DJ, Grines CL, Block E, Ghazzal ZM, et al. Coronary stent restenosis in patients treated with cilostazol. Circulation. 2005;112(18):2826–32.
22. Jeong YH, Hwang JY, Kim IS, Park Y, Hwang SJ, Lee SW, et al. Adding cilostazol to dual antiplatelet therapy achieves greater platelet inhibition than high maintenance doseclopidogrel in patients with acute myocardial infarction: Results of the adjunctive cilostazol versus highmaintenance dose clopidogrel in patients with AMI (ACCEL-AMI) study. Circ Cardiovasc Interv. 2010;3(1):17–26.
23. Ahn Y, Jeong MH, Jeong JW, Kim KH, Ahn TH, Kang WC, et al. Randomized comparison of cilostazol vs clopidogrel after drug-eluting stenting in diabetic patients–clilostazol for diabetic patients in drug-eluting stent (CIDES) trial. Circ J. 2008;72(1):35–9.
24. Suh JW, Lee SP, Park KW, Lee HY, Kang HJ, Koo BK, et al. Multicenter randomized trial evaluating the efficacy of cilostazol on ischemic vascular complications after drug-eluting stent implantation for coronary heart disease results of the CILON-T (Influence of CILostazolbased triple antiplatelet therapy ON ischemic complication after drug-eluting stenT implantation) Trial. J Am Coll Cardiol. 2011;57:280–9.
25. Doo-Soo Jeon MD, Yoo K-D, Park CS, Shin DI, Her SH, et al. The effect of cilostazol on stent thrombosis after drug-eluting stent implantation. Korean Circ J. 2010;40(1):10–5.
26. Rogers KC, Faircloth JM, Finks SW. Use of cilostazol in percutaneous coronary interventions. Ann Pharmacother. 2012;46:839–50.
27. Boersma E, Harrington RA, Moliterno DJ, White H, Théroux P, Van de Werf F, et al. Platelet glycoprotein IIb/IIIa inhibitors in acute coronary syndromes: a meta-analysis of all major randomised clinical trials. Lancet. 2002;359(9302):189–98.
28. Geeganage C, Wilcox R, Bath PMW. Triple antiplatelet therapy for preventing vascular events: a systematic review and meta-analysis. BMC Med. 2010;8:36.
29. Pratt CM. Analysis of the cilostazol safety database. Am J Cardiol. 2001;87(12A):28D–33.
30. Rendell M, Cariski AT, Hittel N, Zhang P. Cilostazol treatment of claudication in diabetic patients. Curr Med Res Opin. 2002;18(8):479–87.
31. Shinohara Y, Katayama Y, Uchiyama S, Yamaguchi T, Handa S, Matsuoka K, et al. Cilostazol for prevention of secondary stroke (CSPS 2): an aspirin-controlled, double-blind, randomised non-inferiority trial. Lancet Neurol. 2010;9(10):959–68. doi:10.1016/S1474-4422(10)70198-8.
32. Kanlop N, Chattipakorn S, Chattipakorn N. Effects of cilostazol in the heart. J Cardiovasc Med (Hagerstown). 2011;12(2):88–95.
33. Lee SW, Park SW, Kim YH, Yun SC, Park DW, Lee CW, et al. A randomized, double-blind, multicenter comparison study of triple antiplatelet therapy with dual antiplatelettherapy to reduce restenosis after drug-eluting stent implantation in long coronary lesions: results from the DECLARE-LONG II (Drug-Eluting Stenting Followed by Cilostazol Treatment Reduces Late Restenosis in Patients with Long Coronary Lesions) trial. J Am Coll Cardiol. 2011;57(11):1264–70.
34. Lee SW, Park SW, Kim YH, Yun SC, Park DW, Lee CW, et al. Comparison of triple versus dual antiplatelet therapy after drug-eluting stent implantation (from the DECLARE-Long trial). Am J Cardiol. 2007;100(7):1103–8.
35. Yang TH, Kim DI, Kim DK, Jang JS, Kim U, Seol SH, et al. Detection of clopidogrel hyporesponsiveness using a point-of-care assay and the impact of additional cilostazol administration after coronary stent implantation in diabetic patients. Korean J Intern Med. 2011;26(2):145–52.
36. Yang TH, Kim DI, Kim JY, Kim IH, Kim KH, Han YC, et al. Comparison of triple anti-platelet therapy (aspirin, clopidogrel, and cilostazol) and double anti-platelet therapy (aspirin and clopidogrel) on platelet aggregation in type 2 diabetic patients undergoing drug-eluting stent implantation. Korean Circ J. 2009;39(11):462–6.
37. Capranzano P, Ferreiro JL, Ueno M, Capodanno D, Dharmashankar K, Darlington A, et al. Pharmacodynamic effects of adjunctive cilostazol therapy in patients with coronary artery disease on dual antiplatelet therapy: impact of high on-treatment platelet reactivity and diabetes mellitus status. Catheter Cardiovasc Interv. 2013;81(1):42–9.
38. Angiolillo DJ, Capranzano P, Goto S, Aslam M, Desai B, Charlton RK, et al. A randomized study assessing the impact of cilostazol on platelet function profiles in patients with diabetes mellitus and coronary artery disease on dual antiplatelet therapy: results of the OPTIMUS-2 study. Eur Heart J. 2008;29:2202–11.
39. Angiolillo DJ, Capranzano P, Ferreiro JL, Ueno M, Capodanno D, Dharmashankar K, et al. Impact of adjunctive cilostazol therapy on platelet function profiles in patients with and without diabetes mellitus on aspirin and clopidogrel therapy. Thromb Haemost. 2011;106(2):253–62.
40. Ha SJ, Kim SJ, Hwang SJ, Woo JS, Kim W, Kim WS, et al. Effect of cilostazol addition or clopidogrel doubling on platelet function profiles in diabetic patients undergoing a percutaneous coronary intervention. Coron Artery Dis. 2013;24(8):690–7.

14

Investigation of the pathophysiology of cardiopulmonary bypass using rodent extracorporeal life support model

Ru-Wen Chang[1], Chien-Ming Luo[2], Hsi-Yu Yu[2,3], Yih-Sharng Chen[3] and Chih-Hsien Wang[2,3*]

Abstract

Background: Extracorporeal life support (ECLS) systems are life-saving devices used for treating patients with severe cardiopulmonary failure. In this study, we implemented a rat model of ECLS without the administration of inotropes or vasopressors.

Methods: The rats underwent 5 min of untreated asphyxial cardiac arrest and were resuscitated by ECLS for 30 min. The right external jugular vein and right femoral artery were separately cannulated to the ECLS outflow and inflow, respectively. Thereafter, ECLS was terminated, wounds were closed, and mechanical ventilation was provided for another 90 min. Subsequently, blood gas and hemodynamic analyses were performed. The plasma levels of C-reactive protein (CRP), interleukin (IL)-6, IL-10, and tumor necrosis factor-alpha (TNF-α) were measured 120 min after reperfusion.

Results: The metabolic rate of lactate in the group of asphyxial cardiac arrest rescued by ECLS was slow; therefore, the pH at 120 min after reperfusion was significantly lower in this group than that in the group of normal rats treated with ECLS. The hemodynamic data showed no between-group differences. The plasma levels of CRP, IL-6, IL-10, and TNF-α increased after ECLS treatment.

Conclusions: We successfully established a rodent ECLS model, which might be a useful approach for studying the pathophysiology induced by ECLS under clinical conditions.

Keywords: Asphyxial cardiac arrest, Extracorporeal life support, Inflammatory response, Rat model

Background

Extracorporeal life support (ECLS) systems preserve adequate blood flow and oxygen supply in both adults [1, 2] and children [3, 4], and they have been described as life-saving devices. Because the components, such as a membrane oxygenator and catheters [5], and driving force of ECLS systems are nonbiological and nonphysiological, their effects on patients have not been completely elucidated. Studies are needed to elucidate the nonbiological and nonphysiological effects of ECLS. Although ECLS models in large animals, such as porcine models [6, 7], are well established because of the equipment, small animal models still have the potential for research in resuscitation studies. Rodent models are more economical when a high number of experiments must be performed. Furthermore, they provide various molecular tools such as genetic knockout or relevant diseases.

For the present study, we designed a rodent ECLS model for the following purposes: 1) to identify whether ECLS can be performed without a blood transfusion or the administration of drugs such as inotropes or vasopressors and by performing only crystalloid priming throughout the experiment; and 2) to measure the plasma levels of C-reactive protein (CRP), interleukin (IL)-6, IL-10, and tumor necrosis factor-α (TNF-α) 120 min after reperfusion.

* Correspondence: wchemail@gmail.com
[2]Department of Surgery, National Taiwan University Hospital, Hsin-Chu Branch, NO. 25, Lane 442, Sec. 1, Jingguo Rd., Hsin-Chu 30059, Taiwan
[3]Cardiovascular Surgery, Department of Surgery, National Taiwan University Hospital, No. 7, Zhongshan S. Rd., Zhongzheng Dist., Taipei 10002, Taiwan
Full list of author information is available at the end of the article

Methods

Animals

Male Wistar–Kyoto rats (450–550 g) were randomly divided into a group of normal rats that did not receive ECLS (sham; n = 11), a group of normal rats treated with ECLS (NC + ECLS; n = 11) and a group of asphyxial cardiac arrest rats rescued by ECLS (CA + ECLS; n = 11). Two rats were housed per cage, and they had free access to Purina chow and water under a 12-h light–dark cycle. The experiments were conducted in accordance with the Guide for the Care and Use of Laboratory Animals, and the study protocol was approved by the Animal Care and Use Committee of National Taiwan University (IACUC number: 20140024).

Anesthesia and surgical preparation

Sodium pentobarbital (Sigma Chemical Co., St. Louis, MO, USA; 50 mg kg^{-1}) was administered intraperitoneally to anesthetize the rats, and intravenous reinjections (35 mg kg^{-1}) were performed every hour. The surgical sites (neck and right and left groin) were shaved, and the lungs were ventilated using a ventilator (Model 131, New England Medical Instruments, Medway, MA, USA). Ventilation was performed with room air through a 14G plastic catheter (B. Braun Medical, Bethlehem, PA, USA) at a tidal volume of 8 mL kg^{-1} and respiratory rate of 70 breaths per min. The rats were placed in the supine position and a rectal temperature probe (TP-K01 and TES-1300, TES Electrical Electronic Corp., Neihu Dist., Taipei, Taiwan) was inserted for the continuous monitoring of rectal temperature. Rectal temperature was maintained at 36 °C by using a circulating warm water blanket (B401H, Firstek Scientific Co. Ltd., Xinzhuang Dist, New Taipei City, Taiwan; TP22G, Gaymar Industries, Inc., Orchard Park, NY, 14,127 USA) and a heating lamp. The electrocardiogram (ECG) of lead II was recorded using a Gould ECG/Biotech amplifier (Gould Electronics, Cleveland, OH, USA).

The surgical sites were shaved and disinfected with betadine. The left femoral artery was cannulated using a Millar catheter (model SPC 320, size 2F; Millar Instrument, Houston, TX, USA) for the continuous monitoring of arterial pressure, and the left femoral vein was cannulated using PE-50 tubing for drug administration throughout the experiment. A 20G IV catheter (B. Braun Medical, Bethlehem, PA, USA) was inserted into the right femoral artery for ECLS inflow and arterial blood sampling. Cannulation of the right external jugular vein for ECLS venous outflow was then performed using a customized template-modified 5-hole 14G catheter, which was advanced to the junction of the right atrium and superior vena cava. This catheter was heparin-locked with 500 UI of heparin to prolong the activated clotting time to longer than 300 s. The arterial blood gas, arterial lactate, and hematocrit (i-STAT CG-4+ and 6+ cartridge, Abbott Point of Care, Princeton, NJ, USA) were determined at the baseline. The same procedure was used for all groups.

Cardiac arrest and ECLS

After instrumentation and the collection of the baseline parameters, a neuromuscular blockade was performed through the intravenous administration of pencuronium bromide (Sigma Chemical Co., St. Louis, MO, USA; 1 mg kg^{-1}) for 5 min. Subsequently, the ventilator was switched off for 5 min to induce asphyxial cardiac arrest. Circulatory arrest was defined as a mean arterial blood pressure (MAP) of <20 mmHg because this pressure is commensurate with the cessation of all tissue blood flow.

The ECLS circuit (Fig. 1) designed for the rats consisted of an open venous reservoir (TERUMO®, Tokyo, Japan; 5-mL syringe), a membrane oxygenator (Micro-1 Rat Oxygenator, Dongguan Kewei Medical Instrument Co., Ltd., Guangdong, China), a heat exchanger (Radnoti Glass Technology Inc., Monrovia, CA, USA), silicone tubing (ID 1.6 mm), and a roller pump (Masterflex, Barrington, IL, USA) that was primed using 19–20 mL of Plasma-Lyte A (Baxter, Deerfield, IL, USA). After 5 min of asphyxia, reperfusion was initiated by starting the ECLS system, which was continued for 30 min.

Discontinuation of ECLS and intensive care unit phase

After 30 min of ECLS, the rats were weaned off the system by removing the right jugular catheter within 5 min, and the incision was closed in two layers by using an absorbable suture for the subcutaneous layer and skin. Arterial samples for blood gas analysis, hematocrit, and lactate were collected at 30, 60, 90, and 120 min after the commencement of reperfusion, defined as the start of ECLS. We did not perform a blood transfusion or administer drugs such as bicarbonate, inotropes, and vasopressors. The pump was primed only with crystalloid throughout the experiment. All rats were humanely euthanized at the end of the experiment.

Estimation of inflammatory response

To estimate the inflammatory response, plasma levels of CRP (Immunology Consultants Laboratory Inc., Portland, OR, USA), IL-6 (BioLegend Inc., San Diego, CA, USA), TNF-α (BioLegend Inc., San Diego, CA, USA), and IL-10 (Abcam, Cambridge, UK) were measured using enzyme-linked immunosorbent assay kits.

Statistical analysis

All data are reported as the mean ± standard error of the mean (SEM). The Mann–Whitney U test was used to compare differences between the groups at the same time points. Kaplan–Meier curves were plotted to depict

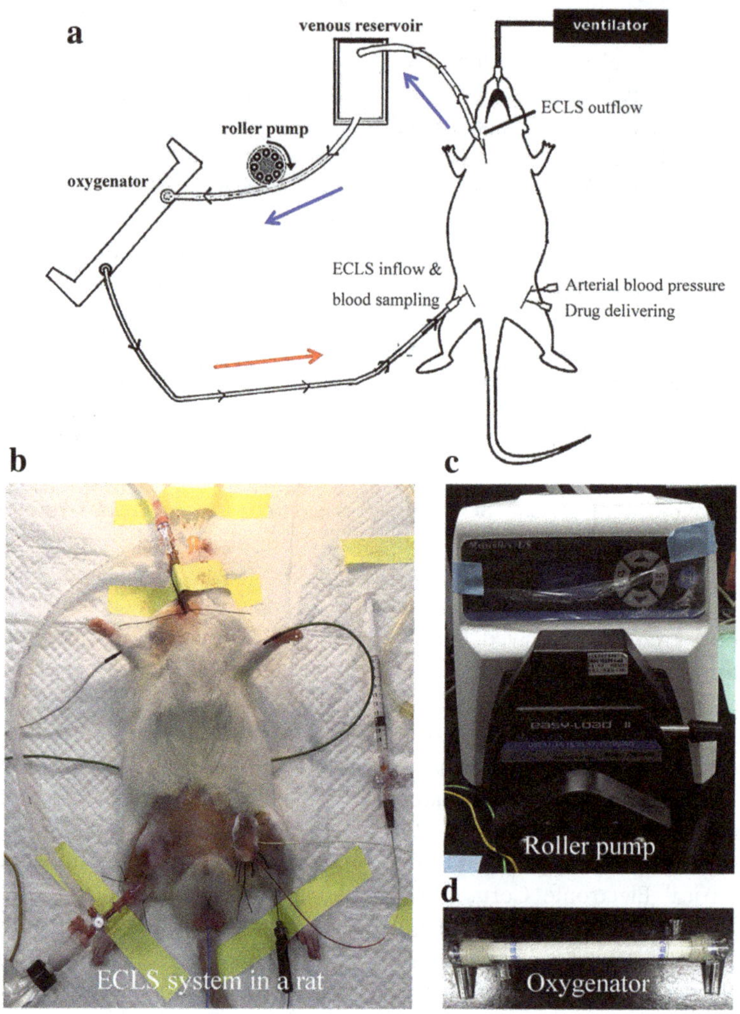

Fig. 1 Rodent extracorporeal life support (ECLS) system. (**a**) schema of the rodent ECLS model; (**b**) demonstration of our rodent ECLS model; (**c**) roller pump; and (**d**) oxygenator

the survival trend. The log-rank test was used to compare the risk between the two groups. In the mortality cases, the survival time was defined as the duration from the baseline to death; among the survivors, the duration was from the baseline to 120 min after the start of reperfusion. Statistical significance was defined as $P < 0.05$.

Results

The Kaplan–Meier curves in Fig. 2 represent the cumulative survival of rats after reperfusion in the NC + ECLS and CA + ECLS groups. Figure 2 shows that not all rats were successfully resuscitated in the CA + ECLS group; therefore, the data for this group depend on the number of rats that survived until 30, 60, 90, or 120 min after reperfusion. Furthermore, the overall survival differed significantly between these two groups ($P = 0.03$).

Surgical preparation time and baseline parameters, namely animal body weight, arterial blood gas, hematocrit, and hemodynamic variables, did not differ between the NC + ECLS and CA + ECLS groups (Tables 1 and 2). The changes in arterial blood gas values after reperfusion during the experiments are presented in Table 2. The ion variable measurements before and after ECLS in the NC + ECLS and CA + ECLS groups are presented in the additional file (Additional file 1: Table S1). At 30 min after reperfusion, the hematocrit decreased to approximately half of the baseline value because the rats in both groups did not receive a blood transfusion during ECLS treatment. After the rats were weaned off the ECLS system, the retained solution in the circuit was reinfused into the rats in the intensive care unit phase; therefore, the hematocrit value gradually increased throughout the experiment. Simultaneously, the increase in MAP after reperfusion also depended on the reinfusion of the retained solution and not on the effects of inotrope or vasopressor administration. The lactate level,

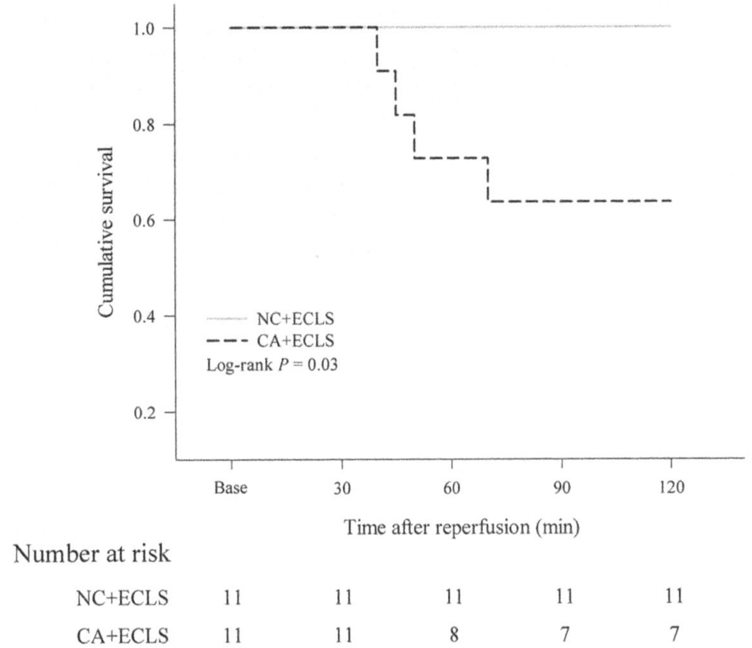

Fig. 2 Kaplan–Meier plot of the survival curves in the NC + ECLS and CA + ECLS groups. CA + ECLS: asphyxial cardiac arrest rats rescued by ECLS; ECLS: extracorporeal life support; NC + ECLS: normal rats treated with ECLS. A significant difference ($P = 0.03$) was observed in the overall survival rate between the CA + ECLS and NC + ECLS groups

which reflects tissue perfusion, decreased in both groups but the decreasing rate was considerably more rapid in the NC + ECLS group (Fig. 3). All the basic parameters in the sham group ($n = 2$) are showed in the additional file (Additional file 2: Table S2).

Comparing the NC + ECLS and CA + ECLS groups at 120 min after reperfusion, the plasma levels of pro-inflammatory cytokines (i.e., IL-6, TNF-α, and CRP) and the anti-inflammatory cytokine (i.e., IL-10) were all significantly lower in the sham group than those in the NC + ECLS and CA + ECLS groups (Fig. 4). There showed no significant differences in IL-6, TNF-α, and CRP levels between NC + ECLS and CA + ECLS groups (Figs. 4a–c); however, the IL-10 levels differed significantly between these two groups (Fig. 4d).

Discussion

In this study, we demonstrated that asphyxial cardiac arrest resuscitated using ECLS in rats was reproducible and enabled the survival of even the rats that were weaned off ECLS. However, the survival rate in the CA + ECLS group was only 63.6%, which was significantly lower than that in the NC + ECLS group. The mechanical-ventilation settings were similar to those in a previous study [8]; the only difference was the inspired gas. Because we used room air instead of higher inspired oxygen fraction as the inspired gas, the levels of blood gases (PaO_2 and $PaCO_2$) in our study were lower than those reported in previous studies [9–12]. However, the blood gas levels in the CA + ECLS and NC + ECLS groups did not exhibit any differences at the same time points in our study.

The rate of the decrease in lactate in the CA + ECLS group was lower than that in the NC + ECLS group. This might have caused the higher mortality rate and lower pH observed in the CA + ECLS group. The inability to metabolize lactate properly, which could cause acidosis in the body, might be a reason for the mortality rate in the CA + ECLS group [13]. Therefore, the adjustment of the acid–base balance appears necessary.

The MAP levels in both groups exhibited their lowest value at 30 min after reperfusion and gradually increased during the remainder of the experiments. Ali et al. used phenylephrine (an α_1 agonist) to augment MAP during the ECLS reperfusion [14] so did in others [15]. By contrast, we used the remaining blood in the ECLS circuit rather than drugs to increase MAP in our study. This not only improves MAP but also could increase hematocrit levels.

In the CA + ECLS and NC + ECLS groups, hematocrit levels were significantly lower after reperfusion than at

Table 1 Comparison of baseline properties between groups

	NC + ECLS ($n = 11$)	CA + ECLS ($n = 11$)	*P*-value
Body weight (g)	472±4	467±5	0.8237
Duration of preparation (min)	103±1	102±1	0.7847

Variables are presented as mean ± SEM. CA + ECLS: asphyxial cardiac arrest rats rescued by ECLS; ECLS: extracorporeal life support; NC + ECLS: normal rats treated with ECLS

Table 2 Arterial blood gas, hematocrit, and hemodynamic variables before and after ECLS

	Baseline	30 min	60 min	90 min	120 min
pHa					
NC + ECLS	7.54±0.01	7.44±0.01	7.38±0.01	7.40±0.01	7.42±0.01
CA + ECLS	7.55±0.01	7.43±0.02	7.33±0.02	7.33±0.02	7.32±0.02*
PaO_2 (mmHg)					
NC + ECLS	92±2	120±3	99±1	89±1	83±1
CA + ECLS	90±1	114±3	102±3	87±4	84±4
$PaCO_2$ (mmHg)					
NC + ECLS	28.3±0.6	18.5±0.3	21.8±0.4	23.6±0.4	24.5±0.5
CA + ECLS	25.9±0.7	19.0±0.8	21.9±1.3	28.6±1.8	27.5±1.9
Base excess (mmol L^{-1})					
NC + ECLS	1.5±0.2	−11.4±0.3	−12.3±0.3	−10.4±0.3	−8.5±0.3
CA + ECLS	0±0.2	−11.5±0.7	−13.8±1.2	−10.1±1.3	-10.7±1.5
Hematocrit (%)					
NC + ECLS	40±0	19±0	21±0	23±0	24±0
CA + ECLS	40±0	17±0	21±0	23±1	25±0
Heart rate (beats min^{-1})					
NC + ECLS	381.8±3.7	348.5±3.8	398.6±2.7	413.4±2.4	429.6±2.2
CA + ECLS	384.9±4.4	367.1±5.1	417.2±3.7	430.6±4.8	419.3±8.9
Mean arterial pressure (mmHg)					
NC + ECLS	121.1±0.9	41.0±0.8	58.9±1.2	72.8±1.2	75.1±1.0
CA + ECLS	113.3±1.3	35.5±1.9	55.6±2.5	73.1±3.0	76.4±3.3

Variables are presented as mean ± SEM. The data depended on the number of surviving rats at each time point. CA + ECLS: asphyxial cardiac arrest rats rescued by ECLS; ECLS: extracorporeal life support; NC + ECLS: normal rats treated with ECLS.
*: $P < 0.05$ when the CA + ECLS group was compared with the NC + ECLS group at the same time point

the baseline, because a blood transfusion was not performed during or after ECLS. Despite the decrease in hematocrit caused by hemodilution, sufficient oxygenation was maintained in both groups. Animal models have been reported to maintain adequate oxygen delivery to satisfy the whole body's oxygen demands without blood product administration when the ventilator was supplied with higher inspired oxygen fraction [10, 12, 16–18]. However, we ventilated only with room air even in the absence of a blood transfusion to maintain acceptable oxygenation.

The results indicated that, compared with the sham group, the plasma levels of the inflammatory cytokines (i.e., IL-6, TNF-α, and CRP) and anti-inflammatory cytokine (i.e., IL-10) were significantly higher in the NC + ECLS and CA + ECLS groups after treatment with ECLS. In the previous study, Fujii et al. demonstrated that the inflammatory responses getting aggravated during ECLS perfusion [8]. Herein, we suggested that a systemic inflammatory response continued to occur in our model even after the extracorporeal circulation was removed. Although the contact of blood with artificial surfaces [19], the nonpulsatile flow caused by the pump [20], and the nonlaminar flow during extracorporeal circulation [21] are possible factors responsible for the inflammatory response during ECLS, they cannot explain the inflammatory response sustained even after the rats were weaned off ECLS.

Extracorporeal circulation has been reported to disrupt the tight junctions of the small intestinal epithelial cells and cause gut barrier dysfunction. Then, because of this gut barrier dysfunction, bacteria in the intestinal lumen might translocate into the blood and increase the blood level of endotoxins such as lipopolysaccharide

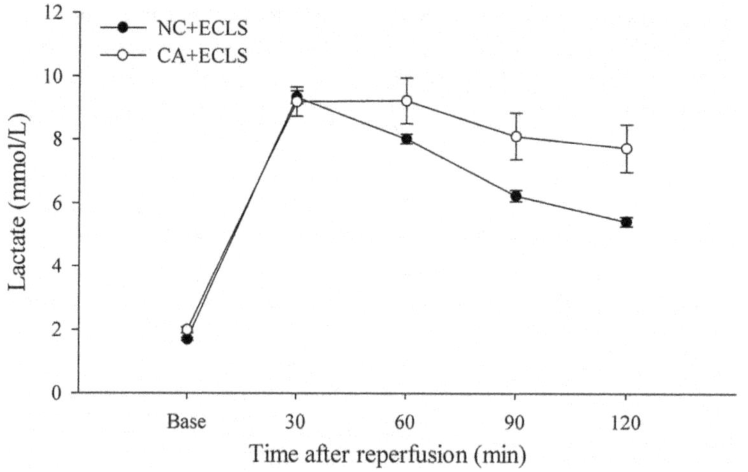

Fig. 3 Lactate level, which is used to describe tissue perfusion, gradually decreased throughout the experiments. The line diagram (mean ± SEM) represents the whole blood lactate levels in both groups. The data shown depended on the number of rats surviving at each time point. CA + ECLS: asphyxial cardiac arrest rats rescued by ECLS; ECLS: extracorporeal life support; NC + ECLS: normal rats treated with ECLS. No significant differences were observed between the CA + ECLS and NC + ECLS groups at the same time points

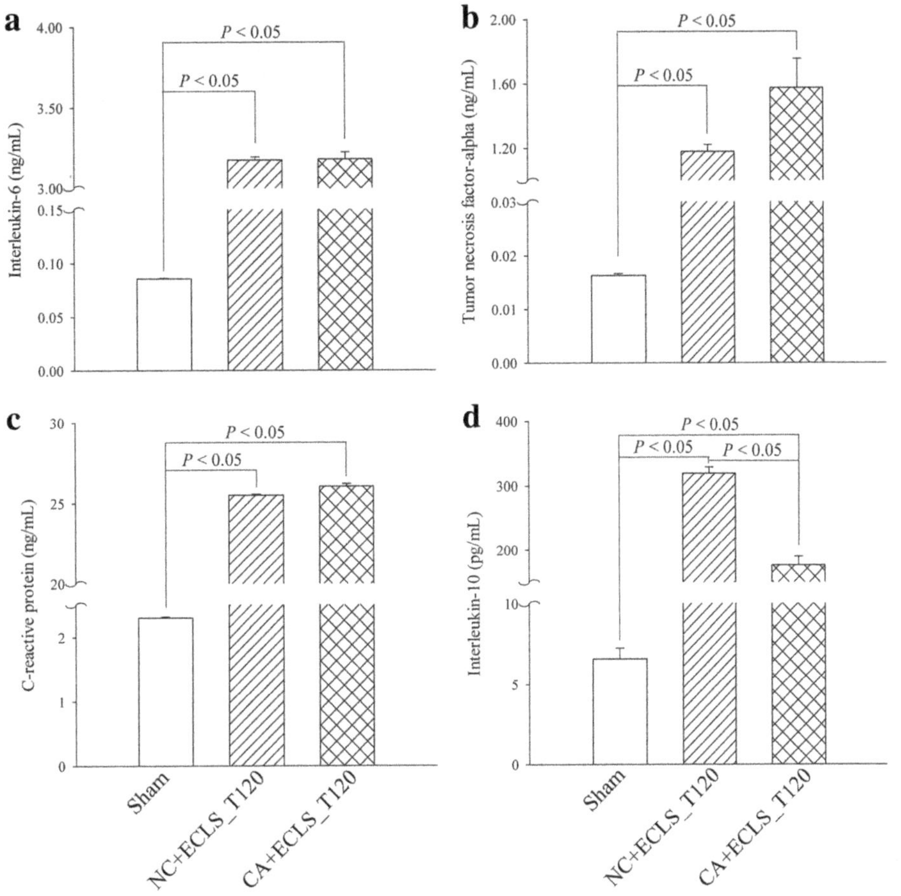

Fig. 4 ECLS treatment increased the plasma levels of pro-inflammatory and anti-inflammatory cytokines compared with the sham group. The pro-inflammatory cytokines were (**a**) interleukin-6 (IL-6), (**b**) tumor necrosis factor-α (TNF-α), and (**c**) C-reactive protein (CRP); (**d**) the anti-inflammatory cytokine was interleukin-10 (IL-10). Bar diagrams (mean ± SEM) depict summarized data. Data represent $n = 11$ in the sham and NC + ECLS groups and $n = 7$ in the CA + ECLS group. CA + ECLS: asphyxial cardiac arrest rats rescued by ECLS; ECLS: extracorporeal life support; NC + ECLS: normal rats treated with ECLS; Sham: normal rats that did not receive ECLS treatment; T120: 120 min after reperfusion

[22, 23]. This bacterial translocation might explain the inflammatory response even after the ECLS was disconnected in our study. In addition, the bacteria can not only induce an inflammatory response but also activate an anti-inflammatory response through stimulation of the vagus nerve [24]. This might explaining the higher level of IL-10 in both ECLS treated groups compared with sham group.

The current model contains some still limitations. Because rodent blood volume is approximately 7% of body weight [25], it is difficult to measure the time dependent performances of the pro-inflammatory and anti-inflammatory cytokines after the rats are weaned off ECLS. The priming volume of our ECLS circuit was approximately 19–20 mL, which accounts for 61% of the blood volume of the rats. However, this was the minimum volume that we could attain in our model. Because we could not miniaturize the circuit, rats are the smallest model that we can operate with ECLS. Moreover, ECLS treatment time in clinical settings is considerably longer than that in our study, and the complex comorbidities seen in patients are difficult to mimic.

Conclusions

In this study, we successfully developed a novel and reproducible miniature rodent ECLS model without blood transfusion or drug administration. We also introduced asphyxial cardiac arrest to our ECLS model and resuscitated the rats successfully. However, the adjustment of the acid–base balance appears necessary, particularly in rats with induced asphyxial cardiac arrest. The proposed model might provide opportunities for studying the mechanism of the pathophysiology of cardiopulmonary bypass without drug effects, even in mutant rats.

Abbreviations
CRP: C-reactive protein; ECLS: Extracorporeal life support; IL: interleukin; MAP: Mean arterial blood pressure; TNF-α: Tumor necrosis factor-alpha

Acknowledgments
Not applicable.

Author contributions
R.W.C. and C.H.W. developed the concept, designed the study, and wrote the manuscript. R.W.C. performed the animal experiments, collected the data, and performed the statistical analysis. C.M.L., H.Y.Y., and Y.S.C. provided funding and advice on the surgical procedure. C.M.L. and H.Y.Y. participated in the data interpretation. C.H.W. supervised this work and critically revised the manuscript. All authors read and approved the final manuscript.

Funding
This study was supported by grants from the National Science Council of Taiwan (MOST 102–2314-B-002-169-MY2), National Taiwan University Hospital, Hsin-Chu Branch (105-HCH018; 105-HCH060), National Taiwan University Hospital (106–16).

Competing interests
The authors have no conflicts of interest relevant to this article.

Author details
[1]Department of Physiology, College of Medicine, National Taiwan University, No. 1, Sec. 1, Ren'ai Rd., Zhongzheng Dist., Taipei 10051, Taiwan.
[2]Department of Surgery, National Taiwan University Hospital, Hsin-Chu Branch, NO. 25, Lane 442, Sec. 1, Jingguo Rd., Hsin-Chu 30059, Taiwan.
[3]Cardiovascular Surgery, Department of Surgery, National Taiwan University Hospital, No. 7, Zhongshan S. Rd., Zhongzheng Dist., Taipei 10002, Taiwan.

References

1. Chen YS, Lin JW, Yu HY, Ko WJ, Jerng JS, Chang WT, Chen WJ, Huang SC, Chi NH, Wang CH, et al. Cardiopulmonary resuscitation with assisted extracorporeal life-support versus conventional cardiopulmonary resuscitation in adults with in-hospital cardiac arrest: an observational study and propensity analysis. Lancet. 2008;372(9638):554–61.
2. Shin TG, Choi JH, Jo IJ, Sim MS, Song HG, Jeong YK, Song YB, Hahn JY, Choi SH, Gwon HC, et al. Extracorporeal cardiopulmonary resuscitation in patients with inhospital cardiac arrest: a comparison with conventional cardiopulmonary resuscitation. Crit Care Med. 2011;39(1):1–7.
3. Huang SC, Wu ET, Chen YS, Chang CI, Chiu IS, Wang SS, Lin FY, Ko WJ. Extracorporeal membrane oxygenation rescue for cardiopulmonary resuscitation in pediatric patients. Crit Care Med. 2008;36(5):1607–13.
4. Topjian AA, Nadkarni VM, Berg RA. Cardiopulmonary resuscitation in children. Curr Opin Crit Care. 2009;15(3):203–8.
5. Schaheen BW, Thiele RH, Isbell JM. Extracorporeal life support for adult cardiopulmonary failure. Best Pract Res Clin Anaesthesiol. 2015;29(2):229–39.
6. Salameh A, Dhein S. Strategies for pharmacological Organoprotection during extracorporeal circulation targeting ischemia-reperfusion injury. Front Pharmacol. 2015;6:296.
7. Keschenau PR, Ribbe S, Tamm M, Hanssen SJ, Tolba R, Jacobs MJ, Kalder J. Extracorporeal circulation increases proliferation in the intestinal mucosa in a large animal model. J Vasc Surg. 2016;64(4):1121–33.
8. Fujii Y, Shirai M, Inamori S, Takewa Y, Tatsumi E. Investigation of the biological effects of artificial perfusion using rat extracorporeal circulation model. Conf Proc IEEE Eng Med Biol Soc. 2014;2014:4483–6.
9. Boller M, Jung SK, Odegaard S, Muehlmatt A, Katz JM, Becker LB. A combination of metabolic strategies plus cardiopulmonary bypass improves short-term resuscitation from prolonged lethal cardiac arrest. Resuscitation. 2011;82(Suppl 2):S27–34.
10. Kim J, Yin T, Yin M, Zhang W, Shinozaki K, Selak MA, Pappan KL, Lampe JW, Becker LB. Examination of physiological function and biochemical disorders in a rat model of prolonged asphyxia-induced cardiac arrest followed by cardio pulmonary bypass resuscitation. PLoS One. 2014;9(11):e112012.
11. Dong GH, Xu B, Wang CT, Qian JJ, Liu H, Huang G, Jing H. A rat model of cardiopulmonary bypass with excellent survival. J Surg Res. 2005;123(2):171–5.
12. Funamoto M, Masumoto H, Takaori K, Taki T, Setozaki S, Yamazaki K, Minakata K, Ikeda T, Hyon SH, Sakata R. Green tea Polyphenol prevents diabetic rats from acute kidney injury after cardiopulmonary bypass. Ann Thorac Surg. 2016;101(4):1507–13.
13. Allen M. Lactate and acid base as a hemodynamic monitor and markers of cellular perfusion. Pediatr Crit Care Med. 2011;12(4 Suppl):S43–9.
14. Ali AA, Downey P, Singh G, Qi W, George I, Takayama H, Kirtane A, Krishnan P, Zalewski A, Freed D, et al. Rat model of veno-arterial extracorporeal membrane oxygenation. J Transl Med. 2014;12:37.
15. Engels M, Bilgic E, Pinto A, Vasquez E, Wollschlager L, Steinbrenner H, Kellermann K, Akhyari P, Lichtenberg A, Boeken U. A cardiopulmonary bypass with deep hypothermic circulatory arrest rat model for the investigation of the systemic inflammation response and induced organ damage. J Inflamm (Lond). 2014;11:26.
16. Zhu X, Ji B, Liu J, Sun Y, Wu S, Zheng Z, Long C, Tang Y. Establishment of a novel rat model without blood priming during normothermic cardiopulmonary bypass. Perfusion. 2014;29(1):63–9.
17. Liam BL, Plochl W, Cook DJ, Orszulak TA, Daly RC. Hemodilution and whole body oxygen balance during normothermic cardiopulmonary bypass in dogs. J Thorac Cardiovasc Surg. 1998;115(5):1203–8.
18. Cao HJ, Sun YJ, Zhang TZ, Zhou J, Diao YG. Penehyclidine hydrochloride attenuates the cerebral injury in a rat model of cardiopulmonary bypass. Can J Physiol Pharmacol. 2013;91(7):521–7.
19. Renne T, Schmaier AH, Nickel KF, Blomback M, Maas C. In vivo roles of factor XII. Blood. 2012;120(22):4296–303.
20. O'Neil MP, Fleming JC, Badhwar A, Guo LR. Pulsatile versus nonpulsatile flow during cardiopulmonary bypass: microcirculatory and systemic effects. Ann Thorac Surg. 2012;94(6):2046–53.
21. Cunningham KS, Gotlieb AI. The role of shear stress in the pathogenesis of atherosclerosis. Lab Investig. 2005;85(1):9–23.
22. Kurundkar AR, Killingsworth CR, McIlwain RB, Timpa JG, Hartman YE, He D, Karnatak RK, Neel ML, Clancy JP, Anantharamaiah GM, et al. Extracorporeal membrane oxygenation causes loss of intestinal epithelial barrier in the newborn piglet. Pediatr Res. 2010;68(2):128–33.
23. McILwain RB, Timpa JG, Kurundkar AR, Holt DW, Kelly DR, Hartman YE, Neel ML, Karnatak RK, Schelonka RL, Anantharamaiah GM, et al. Plasma concentrations of inflammatory cytokines rise rapidly during ECMO-related SIRS due to the release of preformed stores in the intestine. Lab Investig. 2010;90(1):128–39.
24. Sundman E, Olofsson PS. Neural control of the immune system. Adv Physiol Educ. 2014;38(2):135–9.
25. Lee HB, Blaufox MD. Blood volume in the rat. J Nucl Med. 1985;26(1):72–6.

15

In-hospital resource utilization in surgical and transcatheter aortic valve replacement

Jochen Reinöhl[1*], Klaus Kaier[1,5], Anja Gutmann[1], Stefan Sorg[2], Constantin von zur Mühlen[1], Matthias Siepe[2], Hardy Baumbach[4], Martin Moser[1], Annette Geibel[1], Andreas Zirlik[1], Philipp Blanke[3], Werner Vach[5], Friedhelm Beyersdorf[2], Christoph Bode[1] and Manfred Zehender[1]

Abstract

Background: Little is known about preoperative predictors of resource utilization in the treatment of high-risk patients with severe symptomatic aortic valve stenosis. We report results from the prospective, medical-economic "TAVI Calculation of Costs Trial".

Methods: In-hospital resource utilization was evaluated in 110 elderly patients (age ≥ 75 years) treated either with transfemoral (TF) or transapical (TA) transcatheter aortic valve implantation (TAVI, $N = 83$), or surgical aortic valve replacement (AVR, $N = 27$). Overall, 22 patient-specific baseline parameters were tested for within-group prediction of resource use.

Results: Baseline characteristics differed between groups and reflected the non-randomized, real-world allocation of treatment options. Overall procedural times were shortest for TAVI, intensive care unit (ICU) length of stay (LoS) was lowest for AVR. Length of total hospitalization since procedure (THsP) was lowest for TF-TAVI; 13.4 ± 11.4 days as compared to 15.7 ± 10.5 and 21.2 ± 15.4 days for AVR and TA-TAVI, respectively. For TAVI and AVR, EuroScore I remained the main predictor for prolonged THsP ($p < 0.01$). Within the TAVI group, multivariate regression analyses showed that TA-TAVI was associated with a substantial increase in THsP (55 to 61 %, $p < 0.01$). Additionally, preoperative aortic valve area (AVA) was identified as an independent predictor of prolonged THsP in TAVI patients, irrespective of risk scores ($p < 0.05$).

Conclusions: Our results demonstrate significant heterogeneity in patients baseline characteristics dependent on treatment and corresponding differences in resource utilization. Prolonged ThsP is not only predicted by risk scores but also by baseline AVA, which might be useful in stratifying TAVI patients.

Keywords: Transcatheter aortic valve implantation, Aortic valve replacement, Resource utilization, Risk prediction, Cost, Length of stay, Total hospitalization since procedure

Background

Due to the steadily increasing life expectancy in Western countries such as Germany, the prevalence of patients presenting with degenerative calcific aortic valve stenosis (AS) is rapidly increasing. As a result, both the clinical and economic aspects of their treatment are of high interest. The German Aortic Valve Registry (GARY) was initiated as a starting point for the investigation of these issues, and its first published findings confirm the desirability of better data on this subject [1–3].

Since the commercial launch of transcatheter aortic valve implantation (TAVI) in 2007, the technique has been widely adopted by cardiologists and cardiac surgeons, with more than 100,000 procedures performed worldwide by the end of 2013 [4, 5]. The results ofthe PARTNER trial have shown outstanding benefits over a period of 3 years in inoperable and high risk patients with severe AS [6–9]. However, for the technically operable high risk population surgical aortic valve replacement (AVR) continues to be regarded as the gold

* Correspondence: jochen.reinoehl@universitaets-herzzentrum.de
[1]Department of Cardiology and Angiology I, Heart Center Freiburg University, Hugstetter Str. 55, 79106 Freiburg, Germany
Full list of author information is available at the end of the article

standard treatment due to the long-standing clinical experience with the technique. Despite this there is an ongoing debate, notably in the light of the recently updated guidelines on the management of valve disease from the ESC & EACTS, as to where these two therapeutic alternatives should be positioned from both the clinical, and, inevitably, economic perspectives [10].

A better resource utilization is becoming a "real" problem in the medical field. A correct evaluation of the costs has to be done for every new procedure.

Due to the technique's relatively recent introduction into clinical practice, several analyses measuring the in-hospital costs and cost-effectiveness of TAVI have been published in the last two years, and these have been reviewed recently [11–15]. They all present their results for either inoperable (deemed unsafe for surgery) or high-risk patients (where surgery is not ruled out, but not without substantial risk), and overall TAVI is shown as cost-effective versus medical therapy/conservative treatment, however for TAVI versus surgical AVR the results are mixed. Although these studies aimed to make a comparison of the economic aspects of the treatments, they do not directly compare detailed resource usage.

This study sought to define and evaluate preoperative risk factors suitable for the prediction of comparative resource utilization in the treatment of symptomatic AS in elderly patients based on a real world patient cohort enrolled in the "TAVI calculation of costs trial" (TCCT).

Methods

Study design

The TAVI calculation of costs trial (TCCT) was designed as a prospective observational multicenter cohort study on elderly patients with symptomatic AS receiving either AVR or TAVI. This study was approved by the institutional ethics committee (Research Ethics Committee Albert-Ludwigs-Universität Freiburg, Germany, ID: 52/11), and was registred in the German Clinical Trial Register (ID: DRKS00000797). All patients referred between April 2011 and March 2013 to our centers were considered for inclusion into the study. Age above 75 years was deliberately chosen as inclusion criteria with the intention to avoid overwhelming the AVR treatment arm with data on substantially lower risk patients. All treatment decisions were made by a study-independent "heart team" of cardiac surgeons and cardiologists according to best clinical practice. A total of 10 AVR patients that underwent additional coronary artery bypass grafting were excluded from the dataset due to the existence of an additional procedure.

Resource utilization

A primary focus of the study was the use of healthcare resources in treatment. To this end, we examined the complete duration of hospital length of stay (LoS) from admission until final discharge home or to a rehabilitation facility. We approached this by distinguishing two components: 1) procedure-to-discharge LoS; the time from procedure to discharge from the treating centre, generally corresponding to hospital LoS in the literature, and 2) post-discharge LoS; the time from initial treating hospital discharge to final discharge from any other subordinate hospital. From these parameters, we further derived a highly useful overall measure of LoS, the "total hospitalisation since procedure" (THsP); combining procedure-to-discharge LoS and post-discharge LoS. For death prior to discharge, LoS was defined as the time from procedure until the day of death. In addition, all further relevant resource utilization characterized by specific procedural parameters, e.g. duration on ventilator, was also recorded and analyzed.

Statistical analysis

Quantitative continuous variables are described with means ± standard deviations, and quantitative discrete variables with absolute and relative frequencies. Differences between treatment groups were analysed using the non-parametric Wilcoxon rank-sum test or Fisher's exact test. In order to identify suitable within group predictors for in-hospital resource utilization, all baseline parameters were tested against THsP, intensive care unit (ICU) LoS, and time on ventilator. Complete information about resource use can only be retrieved for individuals who are alive at follow-up, but a simple exclusion of individuals with missing information can lead to serious bias in risk prediction. Accordingly, patients who died during hospital stay were censored using right-censored normal regression analyses. In addition, the positive skew of the resource use variables wasaccounted for by application of the natural logarithm of all dependent variables ($\ln(x + 1)$) in the few cases where time on ventilator or ICU LoS were equal to zero). Accordingly, the results may be interpreted as the relative increase of the outcome (percentage changes in the 'Length of hospital stay,' the 'Length of mechanical ventilation' or the 'Length of ICU stay') when comparing the two levels of a binary covariate or a change by 1 unit of a continuous covariate. Mean conditional imputation was applied for missing variables. All analyses were performed using Stata 12 (StataCorp, College Station, TX, USA).

Results

Patient population

The total study population comprised 110 patients undergoing TF-TAVI (n = 60), TA-TAVI (n = 23), and AVR (n = 27).

Baseline demographics and characteristics are provided in Table 1. As treatment decisions were based on clinical judgement according to patient presentation and the decisions of a "heart team", there were substantial differences between groups. AVR patients were significantly younger (p <0.01) and exhibited significantly lower EuroScore I (p <0.01), Euroscore II values (p <0.01) and STS-Scores (p <0.01) than the TAVI patients. Among TAVI patients, patients with a TA approach were, on average, at higher risk than TF-TAVI, although the differences in EuroScore I, EuroScore II and STS score values were not statistically significant (p = 0.065, p = 0.094, p = 0.505, respectively).

There also was a gender imbalance, with a higher proportion of females undergoing TAVI (p = 0.029). This may, however, be explained by the fact that women exhibited significantly higher EuroScore I values (18.62 in comparison to 15.56, p = 0.019). In addition, proBNP (B-type natiuretic peptide) increased in line with EuroScore. Patients with prior CABG were observed in 12 % of TAVI cases and 4 % for AVR. Peripheral vascular disease (PVD) was most frequent in the TA-TAVI groups, 30 % versus 4 % and 17 % for AVR and TF-TAVI.

Resource utilization

AVR and TAVI procedural parameters (timings and staff) and patient LoS are detailed in Table 2. Overall, time in the cathlab or OR was shortest for TAVI and substantially longer for AVR (p <0.01). Both TF and TA-TAVI averaged around two hours (122 and 142 min, respectively), whereas AVR averaged 218 min. Total time, defined as the time a patient was anesthetised, was similarly diverse between TAVI and AVR patients (p <0.01). On average, staff numbers required per procedure were: 3.5 physicians (including one trainee) and 2.7 nurses for TAVI, and 2.7 physicians, 2.0 nurses, and a perfusionist

Table 1 Mean baseline characteristics of TAVI and AVR patients aged ≥ 75 years

	AVR		TAVI						AVR vs. TAVI	
			All		TF-TAVI		TA-TAVI			TF vs. TA-TAVI
	27			83	60		23		*p*-value	*p*-value
Demographics										
Age	78.74	±3.43	82.9	±4.48	82.95	±4.67	82.78	±4.03	p <0.01	0.963
Female	44 %		67 %		68 %		65 %		0.029	0.798
Medical History										
LVEF (%)	50.37	±12.8	50.52	±9.62	51.2	±9.25	48.47	±10.68	0.785	0.257
AVA	0.81	±0.17	0.68	±0.16	0.68	±0.17	0.65	±0.14	p <0.01	0.9796
Renal disease[a]	56 %		64 %		57 %		83 %		0.183	0.043
CAD	37 %		54 %		55 %		52 %		0.183	1.000
Previous MI	11 %		22 %		17 %		35 %		0.272	0.084
Previous PCI	19 %		24 %		23 %		26 %		0.609	0.781
Previous Stroke	4 %		7 %		5 %		13 %		1.000	0.340
Previous CABG	4 %		12 %		8 %		22 %		0.288	0.131
AF	33 %		41 %		33 %		61 %		0.507	0.027
Hypertension	93 %		83 %		85 %		78 %		0.348	0.518
DM	33 %		27 %		25 %		30 %		0.623	0.782
Liver disease	4 %		6 %		5 %		9 %		1.000	0.614
COPD	11 %		16 %		13 %		22 %		0.757	0.336
PVD	4 %		20 %		17 %		30 %		0.068	0.224
Quality of life[b]	0.84	±0.21	0.79	±0.21	0.8	±0.22	0.76	±0.17	0.062	0.134
proBNP (pg/ml)	1474	±1708	4098	±6576	3820	±6111	4805	±7749	0.654	0.760
Risk Scores										
EuroScore I	10.44	±6.21	20.66	±13.05	18.53	±10.16	25.87	±17.49	p <0.01	0.065
EuroScore II	3.54	±3.15	6.77	±5.59	5.83	±4.09	9.04	±7.84	p <0.01	0.094
STS-Score	3.48	±1.57	5.7	±3.36	5.48	±2.88	6.21	±4.35	p <0.01	0.505

Abbreviations: *LVEF* – left ventricular ejection fraction; *AVA* – preoperative aortic valve area; *CAD* – coronary artery disease; *MI* – myocardial infarction: *PCI* – percutaneous coronary intervention; *AF* – atrial fibrillation; *DM* – diabetes mellitus; *COPD* – chronic obstructive pulmonary disease; *PVD* – peripheral vascular disease; *proBNP*–B-type natiuretic peptide. Data are presented as n (%) or mean ± standard deviation

[a]Renal disease defined as (glomerular filtration rate <60 ml/h); [b]Patients quality of life at baseline according to standardized EQ-5D questionnaire

Table 2 Procedural times, staff utilization, patient in-hospital length of stay and discharge behaviour of TAVI and AVR patients aged ≥ 75 years

	TF-TAVI (60)	TA-TAVI (23)	AVR (27)
Procedural resource utilization			
Time cathlab/OR (min.)	122.3 ± 40.5 (118.5)	142.3 ± 96.9 (109)	217.7 ± 48.8 (223)
Staff			
Physician	3.58 ± 0.59 (4)	3.17 ± 0.72 (3)	2.67 ± 0.62 (3)
Nurse	2.55 ± 0.59 (3)	2.91 ± 0.29 (3)	2.04 ± 0.19 (2)
Time anesthesia (min.)	238.3 ± 55.4 (245)	247.5 ± 80.4 (220)	327.9 ± 57.6 (325)
Staff			
Physician	1.0 ± 0.0 (1)	1.96 ± 0.21 (2)	1.93 ± 0.27 (2)
Nurse	1.02 ± 0.34 (1)	0.32 ± 0.02 (0.33)	0.33 ± 0.15 (0.33)
Perfusionists[a]	0 (0)	0 (0)	1.0 ± 0.0 (1)
Post-procedural resource utilization			
Time spent in ICU (hours)	105.0 ± 198.6 (62.7)	105.4 ± 100.4 (66.1)	89.0 ± 131.0 (47.2)
Time on ventilation (hours)	35.8 ± 110.7 (8.6)	35.7 ± 64.6 (9.2)	42.6 ± 115.8 (12.8)
Length of stay (days)			
Procedure to discharge	13.1 ± 11.3 (10)	13.0 ± 6.6 (10)	10.6 ± 4.6 (10)
Post-discharge LoS	0.3 ± 1.4 (0)	8.2 ± 13.6 (0)	5.1 ± 7.0 (4)
Total hospitalisation since procedure	13.4 ± 11.4 (10)	21.2 ± 15.4 (17)	15.7 ± 10.5 (14)
Discharge destination			
Home	46.7 %	13 %	0 %
Rehabilitation	40 %	26.1 %	44.4 %
Hospital	5 %	43.5 %	51.9 %
Nursing Home	3.3 %	0 %	0 %
In-hospital death	5 %	17.4 %	3.7 %

Data are presented as mean ± standard deviation and median in parentheses
[a]In our centers an extracorporeal life-support system and perfusionists are on stand-by for all TAVI procedures

for AVR. Notably, in our centres patients undergoing TAVI are anesthetised in the OR before moving to the cathlab, which substantially increases total time.

Time spent in the ICU varied greatly and was shortest for AVR at 89 h (median 47.2 h). Interestingly, there was very little difference in average ICU stay between TF- and TA-TAVI at 105 h for both. The mean duration of mechanical respiratory support was similar across the groups, around 40 h (median range 8.6–12.8 h). Procedure to discharge LoS was lowest for AVR (10.6 days) and similar for TF-TAVI and TA-TAVI, with 13.1 and 13.0 days respectively. Notably, post-discharge LoS with TA-TAVI and AVR was 8.2 and 5.1 days respectively, whereas for TF-TAVI it was only 0.3 days. The large differences in the mean post-discharge LoS between the different groups is mostly explainable by the fact that TF-TAVI patients were less often discharged to another hospital than TA-TAVI and AVR patients. Average THsP by group, including time spent in subordinate hospitals, therefore was, 13.4 days for TF-TAVI, 15.7 days for AVR, and 21.2 days for TA-TAVI. Accordingly, THsP was different between TF and TA-TAVI patients (p <0.01), but relatively equal between AVR and TAVI patients (p = 0.3058).

Predictors of in-hospital resource use following TAVI

According to univariate regression analyses (see Table 3), significant predictors (p <0.05) for prolonged THsP were: TA procedure, aortic valve area (AVA), history of atrial fibrillation (AF) and/or PVD, as well as higher EuroScore I, EuroScore II and STS Score.

The standard risk scores already cover most of the parameters identified in our calculation as predictive for an increased resource usage. However, neither AVA or AF are included in the cacluation of these scores, and so we hypothesised that they might represent additional variables which could be used by the clinician to predict outcomes. Accordingly, we fitted three multivariate regression models in order to analyse whether the baseline parameters of AVA and AF as well as the access route (TA) are predictors of in-hospital resource use for TAVI, independent of the predictive value of the three risk scores. As shown in Table 4, the TA approach was still associated with a

Table 3 Univariate predictors of in-hospital resource use following TAVI (N = 83)

	Length of THsP (in days)		Length of mechanical ventilation (in hours)		Length of ICU stay (in hours)	
	% change	p-value	% change	p-value	% change	p-value
TA	69.05 %***	(0.000)	65.04 %	(0.158)	4.97 %	(0.820)
Age (per one-year change)	0.81 %	(0.620)	4.57 %	(0.216)	1.64 %	(0.371)
Female	6.16 %	(0.669)	−25.17 %	(0.440)	−4.81 %	(0.813)
Quality of life	−1.06 %	(0.686)	−0.34 %	(0.959)	−1.62 %	(0.589)
LVEF (per one-unit increase)	−1.72 %	(0.085)	−4.60 %*	(0.041)	−2.18 %	(0.139)
AVA (for increase of 0.1 cm2)	−5.62 %*	(0.018)	−8.08 %*	(0.042)	−5.40 %	(0.069)
GFR (per one-unit change)	−0.58 %	(0.060)	−1.26 %	(0.062)	−0.77 %*	(0.031)
CAD	20.20 %	(0.158)	52.20 %	(0.194)	19.72 %	(0.290)
Previous MI	5.50 %	(0.762)	24.23 %	(0.580)	−1.34 %	(0.952)
Previous PCI	17.94 %	(0.305)	−9.61 %	(0.792)	1.21 %	(0.957)
Previous Stroke	46.67 %	(0.304)	29.30 %	(0.390)	31.00 %	(0.451)
Previous CABG	10.74 %	(0.546)	−15.38 %	(0.730)	−10.60 %	(0.673)
AF	34.31 %*	(0.042)	54.96 %	(0.205)	33.51 %	(0.130)
Hypertension	−24.87 %	(0.152)	−60.90 %*	(0.048)	−39.47 %*	(0.016)
DM	7.14 %	(0.668)	11.18 %	(0.797)	−0.63 %	(0.979)
Liver disease	33.78 %	(0.364)	−6.11 %	(0.953)	5.24 %	(0.908)
COPD	−2.25 %	(0.876)	116.19 %	(0.184)	49.18 %	(0.128)
PVD	46.37 %*	(0.021)	44.63 %	(0.441)	33.91 %	(0.282)
EuroScore I (per one-unit change)	1.37 %*	(0.010)	4.76 %***	(0.000)	1.89 %*	(0.014)
EuroScore II (per one-unit change)	2.76 %*	(0.039)	6.82 %	(0.064)	3.05 %	(0.158)
STS Score (per one-unit change)	3.71 %*	(0.032)	10.05 %	(0.109)	6.27 %	(0.068)
proBNP (per 100 pg/ml change)	0.03 %	(0.709)	0.14 %	(0.675)	0.20 %	(0.253)

p-values in parentheses; *p <0.05, **p <0.01, ***p <0.001

substantial (approximately 55 to 61 %) increase in THsP. Moreover, AVA appeared to be an independent predictor of THsP irrespective of which risk-score we adjusted for: Table 4, model (1) contains an adjustment for the EuroScore I, model (2) for the EuroScore II and model (3) for the STS-Score. If we focus on AVA as a predictive factor additional to EuroScore I as shown in model (1), our results indicate that for every reduction in AVA of 0.1 cm^2, the predicted THsP increases by 5.2 %, which is equivalent to almost one additional day of hospitalization (see also Fig. 1).

Predictors of in-hospital resource use following AVR

Similarly, for AVR (see Table 5) a significant predictor in univariate analysis (p <0.05) for prolonged THsP were the STS-Scores. Moreover, a low value of the glomerular

Table 4 Multivariate predictors of Length of hospital stay following TAVI (N = 83)

	Length of hospital stay (THsP)					
	model 1		model 2		model 3	
	% change	p-value	% change	p-value	% change	p-value
TA	54.65 %**	(0.003)	55.89 %**	(0.003)	61.45 %**	(0.001)
AVA (per change of 0.1 cm^2)	−5.20 %*	(0.025)	−5.50 %*	(0.015)	−5.28 %*	(0.022)
AF	21.17 %	(0.171)	20.20 %	(0.197)	18.65 %	(0.241)
EuroScore I (per one-unit change)	0.83 %	(0.067)				
EuroScore II (per one-unit change)			1.42 %	(0.210)		
STS Score (per one-unit change)					1.83 %	(0.220)
N	83		83		83	

p-values in parentheses; *p <0.05, **p <0.01, ***p <0.001

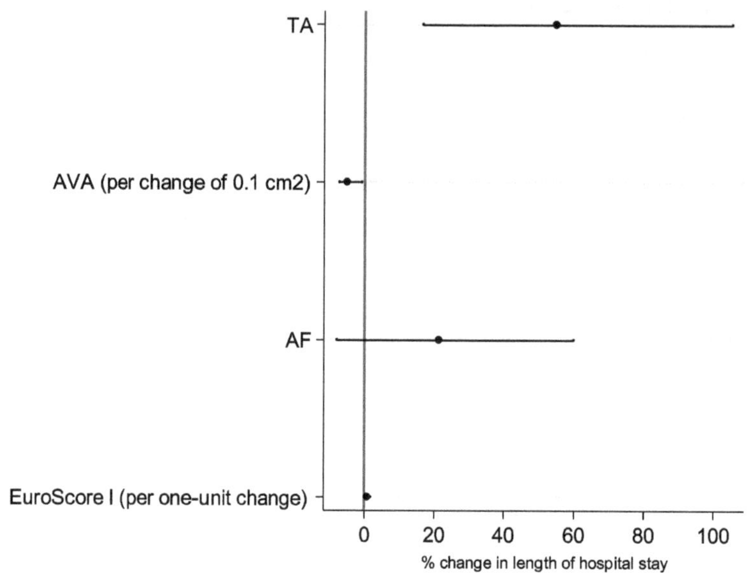

Fig. 1 Multivariate predictors of Length of hospital stay following TAVI (N = 83). Point estimates and confidence intervals of the changes in length of hospital stay (see model (1) in Table 4)

filtration rate at baseline was a predictor for prolonged time on ventilation, whereas patients with a medical history of diabetes spent less time in ICU settings.

Discussion

Our investigation showed that resource utilization differs substantially and significantly between therapy options for severe AS in the elderly, with TF patients experiencing shorter overall LoS (THsP) compared to other options. We hypothesise that the early diagnosis and treatment of symptomatic patients is optimal for reducing healthcare resource utilization and have shown that AVA, as a surrogate for the progress of the disease, is an independent predictor of this. As it is not considered in the three

Table 5 Univariate predictors of in-hospital resource use following AVR (N = 27)

	Length of THsP (in days)		Length of mechanical ventilation (in hours)		Length of ICU stay (in hours)	
	% change	p-value	% change	p-value	% change	p-value
Age (per one-year change)	0.55 %	(0.757)	1.63 %	(0.716)	3.87 %	(0.262)
Female	16.88 %	(0.382)	−33.77 %	(0.370)	−13.76 %	(0.662)
Quality of life[#]	−12.98 %	(0.648)	16.07 %	(0.850)	−3.93 %	(0.962)
LVEF (per one-unit change)	−0.34 %	(0.480)	0.05 %	(0.975)	0.60 %	(0.413)
AVA (per change of 0.1 cm2)	−43.45 %	(0.295)	−86.15 %	(0.134)	−41.02 %	(0.594)
GFR (per one-unit change)	−0.54 %	(0.271)	−2.55 %*	(0.050)	−0.82 %	(0.362)
CAD	−2.46 %	(0.903)	58.88 %	(0.342)	−2.38 %	(0.949)
Previous PCI	−8.61 %	(0.596)	−1.76 %	(0.954)	−17.88 %	(0.565)
AF	1.18 %	(0.943)	87.95 %	(0.157)	49.03 %	(0.203)
Hypertension	−14.53 %	(0.121)	26.49 %	(0.370)	10.45 %	(0.894)
DM	−1.62 %	(0.935)	−20.63 %	(0.549)	−49.49 %*	(0.015)
COPD	25.86 %	(0.480)	−34.82 %	(0.178)	−18.21 %	(0.373)
EuroScore I (per one-unit change)	1.71 %	(0.063)	1.93 %	(0.638)	3.11 %	(0.167)
EuroScore II (per one-unit change)	4.48 %	(0.086)	4.92 %	(0.605)	5.01 %	(0.257)
STS Score (per one-unit change)	9.48 %**	(0.007)	24.86 %	(0.117)	16.30 %	(0.133)
proBNP (per 100 pg/ml change)	0.045 %	(0.721)	0.104 %	(0.712)	0.011 %	(0.958)

p-values in parentheses; *p <0.05, **p <0.01, ***p <0.001

Not tested due to an insufficient number of events: previous MI, previous stroke, previous CABG, liver disease, PV

commonly used risk scores, we suggest that AVA can be an additional predictor of clinical and economic outcomes.

Recently, the national GARY registry has published the first data for TAVI and AVR across Germany. Broadly speaking our results are consistent with this data, certainly in terms of trends between treatments, although the specific measures that are reported in the paper do differ in magnitude. Although no data was given on THsP, the authors do comment in their discussion that "*The length of hospitalization was rather similar* [between the different treatment groups], *and accordingly no critical factor in comparing the techniques*", which may be a point of difference between the two studies [3].

Hospital LoS is a metric that is highly relevant for local and national level decision makers due to its obvious impact on resources and operating logistics within secondary healthcare settings. Not only absolute values are important, but also variability and predictability, in order to improve efficiency. We report highly transparent the length of hospitalisation and show large differences and corresponding variability, with TF-AVI and AVR patients having the shortest LoS. Comparisons with other studies are inherently challenging due to a lack of uniform definitions, variations between healthcare systems, and limited data on alternative, heart-team established strategies. LoS generally ranges between 5 and 13 days for TAVI, [16–18] and 9 and 20 days for AVR [19–22]. But as with other studies, the LoS is not only a consequence of clinical outcomes but also local management practice and, potentially, funding considerations. Without a common definition of LoS that includes stays in other facilities immediately after discharge from the treating centre, it is difficult to compare and interpret the data. We suggest that length of "total hospitalisation since procedure" (THsP) is comprehensive.

As a result of the described risk-selection, comparisons between treatment groups or risk prediction may always be subject to a substantial selection bias. In contrast, within group risk prediction is more appropriate and, according to our univariate and multivariate analyses, TA procedure and AVA were significant and independent predictors of THsP irrespective of the common risk scores. It is well known that TA-TAVI has different outcomes compared with TF-TAVI, and this is due to multiple factors predominantly related to underlying differences which drive the choice of a TA approach rather than the TF route. AVA presents a new concept, which however is probably best interpreted as a marker for worsening medical condition. As the AVA decreases and the stenosis pathology worsens, the effects on the cardiac and circulatory systems, even at the sub-clinical level, lead to a poorer prognosis and the need for more resource utilization for patient recovery. As mentioned above, AVA is not used in the commen risk scores, but parameters associated with the development of degenerative aortic valve stenosis such as chronic kidney failure or patient age are. Thus, when caluclating the risk scores, AVA might have an indirect impact on the result of the risk scores.

Most previous studies focusing on risk prediction for TAVI and/or AVR focus on postoperative factors, such as complications, for predicting clinical and economic outcomes [15, 18, 22–29]. In one of the few exceptions, Green et al. analyzed the association between preoperative frailty status and LoS in elderly patients (mean age 86 years), and showed that a high frailty score was associated with a longer LoS [29]. We examined the impact of self-reported quality of life as this is the only part of this frailty score included in our study, but it didn't show any impact on LoS.

There are multiple benefits to being able to preoperatively predict resource usage for patients. From a hospital perspective it allows the best placement of efforts and optimal planning to achieve the greatest throughput of patients whilst achieving the best clinical outcomes. This is obviously an asset for the hospital as it maximises productivity and limits losses. Efficient planning should enable more procedures whilst maintaining consistent staff levels and should result in fewer cancelled elective procedures as a consequence of unavailability of beds. This also has a direct benefit for the patient, who is more likely to receive optimal planned care and to experience minimal delays in procedures, transfers to other facilities, etc. All of these may be compromised by unexpected resource utilization leading to substandard care resulting from pressures on the system. Finally, the drive towards reducing THsP is also due to the benefit of reducing non-procedural secondary complications such as hospital acquired infections.

Study limitations

Strikingly, within the boundaries of the study design and inclusion/exclusion criteria, there appears to be a number of important differences in patients from either the TAVI and the AVR group. Therefore, it would be highly biased and consequently misleading to make direct comparisons of the results between the groups. As shown in Table 2, outliers strongly affect the force of expression, particularly in small numbers of cases. In contrast to purely medical approaches, however, outliers are of particular interest in health economic considerations. From a societal perspective, outliers influence the overall costs of the treatment. In addition, outliers also affect the gap between actual costs and reimbursement from a hospital perspective and are therefore critical for a number of economic considerations from different perspectives.

Moreover, our initial study design included the enrollment of drug patients, analagous to the conservative treatment arm from PARTNER B, but it was soon evident that these patients were rarely considered inoperable and were typically offered TAVI. This directly reflects the current clinical practice in our, and presumably other centers, and demonstrates the very limited number of patients presenting with a "true" contraindication for TAVI or AVR. It however remains unclear whether these "borderline" patients are a consequence of a shift in perceptions about eligibility for TAVI or surgery, and if so what impact their inclusion will have on mortality and mobidity affecting comparisons between with pivotal studies such as PARTNER.

Conclusion

We present here results from the prospective TAVI Calculation of Costs Trial (TCCT) aimed at evaluating the in-hospital resource use in the treatment of severe aortic valve stenosis in elderly patients. Our findings reveal fundamental differences between patient groups, and different requirements and use of resources. We show that, in addition to the commonly used risk scores, in TAVI patients the preoperative aortic valve area is an independent and so far unknown predictor of hospital length of stay.

Competing interests

The authors declare that they have no competing interests.

Authors' contributions

J R Substantial contributions to conception and design, acquisition and analysis and interpretation of data. Have been involved in drafting the manuscript and have given final approval of the version to be published. K K Substantial contributions to conception and design and analysis and interpretation of data. Have been involved in drafting the manuscript and have given final approval of the version to be published. A G Substantial contributions to conception and design, have been revising the manuscript critically for important intellectual content and have given final approval of the version to be published. S S Substantial contributions to conception and design, have been revising the manuscript critically for important intellectual content and have given final approval of the version to be published. C M Substantial contributions to conception and design, have been revising the manuscript critically for important intellectual content and have given final approval of the version to be published. M S Substantial contributions to conception and design, have been revising the manuscript critically for important intellectual content and have given final approval of the version to be published. M M Substantial contributions to conception and design, have been revising the manuscript critically for important intellectual content and have given final approval of the version to be published. H B Substantial contributions to conception and design, have been revising the manuscript critically for important intellectual content and have given final approval of the version to be published. A G Substantial contributions to conception and design, have been revising the manuscript critically for important intellectual content and have given final approval of the version to be published. A Z Substantial contributions to conception and design, have been revising the manuscript critically for important intellectual content and have given final approval of the version to be published. P B Substantial contributions to conception and design, have been revising the manuscript critically for important intellectual content and have given final approval of the version to be published. W V Substantial contributions to conception and design, have been revising the manuscript critically for important intellectual content and have given final approval of the version to be published. F B Substantial contributions to conception and design, have been revising the manuscript critically for important intellectual content and have given final approval of the version to be published. C B Substantial contributions to conception and design, have been revising the manuscript critically for important intellectual content and have given final approval of the version to be published. M Z Substantial contributions to conception and design, have been revising the manuscript critically for important intellectual content and have given final approval of the version to be published.

Authors' information

Not applicable.

Acknowledegments

The authors express their gratitude to staff members Melanie Avlar, Jutta Schmitz and Christiane Rack for data collection, and thank Gordon Goodall and Pascal Candolfi (both Edwards Lifesciences) for their help in verifying data and manuscript work.

Funding Sources

The project was funded by Edwards Lifesciences SA. However, no restrictions were placed on either the design or the presentation of results, or the interpretation of data. The article processing charge was funded by the German Research Foundation (DFG) and the Albert Ludwigs University Freiburg in the funding programme Open Access Publishing.

Disclosures

JR works as proctor (TF-TAVI) for Edwards Lifesciences SA. HB JR works as proctor (TA-TAVI).

Author details

[1]Department of Cardiology and Angiology I, Heart Center Freiburg University, Hugstetter Str. 55, 79106 Freiburg, Germany. [2]Department of Cardiovascular Surgery, Heart Center Freiburg University, Freiburg, Germany. [3]Department of Diagnostic Radiology, Medical Center-University of Freiburg, Freiburg, Germany. [4]Department of Cardiovascular Surgery, Robert-Bosch-Krankenhaus Stuttgart, Stuttgart, Germany. [5]Center for Medical Biometry and Medical Informatics, Medical Center-University of Freiburg, Freiburg, Germany.

References

1. Beckmann A, Hamm C, Figulla HR, Cremer J, Kuck KH, Lange R, et al. The German Aortic Valve Registry (GARY): a nationwide registry for patients undergoing invasive therapy for severe aortic valve stenosis. Thorac Cardiovasc Surg. 2012;60:319–25.
2. Mohr F. One year results of more than 14,000 patients from the German Aortic Valve Registry. San Francisco, USA: ACC Annual Scientific Session; 2013. oral presentation.
3. Hamm CW, Möllmann H, Holzhey D, Beckmann A, Veit C, Figulla HR, et al. The German Aortic Valve Registry (GARY): in-hospital outcome. Eur Heart J. 2014;35:1588–98.
4. Reinöhl J, von zur Mühlen C, Moser M, Sorg S, Bode C, Zehender M. TAVI 2012: state of the art. J Thromb Thrombolysis. 2012;35:419–35.
5. Mylotte D, Osnabrugge RL, Windecker S, Lefevre T, De Jaegere P, Jeger R, et al. Transcatheter aortic valve replacement in Europe: adoption trends and factors influencing device utilization. J Am Coll Cardiol. 2013;62:210–9.
6. Leon MB, Smith CR, Mack M, Miller DC, Moses JW, Svensson LG, et al. Transcatheter aortic-valve implantation for aortic stenosis in patients who cannot undergo surgery. N Engl J Med. 2010;363:1597–607.
7. Makkar RR, Fontana GP, Jilaihawi H, Kapadia S, Pichard AD, Douglas PS, et al. Transcatheter aortic-valve replacement for inoperable severe aortic stenosis. N Engl J Med. 2012;366:1696–704.
8. Kappadia SR. Three year outcomes of transcatheter aortic valve replacement (TAVR) in "inoperable" patients with severe aortic stenosis: the PARTNER trial. Miami, USA: TCT Conference; 2012. oral presentation.

9. Smith CR, Leon MB, Mack MJ, Miller DC, Moses JW, Svensson LG, et al. Transcatheter versus surgical aortic-valve replacement in high-risk patients. N Engl J Med. 2011;364:2187–98.
10. Vahanian A, Alfieri O, Andreotti F, Antunes MJ, Baron-Esquivias G, Baumgartner H, et al. Guidelines on the management of valvular heart disease (version 2012) The Joint Task Force on the Management of Valvular Heart Disease of the European Society of Cardiology (ESC) and the European Association for Cardio-Thoracic Surgery (EACTS). Eur Heart J. 2012;33:2451–96.
11. Fairbairn TA, Meads DM, Hulme C, Mather AN, Plein S, Blackman DJ, et al. The cost-effectiveness of transcatheter aortic valve implantation versus surgical aortic valve replacement in patients with severe aortic stenosis at high operative risk. Heart. 2013;99:914–20.
12. Indraratna P, Ang SC, Gada H, Yan TD, Manganas C, Bannon P, et al. Systematic review of the cost-effectiveness of transcatheter aortic valve implantation. J Thorac Cardiovasc Surg. 2014;148:509–14.
13. Neyt M, Van Brabandt H, Devriese S, Van De Sande S. A cost-utility analysis of transcatheter aortic valve implantation in Belgium: focusing on a well-defined and identifiable population. BMJ open. 2012;2.
14. Osnabrugge RL, Mylotte D, Head SJ, Van Mieghem NM, Nkomo VT, LeReun CM, et al. Aortic stenosis in the elderly: disease prevalence and number of candidates for transcatheter aortic valve replacement: a meta-analysis and modelling study. J Am Coll Cardiol. 2013;62:1002–12.
15. Reinöhl J, Gutmann A, Kollum M, Von zur Mühlen C, Baumbach H, Avlar M, et al. Transfemoral aortic valve implantation: bleeding events, related costs and outcomes. J Thromb Thrombolysis. 2012;35:469–575.
16. Himbert D, Descoutures F, Al-Attar N, Iung B, Ducrocq G, Detaint D, et al. Results of transfemoral or transapical aortic valve implantation following a uniform assessment in high-risk patients with aortic stenosis. J Am Coll Cardiol. 2009;54:303–11.
17. Webb JG, Altwegg L, Boone RH, Cheung A, Ye J, Lichtenstein S, et al. Transcatheter aortic valve implantation impact on clinical and valve-related outcomes. Circulation. 2009;119:3009–16.
18. Nuis RJ, Piazza N, Van Mieghem NM, Otten AM, Tzikas A, Schultz CJ, et al. In-hospital complications after transcatheter aortic valve implantation revisited according to the valve academic research consortium definitions. Catheter Cardiovasc Interv. 2011;78:457–67.
19. Filsoufi F, Rahmanian PB, Castillo JG, Chikwe J, Silvay G, Adams DH. Excellent early and late outcomes of aortic valve replacement in people aged 80 and older. J Am Geriatr Soc. 2008;56:255–61.
20. Kirsch M, Guesnier L, LeBesnerais P, Hillion ML, Debauchez M, Seguin J, et al. Cardiac operations in octogenarians: perioperative risk factors for death and impaired autonomy. Ann Thorac Surg. 1998;66:60–7.
21. Kolh P, Kerzmann A, Lahaye L, Gerard P, Limet R. Cardiac surgery in octogenarians. Peri-operative outcome and long-term results. Eur Heart J. 2001;22:1235–43.
22. Thourani VH, Myung R, Kilgo P, Thompson K, Puskas JD, Lattouf OM, et al. Long-term outcomes after isolated aortic valve replacement in octogenarians: a modern perspective. Ann Thorac Surg. 2008;86:1458–65.
23. Ledwoch J, Franke J, Gerckens U, Kuck K-H, Linke A, Nickenig G, et al. Incidence and predictors of permanent pacemaker implantation following transcatheter aortic valve implantation: analysis from the German transcatheter aortic valve interventions registry. Catheter Cardiovasc Interv. 2013;82:569–77.
24. Kong WY, Yong G, Irish A. Incidence, risk factors and prognosis of acute kidney injury after transcatheter aortic valve implantation. Nephrology. 2012;17:445–51.
25. Wenaweser P, Pilgrim T, Roth N, Kadner A, Stortecky S, Kalesan B, et al. Clinical outcome and predictors for adverse events after transcatheter aortic valve implantation with the use of different devices and access routes. Am Heart J. 2011;161:1114–24.
26. Tamburino C, Capodanno D, Ramondo A, Petronio AS, Ettori F, Santoro G, et al. Incidence and predictors of early and late mortality after transcatheter aortic valve implantation in 663 patients with severe aortic stenosis. Circulation. 2011;123:299–308.
27. Hayashida K, Lefevre T, Chevalier B, Hovasse T, Romano M, Garot P, et al. Transfemoral aortic valve implantation new criteria to predict vascular complications. JACC Cardiovasc Interv. 2011;4:851–8.
28. Gotzmann M, Pljakic A, Bojara W, Lindstaedt M, Ewers A, Germing A, et al. Transcatheter aortic valve implantation in patients with severe symptomatic aortic valve stenosis-predictors of mortality and poor treatment response. Am Heart J. 2011;162:238–45.
29. Green P, Woglom AE, Genereux P, Daneault B, Paradis JM, Schnell S, et al. The impact of frailty status on survival after transcatheter aortic valve replacement in older adults with severe aortic stenosisA single-center experience. JACC Cardiovasc Interv. 2012;5:974–81.

16

Medium-term outcomes of 78,808 patients after heart valve surgery in a middle-income country

Regina Maria de Aquino Xavier[1*], Vitor Manuel Pereira Azevedo[1], Paulo Henrique Godoy[2], Arn Migowski[1], Antonio Luiz Pinho Ribeiro[3], Rogério Brant Martins Chaves[1], Marcelo Goulart Correia[1], Carolina de Aquino Xavier[4], Lucas de Aquino Hashimoto[5], Clara Weksler[1] and Nelson Albuquerque Souza e Silva[4]

Abstract

Background: Heart valve surgery outcomes are unknown in middle-income countries and thus cannot be used in health system decision making processes. This study estimated in-hospital mortality and medium and long-term survival.

Methods: This was a retrospective study of 78,806 patients who underwent heart valve surgery between 2001 and 2007 in Brazil. Two national databases were used, the Hospital Information System and the Mortality Information System. Kaplan-Meier survival analysis and log-rank tests were performed. Maximum and median follow-up was 7.7 and 2.8 years, respectively (0.002–7.707).

Results: Valve replacement accounted for 69.1% of procedures performed. Mitral stenosis, the most common valve injury, represented 38.9% of the total. In 94.7% of mitral stenosis patients, aetiology was rheumatic heart disease. In-hospital mortality was 7.6% and was higher for women, for patients who had undergone concomitant coronary artery bypass grafting (CABG) and for the elderly. Overall survival was 69.9% at the end of follow-up. Survival was worst among elderly, male and concomitant CABG patients ($P<0.001$).

Conclusions: Rheumatic heart disease is still a major public health problem in Brazil. In-hospital mortality and global survival rates of patients who have undergone heart valve surgery were less satisfactory than those reported in high-income countries. The findings of this study can contribute to guiding decision making processes in middle-income countries similar to Brazil and others concerned with improving the quality of care.

Keywords: Cardiac surgical procedures, Heart valve diseases, Survival analysis, Hospital mortality, Rheumatic heart disease, Medical record linkage, Brazil, Annular repair, cardiac valve

Background

In low and middle-income countries, heart valve disease (HVD) is caused mainly by rheumatic heart disease (RHD) [1–6]. Although incidence of acute rheumatic fever has been declining over recent decades in some of these countries, RHD is still considered a major public health problem worldwide [5]. In high-income countries, HVD remains common, despite decreasing prevalence of RHD, because the decline in inflammatory HVD aetiology has been accompanied by an increase in degenerative valve diseases [7]. Most studies describing HVD patterns have been performed in developed countries, which contain less than 20% of the world's population [4]. Large-scale nation-wide studies in developing countries are scarce [4, 5].

In Brazil, although the incidence of acute rheumatic fever has been reduced in recent decades [8], a large number of patients need to perform heart valve surgery (HVS) to repair or replace valves that have suffered rheumatic injury. In these cases, the mitral or aortic valves, or both simultaneously, are the most affected [9]. Moreover, as in

* Correspondence: aquino1@uol.com.br
[1]Hospital School, National Institute of Cardiology (INC), Ministry of Health, Rua das Laranjeiras 374, Laranjeiras, Rio de Janeiro, RJ, Brazil
Full list of author information is available at the end of the article

high-income countries, population ageing has led to an increased number of injuries caused by cardiac valve degeneration. As a result, Brazil has a double burden of diseases connected with poverty, such as rheumatic fever, and degenerative diseases associated with an aging population [10].

Little is known about HVS patient survival in low- and middle-income countries. Most surgical risk evaluations have been based on high-income country data. Similarly, health managers who need to allocate scarce resources rationally to achieve quality in health services are severely challenged. Moreover, disclosure of variations in cardiac surgery outcomes is known to offer opportunities to improve the quality of health care and to be an essential tool for quality assessment.

This study aims to estimate in-hospital mortality, long-term survival and average length of hospital stay of patients submitted to HVS between 2001 and 2007, from data in the nationwide database of the Brazilian National Health System (*Sistema Único de Saúde, SUS*).

Methods

Study setting and population

This was a retrospective nationwide cohort study of 78,808 consecutive patients who underwent HVS in the SUS from 2001 to 2007. The SUS has 234 hospitals with cardiovascular surgery. It provides universal care for over 200 million people [11] and is the sole coverage for 70% of Brazil's population [12].

In the SUS, hospital records have been processed to an administrative database, the Hospital Information System (*Sistema de Informação Hospitalar*, SIH), since 1979, using International Classification of Diseases (ICD) codes. Mortality information since 1975 is on record in a Mortality Information System (*Sistema de Informação de Mortalidade*, SIM) that covers the whole population nationwide [13]. This mortality data is considered qualitatively reliable and as accurate as that of other countries with long traditions in these statistics [14]. The accuracy of the SIH variables for diagnosis, medical procedures, sex, age group and in-hospital outcomes is considered satisfactory [15].

The study cohort comprised patients submitted to one of the following *SUS* surgical procedures, as they are labelled in the SIH database, from 2001 to 2007:

- Valve replacement (VRp): replacing a heart valve with a biological or mechanical prosthesis;
- Valve repair (VRr): restoring the normal functioning of heart valves without the use of a prosthesis; may use a support ring;
- Multiple valve repair and/or replacement (multiple valve surgeries): repair and/or replacement of more than one heart valve (mitral, aortic, tricuspid or pulmonary) with biological or mechanical prostheses;
- Valve replacement with concomitant coronary artery bypass grafting (concomitant CABG): mitral or aortic valve replacement by biological or mechanical prosthesis and concomitant CABG.

All the HVSs described above were performed by thoracotomy and cardiopulmonary bypass.

We did not select any procedure related exclusively to congenital heart diseases.

The exclusion criteria were the following: records with name field left blank or filled beginning with the words "woman", "man", "stillbirth", "son", "daughter", "newborn" or "unknown" and records with date of birth left blank. After cleaning the SIH and SIM databases, 5026 (6.0%) records were excluded.

Patients in the concomitant CABG group displayed different demographic characteristics from other patients: they were older, entailing degenerative processes towards valvular lesion (although in developing countries, such as Brazil, rheumatic disease cannot be precluded as a concomitant process). Moreover, it should not be forgotten that valve surgery and CABG are two separate procedures, thus extracorporeal time is extended. This group was therefore subjected to statistical sub-analysis as a separate cohort.

The inpatient database provides the following information for each individual patient receiving care: ICD 10.0 code, date of birth, date of admission, date of discharge and date of death (if appropriate), sex, type of surgical procedure, disease by valve, length of stay, discharge status, geographical region of residence and county of residence at time of admission. This database was initially set up for administrative purposes, although several studies have validated its use for research purposes [16]. The death certificate provides basic cause of death (ICD 10.0 code), plus demographic data, such as name, dates of birth and death, geographical region of residence and county of residence and of death.

Study measures

The outcome measures for this study were in-hospital mortality (defined as death during index admission) and time until death during 7-year follow-up. These measures were obtained by probabilistic record linkage [17] using the SIH and SIM databases. The linkage method applied showed 90.6% sensitivity and 100% specificity [18] and was used in a prior study [19].

Patient follow-up was considered for discharges from 1 January 2001, while the cut-off entry date for new records was 30 November, 2007, in order to ensure at least a possible 30 days of observation for all patients in this study. Patients were followed up until death or were censored at 31 December 2007, the last day of the study period.

Probabilistic linkage was performed using the public domain software, RecLink III version 3.1 [17].

Statistical analysis

Descriptive analysis included calculating mean, standard deviation, median and interquartile range (IQR) for continuous variables. Categorical variables were described by counts and relative frequency. Continuous variables were compared between dichotomous groups using Student's t-test for normal distributions and Mann-Whitney, otherwise. For continuous variables with more than two groups and non-normal distribution, the Kruskal-Wallis test was employed. The chi-square test was used to compare categorical variables. The Kolmogorov-Smirnov test rejected the null hypothesis for normal age distribution, therefore the median and interquartile range were used ($p < 0.0001$).

To study in-hospital mortality, univariate and multivariate logistic regression models were performed and odds ratios and their respective 95% confidence intervals (95%CI) were calculated. Multivariate testing was performed in forward stepwise fashion.

Survival curves were constructed with Kaplan-Meier techniques and compared with the log-rank statistic. The Cox proportional hazards model was used and hazard ratios (HRs) and their 95%CIs were reported. Schoenfeld residuals were used to test the proportional hazards assumption [20]. Bivariate Cox proportional hazards regression was performed, followed by multivariate models to estimate the independent effect of the variables previously selected. In the event of violation of the proportional hazard assumption, the Stratified Cox model was employed.

Analyses were performed with STATA software, version 13 (STATA Corp, College Station, Tex.). All statistical tests were two-tailed if not stated otherwise. The alpha level was set at 0.05.

Results

Maximum and median follow-up were 7.7 and 2.8 years, respectively (0.002–7.707). The 78,808 patients included in the study were similarly distributed by sex, with 40,136 (51.0%) females and 38,702 (49.0%) males. Median age was 50.0 (35.9–62.5) years. Most were residents of Brazil's southeast region. Median hospital stay was 10 (7–13, 16–18) days. The most common surgery procedure was VRp, in 54,475 (69.1%) patients. The baseline characteristics of the final cohort are described in Table 1.

Table 1 Demographic characteristics, procedures and length of stay of heart valve surgery patients – 2001 to 2007, Brazil

Variable	Patients ($n = 78{,}808$)
Age (years), median (IQR)	50.0 (35.9–62.5)
Age (years), % by age group	
< 20.0	6.37
20–39.9	25.25
40–59.9	38.61
60–79.9	28.63
≥ 80	1.14
Female, n (%)	40,106 (50.89)
Admission by geographical region of residence, n (%)	
Southeast	36,337 (46.11)
Northeast	14,442 (18.33)
North	2360 (2.99)
Midwest	6919 (8.78)
South	18,750 (23.79)
Length of hospital stay (days), median (IQR)	10 (7–16)
Valve repair	4989 (6.33)
Valve replacement	54,475 (69.12)
Multiple valve repair and/or replacement	12,197 (15.48)
Concomitant CABG	7147 (9.07)

IQR Interquartile range, Concomitant CABG – Valve replacement with concomitant coronary artery bypass graft surgery

Valve injury aetiology, when identified, is shown in Table 2. The most prevalent cause was rheumatic heart disease. The second group was classified as "insufficient aetiology description" (IAD). This group included situations when there is no specific ICD10.0 code to describe the aetiology; for example, degenerative aortic stenosis, probably coded just as "aortic stenosis". IAD group median age was 60.7 years. Median age was lower (44.2 years) in RHD patients than in the remaining cohort (57.5 years) ($p < 0.001$). In mitral stenosis patients, aetiology was RHD in 94.7% ($p < 0.001$). As aetiology was improperly encoded in 35.1% of patients undergoing HVS, this variable was not used in risk assessment.

In-hospital mortality was 7.6% (3585 patients) and overall mortality at close of study period was 22.1% (17,383 patients) from all causes of death. Most causes were classified by ICD codes as diseases of the circulatory system (13,449

Table 2 Frequency and proportion of valve lesion aetiologies in heart valve surgery patients – 2001 to 2007, Brazil

Aetiology	n (%)
Rheumatic heart disease	42,352 (53.74)
Insufficient description of the aetiology	27,585 (35.00)
Infective Endocarditis	7177 (9.11)
Congenital	1354 (1.72)
Prolapsed mitral valve	187 (0.24)
Kawasaki disease or Takayasu arteritis	91 (0.12)
Endomyocardial fibrosis	38 (0.05)
Hypertrophic cardiomyopathy	24 (0.03)
Total	78,808 (100%)

deaths; 77.6%), followed by diseases of the respiratory system (813 deaths; 4.7%).

Table 3 shows a subset of patients ($n = 47,515$) where the type of mitral or aortic valve disease was identified and where there was no concomitant CABG. The most common valve injury encountered was mitral stenosis (38.9%). Patients with combined aortic and mitral lesions were the youngest (median 43.3 years) and those with aortic stenosis were the oldest (median 58.0 years) ($p < 0.001$). Repair was performed predominantly in females (65.9%; $p < 0.0001$).

When stratified by age group, highest in-hospital mortality was observed in patients aged ≥80 years, and the lowest was for those between 20 and 39.9 years ($p < 0.001$). In-hospital mortality rates differed significantly by sex; they were higher among women (7.8% versus 7.3%; $p < 0.001$), although this difference was small (Table 4). In-hospital mortality by valve procedure was 3.5% for VRr, 6.9% for VRp, 8.2% for multiple valve repair and/or replacement and 14.6% for concomitant CABG ($p < 0.001$).

Univariate and multivariate logistic regressions (Tables 5 and 6) were performed to identify independent per-operative predictors for in-hospital mortality. All variables that were significant (<0.10) in univariate analyses were added to the multivariate logistic regression model. Corresponding odds ratios (ORs) and 95%CIs were calculated. Because of their low frequency, the following aetiologies have been grouped as "other": Kawasaki disease, Takayasu arteritis, endomyocardial fibrosis and hypertrophic cardiomyopathy.

The following tables show multivariate analysis by stepwise logistic regression for in-hospital mortality including the variables age and female sex. Table 7 compares concomitant CABG with the other surgeries studied in our cohort. In this comparison, concomitant CABG increases risk (OR = 2.0366). Table 8 compares valve repair against replacement or multiple valve surgeries. In this comparison, repair reduces risk (OR = 0.4586).

Shortest hospital stays were for repair procedures (median = 9 days) ($p < 0.001$) and showed no difference when analysed by sex ($p = 0.21$). They were shorter for patients who died during index procedure admission (7 days) than for survivors (10 days) ($p < 0.001$). Significantly longer hospital stays were observed among patients who underwent concomitant CABG (11 days) and those over 80 years old (12 days).

Overall survival of HVS patients is shown in Table 9 and Fig. 1a. There were 78,808 HVS patients, and survival was 69.9% (69.38–70.47%) at the end of follow-up time. Table 10 shows overall survival of patients with rheumatic heart disease. Figure 1b shows survival by

Table 3 Frequency and proportion of valve disease types in non-concomitant coronary artery bypass graft surgery in heart valve surgery patients – 2001 to 2007, Brazil

Type of valve disease	n (%)
Double aortic lesion	1980 (4.17)
Double mitral lesion	2097 (4.41)
Aortic stenosis	7019 (4.77)
Mitral stenosis	18,471 (38.88)
Aortic regurgitation	5241 (11.03)
Mitral regurgitation	8985 (18.91)
Aortic + Mitral lesion	3722 (7.83)
Total	47,515

Table 4 Frequency and proportion of in-hospital mortality, by age group, in heart valve surgery patients – 2001 to 2007, Brazil

Age, by age group	Living, n (%)	Deceased, n (%)	Total, n
<19.9	4756 (94.78)	262 (5.22)	5018
20–39.9	19,175 (96.37)	723 (3.63)	19,898
40–59.9	28,400 (93.34)	2027 (6.66)	30,427
60–79.9	19,776 (87.64)	2788 (12.36)	22,564
≥80	735 (81.58)	166 (18.42)	901
Total	72,842 (92.43)	5966 (7.57)	78,808

Table 5 Univariate analysis by logistic regression of in-hospital mortality in heart valve surgery patients – 2001 to 2007, Brazil

Variable	OR	95% CI	P
Age (years)	1.0338	1.0316–1.0361	<0.001
Female	1.1410	1.0669–1.2204	<0.001
Procedures:			
Repair (reference)			
Replacement	2.2512	1.8015–2.8131	<0.001
Multiple valve repair and/or replacement	4.0268	3.1990–5.0688	<0.001
Concomitant CABG	7.1102	5.6444–8.9565	<0.001
Any valve surgery (reference)			
Concomitant CABG	2.8941	2.6606–3.1481	<0.001
Type of valve disease:			
Aortic regurgitation (reference)			
Mitral stenosis	1.1293	0.9488–1.3441	0.171
Double mitral lesion	1.1743	0.8905–1.5485	0.255
Mitral regurgitation	1.2343	1.0217–1.4912	0.029
Aortic stenosis	1.2492	1.0266–1.5200	0.026
Aortic + Mitral lesion	1.3667	1.0924–1.7097	0.006
Double aortic lesion	1.4375	1.1060–1.8684	0.007
Aetiology			
Rheumatic heart disease (reference)			
Congenital	1.4653	1.1358–1.8905	0.003
Infective Endocarditis	1.5525	1.3796–1.7470	<0.001
Other	1.8162	1.1524–2.8622	0.010
Insufficient description of aetiology	1.9407	1.8058–2.0857	<0.001

OR Odds ratio Concomitant CABG – Valve replacement with concomitant coronary artery bypass graft surgery

Table 6 Multivariate analysis, by logistic regression, for overall in-hospital mortality, by age and sex, in heart valve surgery patients – 2001 to 2007, Brazil

Procedures:	OR	95% CI	*P*
Valve repair (reference)			
Valve replacement	2.0728	1.7740–2.4219	<0.001
Multiple valve repair and/or replacement	2.5011	2.1202–2.9507	<0.001
Concomitant CABG	4,7693	4.0410–5.6288	<0.001
Any valve surgery (reference)			
Concomitant CABG	2.3070	2.1472–2.4789	<0.001
Type of valve disease:			
Aortic regurgitation (reference)			
Mitral stenosis	1.1350	0.9997–1.2886	0.051
Double mitral lesion	1.0072	0.8147–1.2451	0.947
Mitral regurgitation	1.1392	0.9907–1.3100	0.067
Aortic stenosis	1.1013	0.9513–1.2751	0.196
Aortic + Mitral lesion	1.1950	1.0089–1.4152	0.039
Double aortic lesion	1.1744	0.9577–1.4403	0.123
Aetiology			
Rheumatic heart disease (reference)			
Congenital	1.5601	1.2879–1.8899	<0.001
Infective Endocarditis	2.4386	2.2524–2.6404	<0.001
Other	3.2313	2.4241–4.3073	<0.001
Insufficient description of aetiology	1.4989	1.4137–1.5892	<0.001

OR odds ratio Concomitant CABG – Valve replacement with concomitant coronary artery bypass surgery

procedure: at 1 and 5 years, this was 92.5% (95%CI 91.8–93) and 85.3% (95%CI 84.2–86.4) for valve repair; 85.7% (95%CI 85.4–86.0) and 75.5% (95%CI 75.1–76) for valve replacement; 83.8% (95%CI 83.1–84.4) and 74.4% (95%CI 73.4–75.5) for multiple valves surgery; and 72.2 (95%CI 71.1–73.2) and 58.1% (95%CI 56.2–60) for concomitant CABG. Survival, by type of valvular lesion showed no differences.

Survival was observed to differ significantly by sex (Fig. 2a). Long-term survival by sex at year 1 and 5 was, respectively, 85.0% and 76.5% for females and 84.2% and 72.5% for males.

Table 7 \Multivariate analysis, by stepwise logistic regression, for in-hospital mortality of heart valve surgery patients – 2001 to 2007, Brazil

Variables	OR	95% CI	*P*
Age (year)	1.0302	1.0279–1.0325	<0.001
Female	1.3051	1.2180–1.3975	<0.001
Concomitant CABG	2.0366	1.8643–2.2249	<0.001

OR Odds ratio Concomitant CABG – Valve replacement with concomitant coronary artery bypass surgery

Table 8 Multivariate analysis, by stepwise logistic regression, for in-hospital mortality of heart valve surgery patients, except CABG – 2001 to 2007, Brazil

Variables	OR	95% CI	*P*
Age (year)	1.0289	1.0264–1.0314	<0.001
Female	1.2776	1.1835–1.3789	<0.001
Valve repair	0.4586	0.3670–0.5731	<0.001

OR – odds ratio

Significant differences by age group are illustrated in Fig. 2b. Survival was worst among patients aged ≥80 years and best in the 20 to 39 year age group. Survival rates after year 1 and 5 of follow-up were, respectively, 64.7%, and 46.4% in the ≥80 year age group and 91.5% and 85.1% in the 20 to 39 year group.

Long-term survival rates differed significantly between patients who underwent HVS and concomitant CABG and those who underwent HVS only (Fig. 3a): at years 1 and 5 of follow-up, these were, respectively, 72.1% and 58.1%, against 85.9% and 76.0%.

Figure 3b shows long-term survival of patients submitted to HVS with non-concomitant CABG. Long-term survival rates for VRp and multiple valve surgery were similar at year 1 (85.7% versus 83.8%) and year 5 (75.5% versus 74.4%) of follow-up, while VRr returned highest long-term survival rates (92.5% and 85.3%), respectively.

The proportional hazard assumption was violated for sex and geographical region of residence; accordingly, these variables were stratified in multivariate survival analysis. For the other variables, the proportional hazard assumption was satisfied 30 days after hospital discharge; thus this is the timeframe considered in multivariate analysis. Patients who underwent valve surgery with concomitant CABG showed greater risk than those who underwent valve surgery alone (HR 1.3123; 95%CI 1.2271–1.4033; $p < 0.0001$), while patient age contributed, as secondary factor, to increases in this set (HR 1.0216; 95%CI 1.0203–1.0229; $p < 0.0001$). Non-concomitant CABG patients submitted to valve repair showed lower risk than those with VRp or multiple surgeries (HR 0.6937; 95%CI 0.6296–0.7645; $p < 0.0001$), but age

Table 9 Overall survival of heart valve surgery patients – 2001 to 2007, Brazil

Time (years)	Survival Function (%)	Standard Error (%)	95% CI (%)
1	84.62	0.13	84.37–84.87
2	81.98	0.14	81.70–82.25
3	79.49	0.15	79.19–79.78
4	77.12	0.17	76.79–77.44
5	74.54	0.18	74.18–74.90
6	72.06	0.21	71.64–72.47
7	69.93	0.28	69.38–70.47

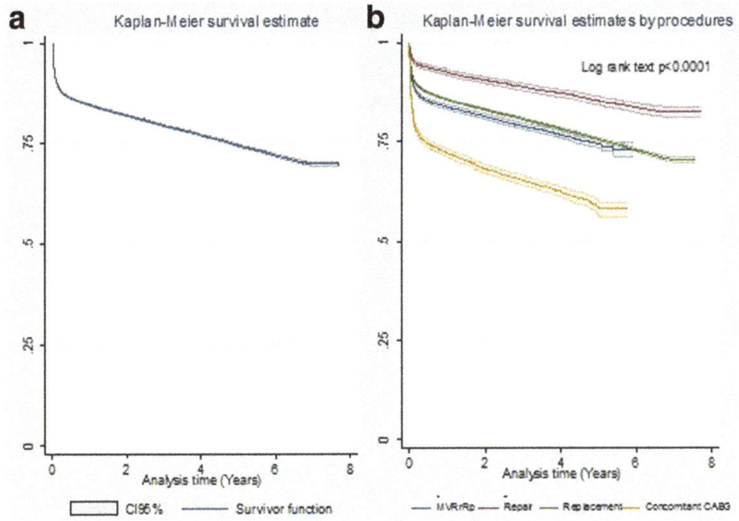

Fig. 1 a Overall survival of heart valve surgery patients – 2001 to 2007; (**b**) Long-term survival of heart valve surgery patients, by procedure type

contributed, as a secondary factor, to increases in this set (HR 1.0209; 95%CI 1.0195–1.0222; $p < 0.0001$).

Discussion

To the best of our knowledge, this retrospective HVS cohort, comprising 78,808 patients, is one of the largest ever published. Sex distribution was balanced. Valve replacement accounted for 69.1% of procedures performed. The most common valve injury was mitral stenosis (38.9% of the total). In 94.7% of mitral stenosis patients, aetiology was rheumatic heart disease. In-hospital mortality was 7.6% and was higher for females who had undergone the concomitant CABG procedure and for the elderly. Overall survival was 69.9% at the end of follow-up time. Survival was worst among elderly, male and concomitant coronary artery bypass grafting patients. Median age was 50.0 years, a lot younger than in studies in developed countries, such as in the Euro Heart Survey on Valvular Heart Disease, where mean age was 64 years [21]. Proportions of valve lesion types and aetiologies were also different from most published studies based on North American and European populations [22–24]. In the "valve lesion identified" subset of the study population, mitral stenosis was the most frequent lesion. RHD was the most prevalent aetiology, accounting for more than half of the subjects studied. This finding is similar to those of other studies in lower- and middle-income countries [10, 25–27].

Table 10 Overall survival of heart valve surgery patients with rheumatic heart disease – 2001 to 2007, Brazil

Time (years)	Survival Function (%)	Standard Error (%)	95% CI (%)
1	93.73	0.12	93.48–93.97
2	91.55	0.14	91.27–91.83
3	89.57	0.17	89.25–89.89
4	87.50	0.19	87.13–87.87
5	85.24	0.22	84.80–85.67
6	83.07	0.28	82.52–83.61
7	81.35	0.40	80.55–82.11

Rheumatic fever is the leading cause of mitral stenosis worldwide and, in 40% of cases, it presents as a single lesion [28]. In our cohort, the aetiology underlying 94.7% of mitral stenosis lesions was RHD. VRp accounted for more than two thirds of procedures, while multiple valve surgery accounted for 15.48%. Multiple valve surgery was observed more frequently than reported in the literature (3–14%) [29], which probably relates to the prevalence of RHD in our cohort (53.7%).

In developing countries, although repair procedures offer the advantage of averting long-term anticoagulation therapy and achieve better outcomes, VRp is usually performed more than VRr in cases of rheumatic disease [25, 30, 31]. Patients are less likely to be suitable for VRr in developing countries, where waiting times are long and RHD is common; as a result, access to surgery tends to occur at an advanced stage of disease. The likelihood of successful mitral repair is associated with the timing of surgical referral, annual volume and expertise of cardiac surgery centres, underlying aetiologies and type of lesion [26, 27]. In RHD, valve repair may be rendered impossible, even for experienced surgeons, by various degrees of fibrotic process, involvement of *chordae tendineae* and calcification of the mitral leaflets or annulus [25]. In developed countries, at institutions with good performance, valve repair is standard therapy for most patients with mitral regurgitation [32]. Note, however, that the

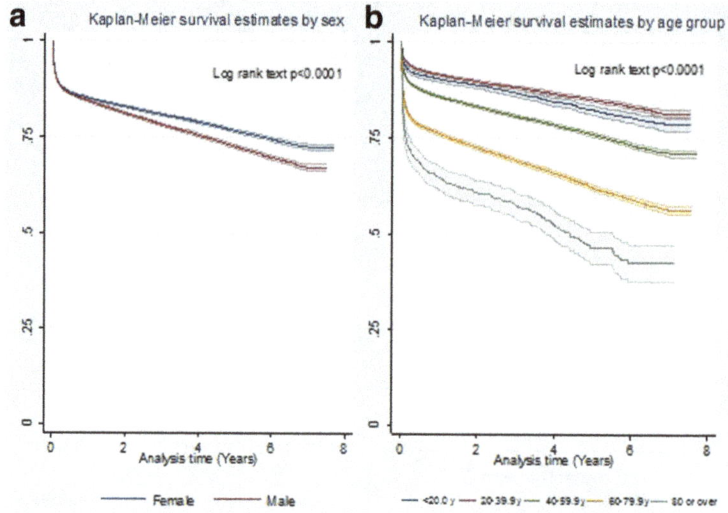

Fig. 2 Long-term survival of heart valve surgery patients – 2001 to 2007: **a**) by sex; (**b**) by age group

most common aetiologies for valve dysfunction in low- and middle-income countries are different from those studied and often published in developed countries. Accordingly, valve repair entails different levels of challenge and outcomes in these different real settings. Although overall survival has been better among RHD patients than among those with valve lesions with other aetiologies (probably as a result of younger age and fewer comorbidities), valve lesions from rheumatic fever are still a undesirable outcome since RHD is largely avoidable by means of primary and secondary prevention.

Valve injury aetiology was not clearly stated in some groups of our cohort and hence we classified it as "insufficient aetiology description". The lack of a specific ICD 10.0 code may be one of the underlying causes of insufficient coding. In Brazilian public health databases, the "diagnosis" field draws on the ICD 10.0 codex to classify diseases and other health problems. In the literature, degenerative aetiology plays a very important role in other HVS cohorts [33, 34]. Although this study population is younger, it must be assumed that many patients grouped as "insufficient aetiology description" presented injuries caused by a degenerative process of the heart valves. The median age of these miscoded patients was 60.7 years, in contrast to the remaining group where the median was 44.2 years. Corroborating this assumption, almost 80% of patients over

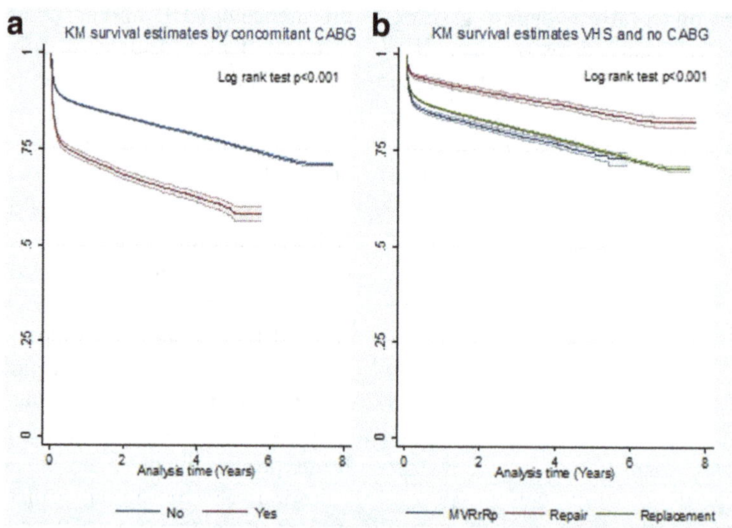

Fig. 3 Long-term survival of heart valve surgery patients: **a**) with concomitant coronary artery bypass grafting (CABG); and **b**) heart valve surgery (HVS) with non-concomitant coronary artery bypass grafting (CABG)

80 years old were classified as "aetiology insufficiently described". In addition, the proportion of Brazil's population over 65 years old was 4.0% in 1980, increasing to 7.4% in 2010. Life expectancy in Brazil increased 10 years in that period and, therefore, aging-related diseases can be expected to emerge [35].

Note also that, in one of the few studies evaluating the burden of HVD in developing countries, the most frequent aetiology was RHD (60.3%), in line with this study, while degenerative valve disease, detected in 15% of patients, was the second most common aetiology [10].

Overall in-hospital mortality was 7.6%, but higher for female patients who had undergone concomitant CABG and for the elderly. Concomitant CABG increases mortality substantially [22, 29, 33]. Here, the study population was younger (age has been identified as an important independent predictor of HVS outcomes in adults) [29, 33, 34]. This study involved more patients than those of Leavitt (1057) and Nicolini (1167), although the number of concomitant CABG surgeries was smaller and involved a younger population. Leavitt and Nicolini reported overall in-hospital mortality of 15.5% and 6.9%, respectively. Hannan (14,190) reported 3.3% for CCV without concomitant CABG and 18.7% for multiple valve surgery with concomitant CABG. Both Hannan and Nicolini observed that in-hospital mortality rates were better for VRr than for replacements, similar what is reported in other studies [22, 36–39]. Ribeiro [40] reported cardiac surgery in-hospital mortality in Brazil as 8.9%, from 2000 to 2003; this was not solely for HVS, however, but included other procedures.

Unlike other published studies [22, 29, 33], this study found better overall long-term survival for women. Although VRr was performed more often in women, it cannot explain this favourable result, because VRr contributed only 6.3% of total procedures. In this study, overall long-term survival rates at 1 and 5 years were 84.6% and 74.5%, which are lower than those reported for a double valve surgery cohort, showing that our outcomes seem to be less satisfactory [29]. Seventy per cent of patients were alive at close of follow-up, which agrees with a previous study with similar procedure mix [41]. Long-term survival for VRr was better than for replacements, as reported in another study [39], but different from Leavitt and Nicolini. The latter author does not supported the theory that, for patients undergoing HVS, VRr is better than replacement. He reported comparable long-term survival at 5 years for VRr and replacement. Different outcomes in different studies can probably be ascribed to cohorts with different demographic characteristics, comorbidities, valve lesion aetiologies, surgeons' skills and repair techniques, especially in observational studies such as this.

The group of patients who underwent multiple valve surgery comprised a great diversity of clinical features and possible combinations of surgeries, making it difficult to analyse this group in comparison with the VRp group, although they displayed similar results and no statistically significant difference in long-term survival.

Concomitant CABG reduced long-term survival considerably. For patients who underwent concomitant CABG, long-term survival at years 1 and 5 of follow-up was, respectively, 72.1% and 58.1% and, for those who underwent HVS alone, 85.9% and 76.0%.

These rates were similar to those reported in the literature [29, 32, 42, 43]. Hannan and Nicolini have observed that patients who underwent HVS and concomitant CABG were older, had more comorbidities and had more often undergone other previous cardiovascular surgeries. These features could account for lower overall survival.

Taken together with the in-hospital mortality rates and long-term survival found here, length of hospital stay for repair procedures reinforces the assumption that, in Brazil, patients selected for VRr procedures are likely to present better valve and general health status than those submitted to other procedures, which is in line with other studies [34, 39]. Comorbidities and old age predicted lesser likelihood of repair, although good results have been reported for elderly patients undergoing mitral valve surgery, especially mitral VRr, in a large series [34]. Gillinov observed that mitral valve repair was more likely to be performed if valve leaflets were morphologically normal, with functional mitral valve regurgitation, while mitral valve replacement was more often performed in the event of preoperative atrial fibrillation, severe mitral valve stenosis and calcified mitral leaflets or if a mechanical aortic prosthesis was in place [39].

It is clear that old age influences in-hospital mortality, length of hospital stay and long-term survival of patients undergoing HVS. This was also found in this study (OR = 1.0338 for each additional year during hospitalisation). In-hospital mortality was the highest, length of hospital stay, the longest and long-term survival at year 5 of follow-up, the shortest for patients older than 80 years, in agreement with other studies [33, 34, 41, 44].

Length of hospital stay was similar by sex [33] and shorter in patients who died during index procedure admission than in survivors. Most in-hospital deaths (53.9%) occurred up to day 7 of hospitalisation and 25.03% up to day 2. These rates suggest that half of patients died in the operating theatre or in the very early postoperative period. This finding serves to highlight the need to improve the quality of surgical care during the operation or to improve the appropriateness of surgical indications for HVS in Brazil.

The scarcity of long-term survival series drawn from large databases in middle-income countries makes it difficult to compare between studies of populations exposed to similar risk factors and similar patterns of diseases, which reinforces the importance of our findings.

This study was based on a nationwide cohort of patients in the real world setting, which is its main strength. Nevertheless, its conclusions should be read in the light of certain limitations. The two large databases employed offered few clinical variables. This means that we were unable to identify all possible confounding variables. We adjusted for all the available variables, but we should not underestimate the possibility that the omission of important covariates may affect our results.

The limitations of the present study include also the inherent constraints of retrospective, nonrandomised data collection. Although case matching and multivariate analysis can help to account for some differences in the groups, the effects of unmeasured variables affecting selection of therapy may confound the analysis.

Conclusions

In Brazil at the beginning of the twenty-first century, the most common valve lesion is still mitral stenosis, while the most common underlying aetiology is rheumatic heart disease. Single valve replacement accounts for the overwhelming majority of the procedures performed, whereas only a very small number of patients with heart valve diseases benefited from valve repairs. In-hospital mortality and overall survival rates of patients who have undergone heart valve surgery were less satisfactory than those reported in high-income countries. The findings of this study can help guide decision-making processes in middle-income countries similar to Brazil and those concerned with improving the quality of care.

Abbreviations

CABG: Coronary artery bypass grafting; CI: Confidence interval; HR: Hazard ratio; HVD: Heart valve disease; HVS: Heart valve surgery; ICD: International Classification of Diseases; IQR: Interquartile range; OR: Odds ratio; RHD: Rheumatic Heart Disease; SIH: Brazilian Hospital Database; SIM: Brazilian National Mortality Database; SUS: Brazilian National Health System; VRp: Valve replacement; VRr: Valve repair

Acknowledgements

ALPR was supported in part by CNPq (research fellowship number 310679/2016-8), FAPEMIG (PPM-00428-17) and is a member of the National Institute of Science and Technology for Health Technology Assessment (IATS) CNPq/465518/2014-1).

Funding

None.

Authors' contributions

RMAX undertook the literature review. RMAX, VMPA and NASS contributed to the study conception and design. VMPA, RBMC, CW and RMAX performed data cleaning. RMAX, CAX, LAH and RBMC contributed to data acquisition. VMPA, RMAX, MGC and RBMC performed statistical analysis. RMAX, VMPA, RBMC, AM, NASS, PHG, ALPR and CW contributed to data interpretation. RMAX, VMPA, ALPR and AM drafted the manuscript. All authors read, critically revised and approved the final manuscript and are accountable for all aspects of the work.

Competing interests

The authors declare that they have no competing interests.

Author details

[1]Hospital School, National Institute of Cardiology (INC), Ministry of Health, Rua das Laranjeiras 374, Laranjeiras, Rio de Janeiro, RJ, Brazil. [2]Hospital Naval Marcílio Dias, Rio de Janeiro, Brazil. [3]University Hospital and School of Medicine - Universidade Federal de Minas Gerais (UFMG), Minas Gerais, Brazil. [4]University Hospital and School of Medicine, Federal University of Rio de Janeiro (UFRJ), Rio de Janeiro, Brazil. [5]Hospital Municipal Salgado Filho, Rio de Janeiro, Brazil.

References

1. Gaziano JM. Global Burden of Cardiovascular Disease. In: Braunwald E, Zipes D, Libby P, editors. Heart Disease. 8th ed. New York: WB Saunders, Elsevier; 2007. p. 1–34.
2. Boudoulas KD, Borer JS, Boudoulas H. Etiology of valvular heart disease in the 21st century. Cardiology. 2013;126:139–52.
3. World Health Organ Tech Rep Ser. Rheumatic fever and rheumatic heart disease. 2004;923:1–122
4. Iung B, Vahanian A. Epidemiology of valvular heart disease in the adult. Nat Rev Cardiol. 2011;8:162–72.
5. Carapetis JR. Rheumatic heart disease in developing countries. N Engl J Med. 2007;357:439–41.
6. Iung B, Vahanian A. Epidemiology of acquired valvular heart disease. Can J Cardiol. 2014;30:962–70.
7. Horstkotte D, Niehues R, Strauer BE. Pathomorphological aspects, aetiology and natural history of acquired mitral valve stenosis. Eur Heart J. 1991;12:55–60.
8. Azevedo VMP, Müller RE, Kaufman R, Santos MA, Chaves RBM, Migowski A, Pinheiro MC, Xavier RMI. Rheumatic fever in Brazilian young adults an already controlled disease? An overview about the last 21 years epidemiological data. Global Heart. 2014;9(1, suppl):e259.
9. Otto CM, Bonow RO. Valvular heart disease. In: Braunwald E, Zipes D, Libby P, editors. Heart Disease. 8 ed. New York: WB Saunders, Elsevier; 2007. p. 1625–1712.
10. Ribeiro GS, Tartof SY, Oliveira DW, Guedes AC, Reis MG, Riley LW, Ko AI. Surgery for valvular heart disease: a population-based study in a Brazilian urban center. PLoS One. 2012;7:e37855.
11. IBGE. Estimativas da população residente no Brasil e unidades da Federação com data de referência em 1° de julho de 2014. Rio de Janeiro: IBGE. 2014:135.
12. IBGE. Um panorama da saúde no Brasil: acesso e utilização dos serviços, condições de saúde e fatores de risco e proteção à saúde 2008. Rio de Janeiro: IBGE. 2010:245.
13. Sistema de Informações Hospitalares do SUS (SIH/SUS) [Internet]. 2015 [cited 04 March 2015]. Available from: http://tabnet.datasus.gov.br/cgi/deftohtm.exe?sih/cnv/nruf.def.
14. Laurenti R, de Mello Jorge MH, Gotlieb SL. Underlying cause-of-death mortality statistics: considering the reliability of data. Rev Panam Salud Publica. 2008;23:349–56.
15. Escosteguy CC, Portela MC, De A MR, De Vasconcellos MT. The Brazilian hospital information system and the acute myocardial infarction hospital care. Rev Saude Publica. 2002;36:491–9.
16. Abreu CD, Xavier RM, Nascimento JS, Ribeiro AL. Long-term outcome after cardiac resynchronization therapy: a nationwide database. Int J Cardiol. 2012;155:492–3.
17. Camargo KR Jr, Coeli CM. Reclink: an application for database linkage implementing the probabilistic record linkage method. Cad Saude Publica. 2000;16:439–47.
18. Migowski A, Chaves RB, Coeli CM, Ribeiro AL, Tura BR, Kuschnir MC, Azevedo VM, Floriano DB, Magalhães CA, Pinheiro MC, Xavier RM. Accuracy of probabilistic record linkage in the assessment of high-complexity cardiology procedures. Rev Saude Publica. 2011;45:269–75.
19. Migowski A, Ribeiro AL, Carvalho MS, Azevedo VM, Chaves RB, Hashimoto LA, Xavier CA, Xavier RM. Seven years of use of implantable cardioverter-defibrillator therapies: a nationwide population-based assessment of their effectiveness in real clinical settings. BMC Cardiovasc Disord. 2015;15:22.
20. Kleinbaum DGKM. Survival analysis: a self-learning text. 3rd ed. USA: Springer; 2012. 695 p.

21. Iung B, Baron G, Butchart EG, Delahaye F, Gohlke-Barwolf C, Levang OW, Tornos P, Vanoverschelde JL, Vermeer F, Boersma E, Ravaud P, Vahanian A. A prospective survey of patients with valvular heart disease in Europe: the euro heart survey on Valvular heart disease. Eur Heart J. 2003;24:1231–43.
22. Boudoulas KD, Ravi Y, Garcia D, Saini U, Sofowora GG, Gumina RJ, Sai-Sudhakar CB. Type of Valvular heart disease requiring surgery in the 21st century: mortality and length-of-stay related to surgery. Open Cardiovasc Med J. 2013;7:104–9.
23. Go AS, Mozaffarian D, Roger VL, Benjamin EJ, Berry JD, Blaha MJ, Dai S, Ford ES, Fox CS, Franco S, Fullerton HJ, Gillespie C, Hailpern SM, Heit JA, Howard VJ, Huffman MD, Judd SE, Kissela BM, Kittner SJ, Lackland DT, Lichtman JH, Lisabeth LD, Mackey RH, Magid DJ, Marcus GM, Marelli A, Matchar DB, DK MG, Mohler ER 3rd, Moy CS, Mussolino ME, Neumar RW, Nichol G, Pandey DK, Paynter NP, Reeves MJ, Sorlie PD, Stein J, Towfighi A, Turan TN, Virani SS, Wong ND, Woo D, Turner MB. Heart disease and stroke statistics–2014 update: a report from the American Heart Association. Circulation. 2014;129:e28–e292.
24. Nkomo VT, Gardin JM, Skelton TN, Gottdiener JS, Scott CG, Enriquez-Sarano M. Burden of valvular heart diseases: a population-based study. Lancet. 2006 Sep 16;368:1005–11.
25. Bakir I, Onan B, Onan IS, Gul M, Uslu N. Is rheumatic mitral valve repair still a feasible alternative?: indications, technique, and results. Tex Heart Inst J. 2013;40:163–9.
26. Bolling SF, Li S, O'Brien SM, Brennan JM, Prager RL, Gammie JS. Predictors of mitral valve repair: clinical and surgeon factors. Ann Thorac Surg. 2010;90: 1904–11. discussion 12
27. Russell EA, Tran L, Baker RA, Bennetts JS, Brown A, Reid CM, Tam R, Walsh WF, Maguire GPA. Review of valve surgery for rheumatic heart disease in Australia. BMC Cardiovasc Disord. 2014;14:134.
28. Kirklin JKKN, Blackstone EH, Hanley FL. Cardiac surgery: morphology, diagnostic criteria, natural history, techniques, results and indications. 4th ed. Elsevier Saunders: USA; 2013.
29. Nicolini F, Agostinelli A, Fortuna D, Contini GA, Pacini D, Gabbieri D, Zussa C, Pigini F, De Palma R, Gherli T. Outcomes of patients undergoing concomitant mitral and aortic valve surgery: results from an Italian regional cardiac surgery registry. Interact Cardiovasc Thorac Surg. 2014;19:763–70.
30. Waller B, Howard J, Fess S. General concepts in the morphologic assessment of operatively excised cardiac valves – part I. Clin Cardiol. 1994;17:41–6.
31. Kikon M, Dutta Choudhury K, Prakash N, Gupta A, Grover V, Kumar Gupta V. Mitral valve replacement in a young pregnant woman: a case report and review of literature. Res Cardiovasc Med. 2014;3:e17561.
32. Thourani VH, Weintraub WS, Guyton RA, Jones EL, Williams WH, Elkabanni S, Craver JM. Outcomes and long-term survival for patients undergoing mitral valve repair versus replacement: effect of age and concomitant coronary artery bypass grafting. Circulation. 2003 Jul 22;108:298–304.
33. Leavitt BJ, Baribeau YR, DiScipio AW, Ross CS, Quinn RD, Olmstead EM, Sisto D, Likosky DS, Cochran RP, Clough RA, Boss RA Jr, Kramer RS, O'Connor GT. Outcomes of patients undergoing concomitant aortic and mitral valve surgery in northern new England. Circulation. 2009;120:S155–62.
34. Vassileva CM, Mishkel G, McNeely C, Boley T, Markwell S, Scaife S, Hazelrigg S. Long-term survival of patients undergoing mitral valve repair and replacement: a longitudinal analysis of Medicare fee-for-service beneficiaries. Circulation. 2013;127:1870–6.
35. IBGE. Projeção da população do Brasil por sexo e idade 1980-2050, Revisão 2008. Rio de Janeiro: IBGE; 2008.
36. Urban M, Pirk J, Szarszoi O, Skalsky I, Maly J, Netuka I. Mitral valve repair versus replacement in simultaneous aortic and mitral valve surgery. Exp Clin Cardiol. 2013;18:22–6.
37. Hannan EL, Racz MJ, Jones RH, Gold JP, Ryan TJ, Hafner JP, Isom OW. Predictors of mortality for patients undergoing cardiac valve replacements in New York state. Ann Thorac Surg. 2000;70:1212–8.
38. Hellgren L, Kvidal P, Stahle E. Improved early results after heart valve surgery over the last decade. Eur J Cardiothorac Surg. 2002;22:904–11.
39. Gillinov AM, Blackstone EH, Cosgrove DM 3rd, White J, Kerr P, Marullo A, McCarthy PM, Lytle BW. Mitral valve repair with aortic valve replacement is superior to double valve replacement. J Thorac Cardiovasc Surg. 2003;125:1372–87.
40. Ribeiro AL, Gagliardi SP, Nogueira JL, Silveira LM, Colosimo EA, Lopes do Nascimento CA. Mortality related to cardiac surgery in Brazil, 2000-2003. J Thorac Cardiovasc Surg. 2006;131:907–9.
41. Mohty D, Enriquez-Sarano M. The long-term outcome of mitral valve repair for mitral valve prolapse. Curr Cardiol Rep. 2002;4:104–10.
42. Gopaldas RR, Bakaeen FG, Dao TK, Coselli JS, LeMarie SA, Huh J, Chu D. Outcomes of concomitant aortic valve replacement and coronary artery bypass grafting at teaching hospitals versus nonteaching hospitals. J Thorac Cardiovasc Surg. 2012 Mar;143:648–55.
43. Saxena A, Dinh D, Smith JA, Reid CM, Shardey GC, Newcomb AE. Excellent short-and long-term outcomes after concomitant aortic valve replacement and coronary artery bypass grafting performed by surgeons in training. The journal of the thoracic and. Cardiovasc Surg. 2013 Feb;145:334–40.
44. Avery GJ 2nd, Ley SJ, Hill JD, Hershon JJ, Dick SE. Cardiac surgery in the octogenarian: evaluation of risk, cost, and outcome. Ann Thorac Surg. 2001;71:591–6.

17

Role of elevated red cell distribution width on acute kidney injury patients after cardiac surgery

Zhouping Zou[1,2,3,4†], Yamin Zhuang[5†], Lan Liu[5†], Bo Shen[1,2,3,4], Jiarui Xu[1,3,4], Wuhua Jiang[1,3,4], Zhe Luo[5], Jie Teng[1,2,3,4,6,7*], Chunsheng Wang[8] and Xiaoqiang Ding[1,2,3,4,6,7*]

Abstract

Background: The aim of the study was to explore associations between elevated red cell distribution width (RDW) and acute kidney injury (AKI) in patients undergoing cardiac surgery (CS-AKI).

Methods: Preoperative, intraoperative and postoperative data of 10,274 patients undergoing cardiac surgery, including demographic data, were prospectively collected from January 2009 to December 2014. Propensity score matching was used on the basis of clinical characteristics and preoperative variables. An elevated RDW was defined as the difference between RDW 24 h after cardiac surgery and the latest RDW before cardiac surgery.

Results: A total of 10,274 patients were included in the unmatched cohort, and 3146 patients in the propensity-matched cohort. In the unmatched cohort, the overall CS-AKI incidence was 32.8% ($n = 3365$) with a hospital mortality of 5.5% ($n = 185$). In the propensity-matched cohort, the elevated RDW in AKI patients was higher than in patients without AKI (0.3% (0.0%, 0.7%) vs 0.5% (0.1, 1.1%), $P < 0.001$) and the elevated RDW incidences were 0.4% (0.1%, 0.9%), 0.6% (0.2%, 1.1%) and 1.1% (0.3%, 2.1%) in stage 1, 2 and 3 AKI patients ($P < 0.001$). Among propensity-matched patients with CS-AKI, the level of elevated RDW in non-survivors was higher than in survivors [1.2% (0.5%, 2.3%) vs 0.5% (0.1%, 1.0%), $P < 0.001$] and a 0.1% increase in elevated RDW was associated with a 0.24% higher risk of within-hospital mortality in patients with CS-AKI. Estimating the receiver-operating characteristic (ROC) area under the curve (AUC) showed that an elevated RDW had moderate discriminative power for AKI development (AUC = 0.605, 95% CI, 0.586–0.625; $P < 0.001$) and hospital mortality (AUC = 0.716, 95% CI, 0.640–0.764; $P < 0.001$) in the propensity-matched cohort.

Conclusions: An elevated RDW might be an independent prognostic factor for the severity and poor prognosis of CS-AKI.

Keywords: Acute kidney injury, Cardiac surgery, Prognosis, Red cell distribution width

Background

Red blood cell distribution width (RDW), which is a marker that describes the morphology of red blood cells and is routinely reported in complete blood counts, is a measurement of erythrocyte variability and heterogeneity. RDW can be expressed either in absolute values (RDW-SD) or as a percentage (RDW %); the latter approach is more widely used in routine laboratory practice. RDW s together with the value of mean corpuscular volume (MCV) to classify, diagnose and differentiate the causes of anemia, especially iron-deficiency anemia [1]. Recently, several studies have shown that a high RDW level is a strong independent predictor of increased morbidity and mortality in patients with heart failure, myocardial infarction, paroxysmal atrial fibrillation, primary biliary cirrhosis, chronic hepatitis C, pulmonary embolism, chronic obstructive pulmonary disease (COPD), leukoaraiosis and drug-eluting stent restenosis [2–9]. However, there is limited research regarding the potential association between elevated RDW and the development, severity and prognosis of AKI associated with cardiac surgery (CS-AKI). The present study investigated the potential association between elevated RDW and the development

* Correspondence: teng.jie@zs-hospital.sh.cn; ding.xiaoqiang@zs-hospital.sh.cn
†Zhouping Zou, Yamin Zhuang and Lan Liu contributed equally to this work.
[1]Department of Nephrology, Zhongshan Hospital, Shanghai Medical College, Fudan University, No 180 Fenglin Road, Shanghai 200032, China

and prognosis of CS-AKI patients in order to identify a novel biomarker for the early diagnosis, clinical severity and prognosis of CS-AKI.

Methods

Study population

We retrospectively analyzed data from patients who underwent cardiac surgery from January 2009 to December 2014 in the Zhongshan Hospital affiliated to Fudan University and matched them 1:1 based on propensity scoring. The criteria for exclusion were: age (< 18 years), anemia (hemoglobin < 120 g/L for males; hemoglobin < 110 g/L for females), solitary kidney or history of kidney transplants, severe renal dysfunction with estimated glomerular filtration rate (eGFR) ≤ 30 mL/min/1.73 m^2 at baseline; preoperative circulatory assist devices, preoperative renal replacement therapy (RRT) or those undergoing a heart transplant; insufficient examination results at baseline.

AKI and RDW definitions

AKI was defined according to the Kidney Disease Improving Global Outcomes (KDIGO) [10] criteria as described recently [11]: 1) Increase in serum creatinine (Scr) by ≥0.3 mg/dL (≥ 26.5 μmol/L) within 48 h; 2) Increase in Scr to ≥1.5 times baseline, which is known or presumed to have occurred within the prior 7 days; 3) Urine volume < 0.5 mL/kg/h for 6 h and staged according to the Scr and urine output. An elevated RDW was defined as the difference between the RDW value 24 h after cardiac surgery and the latest RDW value before cardiac surgery. The reference range for RDW value was 11.0–16.0% at the Zhongshan Hospital affiliated to Fudan University.

Clinical trial design and methods

Informed consent was provided by all of the patients according to hospital guidelines. At admission, baseline blood testing, echocardiography and electrocardiography were performed. Recorded clinical data were preoperative baseline characteristics and blood tests, complications, preoperative renal function (determined by the latest serum creatinine value before cardiac surgery) as well as perioperative data about cardiac functions according to the 1994 New York Heart Association (NYHA) classification and intraoperative variables which included cardiac output data derived from echocardiography, cardiopulmonary bypass (CPB) and aortic cross-clamp (ACC) durations in minutes, as well as types of surgery. The recorded postoperative variables were mechanical ventilation duration and urine output during the first post-surgery 24 h as well as AKI incidence and stage in addition to hospital mortality.

Outcomes

The primary endpoint was the occurrence of AKI. The secondary endpoint was all cause of mortality.

Statistical analysis

All statistical analyses were performed using SPSS Statistics for Windows (Version 22.0. Armonk, NY: IBM Corp). Propensity score matching was used to adjust for observed differences in characteristics of patients with and without AKI. Comparisons of the differences in the baseline characteristics were performed using a Student's *t*-test for parametric data and a Mann-Whitney U-test for non-parametric data. Categorical variables were compared using a chi-square test or Fisher's exact test.

Associations of pre-, intra-, post-operative and demographic data were tested with Wilcoxon rank-sum or two-sample *t*-tests for continuous and a Pearson $\chi 2$ test for categorical variables. Continuous variables are presented as mean ± standard deviation or median (interquartile range [IQR]) and categorical variables are shown as frequency counts (%). A multivariable logistic regression model was used for estimation of unadjusted and adjusted odds ratios (ORs). Pearson's and Spearman correlation tests were used to determine the correlation between variables. Receiver operator characteristic (ROC) curves were constructed to analyze the discriminating power of elevated RDW for predicting the development of AKI and all-cause hospital mortality. ROC curve analysis statistics were determined with area under the curve (AUC) (95% CI) estimated by bootstrapping. Two-tailed P-values < 0.05 were considered to be statistically significant for all analyses.

Results

Patient characteristics of the study population

Unmatched cohort

A total of 10,274 patients undergoing cardiac surgery were enrolled; most were men (56.7%). The overall CS-AKI incidence was 32.8% ($n = 3365$) with a hospital mortality of 5.5% ($n = 185$). The mean age at hospital admission was 53.3 years (± SD 13.9). The mean age, proportion of males mean body mass index (BMI), hemoglobin, white blood cells (WBC), serum creatinine (SCr), blood urea nitrogen (BUN), serum uric acid (SUA), CPB time, elevated RDW, preoperative proportions of hypertension, diabetes mellitus (DM), coronary angiography, chronic heart failure (NYHA > II), aortic cross-clamp (ACC) time were increased in the AKI group, whereas baseline albumin was decreased (Table 1).

Risk factors for the development of CS-AKI

All the variables recorded in Table 1 were put into a univariate logistic regression model and the detailed results are presented in Table 2. The odds ratios of CS-AKI in the unmatched cohort for the independent risk factors that were computed from the multivariate logistic regression model are shown in Table 3. The independent risk factors that were computed from the multivariate logistic regression

Table 1 Comparison of the Demographic and Baseline Characteristics of unmatched and matched AKI and non-AKI groups

	Unmatched Cohort (*n* = 10,274)		*P*-value	Matched Cohort (*n* = 3146)		*P*-value
	Non-AKI group (*n* = 6909)	AKI group (*n* = 3364)		Non-AKI group (*n* = 1573)	AKI group (*n* = 1573)	
Age (years)	51.7 ± 14.0	56.8 ± 12.3	< 0.001	54.6 ± 12.0	54.4 ± 12.1	0.782
Male, sex	3584 (51.9%)	2233 (66.6%)	< 0.001	966 (61.4%)	913 (58.0%)	0.059
Comorbidities						
Hypertension	1748 (25.3%)	1177 (35%)	< 0.001	422 (26.8%)	457 (29.1%)	0.177
DM	628 (9.1%)	386 (11.5%)	< 0.001	139 (8.8%)	151 (9.6%)	0.498
Creatinine, μmol/L	75.7 ± 20.6	83.6 ± 29.5	< 0.001	77.1 ± 17.3	77.8 ± 19.7	0.325
eGFR	93.0 ± 22.1	87.3 ± 25.3	< 0.001	91.5 ± 20.7	91.0 ± 24.1	0.566
BUN	6.1 ± 2.1	7.0 ± 2.8	< 0.001	6.2 ± 1.9	6.3 ± 1.8	0.063
Albumin baseline	40.6 ± 3.3	40.1 ± 3.3	< 0.001	40.0 ± 3.4	39.9 ± 3.5	0.162
Hemoglobin, g/dL	136.5 ± 14.6	137.3 ± 15.9	0.005	134.7 ± 17.0	133.6 ± 18.7	0.093
WBC, 1000/μL	6.4 ± 2.0	6.5 ± 2.2	0.033	6.4 ± 2.4	6.4 ± 2.0	0.532
Elevated RDW, %	0.3 (0.0, 0.6)	0.5 (0.1,1.0)	< 0.001	0.3 (0.0,0.7)	0.5 (0.1,1.1)	< 0.001
Platelet fl	188.8 ± 56.7	177.3 ± 56.4	< 0.001	189.2 ± 62.1	178.2 ± 58.7	< 0.001
BMI, kg/m^2	22.9 ± 3.0	23.5 ± 3.2	0.013	22.6 ± 3.2	23.3 ± 3.7	< 0.001
SUA	351.0 ± 104.7	394.0 ± 138.6	< 0.001	355.6 ± 101.0	377.0 ± 108.6	< 0.001
NYHA functional class						
I-II	3420 (49.5%)	1370 (40.7)	< 0.001	755 (48.0%)	610 (38.8%)	< 0.001
III-IV	3489 (50.5%)	1995 (59.3)	< 0.001	818 (52.0%)	963 (61.2%)	< 0.001
LVEF%	62.4 ± 8.3	61.4 ± 19.3	0.071	62.1 ± 8.1	61.3 ± 9.4	0.092
CPB time (min)	81.0 (65.0, 105.0)	101.0 (78.0, 128.0)	< 0.001	80.5 (65.0,105.0)	99.0 (78.0,126.0)	< 0.001
ACC time (min)	48.0 (36.0, 67.0)	58.0 (43.0, 78.0)	< 0.001	48.0 (37.0,67.0)	55.0 (41.0,78.0)	< 0.001
Pre-operative coronary angiography n (%)	2543 (36.8)	1528 (45.4)	< 0.001	690 (43.9%)	617 (39.2%)	0.009
Time interval between coronary angiogram and cardiac surgery (days)	4 (2, 6)	4 (2, 6)	0.212	3 (2,6)	3 (2,6)	0.981

AKI acute kidney injury, *BMI* body mass index, *DM* diabetes mellitus, *WBC* white blood cell, *RDW* red cell distribution width, *BUN* blood urea nitrogen, *eGFR* estimated glomerular filtration rate *SUA* serum uric acid, *NYHA* New York Heart Association, *LVEF* left ventricular ejection fraction, *CPB* cardiopulmonary bypass, *ACC* Aortic cross-clamp

model were age (OR = 1.036, 95% CI: 1.029–1.042, *P* < 0.001), male (OR = 1.873, 95% CI: 1.622–2.164, *P* < 0.001), BMI (OR = 1.035, 95% CI: 1.016–1.055, *P* < 0.001), elevated RDW (OR = 1.302, 95% CI: 1.209–1.401, *P* < 0.001), BUN (OR = 1.076, 95% CI: 1.041–1.112, *P* < 0.001), SUA (OR = 1.002, 95% CI: 1.001–1.003, *P* < 0.001), CPB time (additional 30 min) (OR = 1.627 95% CI: 1.491–1.775, *P* < 0.001).

The association between elevated RDW and the development and prognosis of CS-AKI

The AKI group had a higher level of elevated RDW than the non-AKI group[0.5% (0.1%, 1.0%) vs 0.3% (0, 0.6%), *P* < 0.001]. Each 0.1% increment in elevated RDW was associated with a 1.1% higher risk of CS-AKI. The elevated RDW were 0.4% (0.1%, 0.9%), 0.5% (0.2%, 1.0%), 0.8% (0.3%, 1.7%) in stages 1, 2 and 3 of AKI, respectively. An increment in elevated RDW was associated with having a higher stage of AKI (*P* = 0.02). The patients were divided into two groups according to whether the RDW baseline was ≥16.0%. The incidence of CS-AKI in the RDW group (> 16.0%) was significantly higher than in the RDW group (≤ 16.0%, 33.9% vs 38.4%, *P* < 0.001). The adjusted odds ratio of CS-AKI development in the RDW group > 16.0% was 1.67-fold, compared with RDW ≤ in the 16.0% group. Among patients with CS-AKI, the level of elevated RDW in non-survivors was higher than survivors[1.1% (0.4%, 2.0%) vs 0.4% (0.1%, 0.9%), *P* < 0.001]. There was no significant difference in elevated RDW between non-survivors and survivors without CS-AKI [0.4% (− 0.1%, 0.9%) vs 0.3% (0.0, 0.6%), *P* = 0.875]. A 0.1% increase in elevated RDW was associated with a 0.24% higher risk of within-hospital mortality in those patients with CS-AKI.

Table 2 Univariate logistic regression analysis of risk factors for CS-AKI

	Before Propensity Matching			After Propensity Matching		
	OR	95%CI	*P*-value	OR	95%CI	*P*-value
Age	1.030	1.027–1.034	< 0.001	0.999	0.993–1.005	0.782
Male	1.825	1.680–1.994	< 0.001	0.869	0.754–1.002	0.754
BMI	1.066	1.051–1.081	< 0.001	1.063	1.037–1.090	< 0.001
HTN	1.588	1.452–1.736	< 0.001	1.117	0.956–1.305	0.164
DM	1.305	1.145–1.487	< 0.001	1.095	0.860–1.395	0.46
Pre-operative coronary angiography	1.421	1.313–1.553	< 0.001	0.826	0.717–0.952	0.08
Hb	1.004	1.001–1.007	< 0.001	0.997	0.993–1.001	0.093
WBC	1.019	1.002–1.042	< 0.001	0.990	0.958–1.022	0.533
Plt	0.996	0.996–0.997	0.633	0.997	0.996–0.998	0.601
Elevated RDW	1.497	1.419–1.578	< 0.001	1.192	1.126–1.262	< 0.001
BUN	1.178	1.147–1.193	< 0.001	1.036	0998–1.076	0.064
Scr	1.015	1.013–1.017	< 0.001	1.002	0.998–1.006	0.325
eGFR	0.989	0.987–0.991	0.002	0.999	0.996–1.002	0.004
UA	1.003	1.003–1.004	< 0.001	1.002	1.001–1.003	< 0.001
Alb	0.954	0.941–0.965	< 0.001	0.986	0.996–1.006	0.162
CPB time (every 30 min)	1.498	1.439–1.559	< 0.001	1.490	1.385–1.603	< 0.001
ACC time (every 20 min)	1.295	1.248–1.343	< 0.001	1.253	1.176–1.336	< 0.001

AKI acute kidney injury, *BMI* body mass index, *HTN* hypertension, *DM* diabetes mellitus, *Hb* hemoglobin, *WBC* white blood cell, *Plt* platelet, *RDW* red cell distribution width, *BUN* blood urea nitrogen, *Scr* serum creatinine, *eGFR* estimated glomerular filtration rate, *SUA* serum uric acid, *CPB* cardiopulmonary bypass, *ACC* Aortic cross-clamp

Bivariate correlation analyses of elevated RDW and various clinical and laboratory parameters of the study population in the unmatched cohort

The results of bivariate correlation analyses showed that there was a positive correlation between elevated RDW and age ($r = 0.188$, $P < 0.001$), HTN ($r = 0.080$, $P < 0.001$), DM ($r = 0.052$, $P < 0.001$), BUN($r = 0.039$, $P < 0.001$), CPB time ($r = 0.159$, $P < 0.001$), ACC time ($r = 0.136$, $P < 0.001$), AKI stage ($r = 0.171$, $P < 0.001$) and a negative correlation with male ($r = -0.096$, $P < 0.001$), BMI($r = -0.045$, $P = 0.01$), hemoglobin ($r = -0.147$, $P < 0.001$), Albumin ($r = -0.047$, $P < 0.001$), and eGFR ($r = -0.105$, $P < 0.001$) (see Table 4).

Table 3 Multivariate logistic regression analysis of risk factors for CS-AKI in the unmatched Cohort

	OR	*95% CI*	*P*-value
Age	1.036	1.029 1.042	< 0.001
Male	1.873	1.622–2.164	< 0.001
BMI	1.035	1.016–1.055	< 0.001
Elevated RDW	1.302	1.209–1.401	< 0.001
BUN	1.076	1.041–1.112	< 0.001
SUA	1.002	1.001–1.003	< 0.001
CPB time (every 30 min)	1.627	1.491–1.775	< 0.001

AKI acute kidney injury, *BMI* body mass index, *RDW* red cell distribution width, *BUN* blood urea nitrogen, *SUA* serum uric acid, *CPB* cardiopulmonary bypass

Propensity-matched cohort

Propensity score matching created a matched cohort of 1573 in each group. In this matched cohort, few differences remained in non-AKI and AKI groups (Table 1). The results of univariate logistic regression model are presented in Table 2. The odds ratios of CS-AKI in the matched cohort for the independent risk factors that were computed from the multivariate logistic regression model are shown in Table 5. In the matched cohort, the elevated RDW in AKI patients was higher than in patients without AKI (0.3% (0.0%, 0.7%) vs 0.5% (0.1, 1.1%), $P < 0.001$). The elevated RDW incidences were 0.4% (0.1%, 0.9%), 0.6% (0.2%, 1.1%) and 1.1% (0.3%, 2.1%) in stage 1, 2 and 3 AKI patients ($P < 0.001$). Among patients with CS-AKI, the level of elevated RDW in non-survivors was higher than in survivors [1.2% (0.5%, 2.3%) vs 0.5% (0.1%, 1.0%), $P < 0.001$] and a 0.1% increase in elevated RDW was associated with a 0.24% higher risk of within-hospital mortality in patients with CS-AKI.

Receiver-operating characteristic curve analysis for prediction of the development and prognosis of CS-AKI in the matched cohort by elevated red cell distribution width level

To assess discrimination of RDW for all causes of hospital mortality, we used receiver-operating characteristic (ROC) analysis and determined the area under the curve (AUC). The cut-off value of elevated RDW for predicting CS-AKI

Table 4 Bivariate correlation analyses of elevated RDW and various clinical and laboratory parameters of the study population in the umatched Cohort

	r	*P*-value
Age	0.188	< 0.001
Male	−0.096	< 0.001
BMI	−0.045	0.01
HTN	0.098	< 0.001
DM	0.052	< 0.001
Hb	−0.147	< 0.001
WBC	−0.010	0.292
Alb	−0.047	< 0.001
BUN	0.039	< 0.001
SCr	0.020	0.040
eGFR	−0.105	< 0.001
SUA	−0.010	0.292
CPB time	0.159	< 0.001
ACC time	0.136	< 0.001
AKI stage	0.171	< 0.001

BMI body mass index, *HTN* hypertension, *DM* diabetes mellitus, *Hb* hemoglobin, *WBC* white blood cell, *Alb* albumin, *BUN* blood urea nitrogen, *SCr* serum creatinine, *eGFR* estimated glomerular filtration rate, *SUA* serum uric acid, *CPB* cardiopulmonary bypass, *ACC* Aortic cross-clamp, *AKI* acute kidney injury

was 0.30%. The AUC value was 0.605 (95% CI: 0.586–0.625, $P < 0.001$) and the sensitivity, specificity, positive likelihood ratio and negative likelihood ratio of elevated RDW were 51.6%, 63.3%, 1.41 and 0.76, respectively.

Elevated RDW had moderate discriminative power for predicting the death of CS-AKI patients. The cut-off value of elevated RDW for predicting death of CS-AKI patients was 0.75%; AUC value 0.716 (95% CI: 0.640–0.764, $P < 0.001$) and the sensitivity, specificity, positive likelihood ratio and negative likelihood ratio of elevated RDW were 71.4%, 65.5%, 1.53 and 0.83, respectively.

Discussion

The main finding of the present study was the establishment of an independent association between elevated RDW and in-hospital mortality with CS-AKI. An elevated RDW remains a significant predictor for the severity and mortality of CS-AKI patients following multivariable adjustments. However, there was no clear evidence to show that the elevated RDW was a significant predictor for the development of CS-AKI and there was no significant effect modification between an elevated RDW and in-hospital mortality in those patients without CS-AKI.

Table 5 Multivariate logistic regression analysis of risk factors for CS-AKI in the matched Cohort

	OR	*95% CI*	*P*-value
BMI	1.078	1.046–1.111	< 0.001
Elevated RDW	1.159	1.074–1.251	< 0.001
eGFR	1.006	1.001–1.010	0.015
SUA	1.002	1.001–1.003	< 0.001
CPB time (every 30 min)	1.493	1.363–1.635	< 0.001

AKI acute kidney injury, *BMI* body mass index, *RDW* red cell distribution width, *eGFR* estimated glomerular filtration rate, *SUA* serum uric acid, *CPB* cardiopulmonary bypass

A previous study showed that RDW is a strong and independent prognostic predictor of mortality and morbidity in patients with CKD, which described RDW changes in CKD patients undergoing hemodialysis for the first time [12]. Recent research indicates that a higher RDW was independently associated with increased cardiovascular disease (CVD) mortality in peritoneal dialysis (PD) and in end stage renal disease (ESRD) patients [13, 14]. Mario Sičaja et al. found that for each 1% point increase in the RDW level the one-year all cause mortality risk was increased by 54% in patients requiring chronic dialysis [15].

Recent clinical research on RDW and AKI have focused on RDW and contrast-induced AKI in percutaneous coronary interventions (CI-AKI). The results showed that RDW has become a recent target of investigations into new predictors of kidney function and mortality after percutaneous coronary interventions (PCI) [2, 16–18]. The study by Atsushi Mizuno et al. analyzed 102 patients with ST-elevation myocardial infarction and found that RDW was an independent variable predicting CI-AKI and has additional value to the Mehran risk score for predicting contrast-induced (CI)-AKI [19]. Other researchers have investigated the association between RDW and CI-AKI and suggested that RDW was associated independently with the development of CI-AKI and may well be a useful marker in CI-AKI risk stratification [16, 20].

To the best of our knowledge, our study is the first research in the literature that has explored the association between elevated RDW and CS-AKI. However, it needs more research to establish an association between elevated RDW and CS-AKI incidence. The mechanisms underlying the association between higher RDW and poor prognosis have not been clearly determined. Several possible explanations can be considered in cardiac surgery patients. Hemolysis, blood loss, hypothermia, ischemia, and perfusion injury as well as neutrophil activation during CPB play a pivotal role in oxidative stress and the associated activation of inflammation. In particular, ischemia and reperfusion injury during cardiac surgery can lead to the generation of pro-inflammatory mediators [21–24]. In our research, the results of bivariate correlation analyses showed that there was a positive correlation between elevated RDW and the CPB and ACC times. Inflammation may play a role in the regulation of RDW by direct myelo-suppression of erythroid precursors, decreasing erythropoietin production, reducing the bioavailability of iron and by promoting erythropoietin resistance and red cell apoptosis [25–29].

Related research [30–34] has demonstrated that oxidative stress increases anisocytosis by disrupting erythropoiesis and altering blood cell membrane deformability and thus the red blood cell circulation lifetime, ultimately leading to an increase in RDW. In addition, during CPB, ischemia and reperfusion play a pivotal role in oxidative stress by initiating a series of biochemical events [22]. However, in our study, we were not able to adjust the analysis to include inflammatory markers, C-reactive protein (CRP) and other factors, as these were not routinely measured at patient admission.

The renin-angiotensin-aldosterone system (RAAS) is activated by arterial underfilling caused by CPB, heart failure, shock and so on after cardiac surgery. The activation of the RAAS system and adrenergic hormone release could cause increased RDW with erythropoiesis, resulting in a poor prognosis [34]. There is evidence suggesting that angiotensin II acts as a growth factor for erythroid precursors as well as an erythropoietin secretagogue resulting in an increment in RDW due to macrocytosis from skipped cell divisions [35].

RDW is increased in conditions such as malnutrition and deficiencies such as in vitamin B12 [36], iron [37] or folic acid [38], increased red cell destruction (such as hemolysis), or after blood transfusion. Previous research has reported that RDW was correlated negatively with nutrition in heart failure [39] and HD patients [13]. This latter study showed that elevated RDW was negatively correlated with the albumin level. Patients with malnutrition have a higher risk of infection and adverse outcomes and elevated RDW and poor prognosis may relate to the fact that there is an interaction between malnutrition and inflammation.

The present research work has several limitations. First, it was a retrospective design from a single central pool of patients. Second, we did not measure hematopoietic factors (including iron, vitamin B12, folate, etc.) that may influence RDW. Third, though neurohumoral activation and inflammation may be a mechanistic link between elevated RDW and poor outcomes, we did not assess laboratory markers including CRP, other pro-inflammatory cytokines, norepinephrine and angiotensin II. Despite these limitations, a major strength of the present study is that it had a sufficient number of patients undergoing cardiac surgery to ensure adequate reliability of our incidence and mortality estimates. Future studies of a larger cohort of single center pool patients will be required to confirm the results of the present investigation.

Conclusion

The results of the present study suggest, that an elevated RDW might be an independent prognostic factor for the severity and poor prognosis of CS-AKI.

Abbreviations

ACC: Aortic cross-clamp; AKI: Acute kidney injury; AUC: Area under the curve; BMI: Body mass index; BUN: Blood urea nitrogen; CI-AKI: AKI in percutaneous coronary interventions; COPD: Chronic obstructive pulmonary disease; CPB: Cardiopulmonary bypass; CRP: C-reactive protein; CS-AKI: AKI in patients undergoing cardiac surgery; CVD: Cardiovascular disease; DM: Diabetes mellitus; eGFR: Estimated glomerular filtration rate; ESRD: End stage renal disease; IQR: Interquartile range; KDIGO: Kidney Disease Improving Global Outcomes; LOS: Length-of-stay; MCV: Mean corpuscular volume; ORs: Odds ratios; PCI: Percutaneous coronary interventions; PD: Peritoneal dialysis; RAAS: Renin-angiotensin-aldosterone system; RDW: Red cell distribution width; ROC: Receiver-operating characteristic; RRT: Renal replacement therapy; Scr: Serum creatinine; SUA: Serum uric acid; WBC: White blood cells

Funding

The work was supported by The Project of Shanghai Municipal Commission of Health and Family Planning [grant number 15GWZK0502]; The Projects of Science and Technology Commission of Shanghai Municipality [grant number 14DZ2260200]; The Project of Shanghai Key Laboratory of Kidney and Blood Purification [grant number 17140902300].

Authors' contributions

ZZ, YZ, LL, JT and XD were responsible for the conception and design of the study. ZZ, YZ, LL, BS, JX, WJ, ZL and JT were responsible for acquisition and analysis of data; furthermore, ZZ, BS, JX, WJ and ZL were in charge of statistical analysis. ZZ, YZ and LL drafted the manuscript; JT, CW and XD revised and commented the draft. All authors read and approved the final version of the manuscript.

Competing interests

The authors declare that they have no competing interests.

Author details

[1]Department of Nephrology, Zhongshan Hospital, Shanghai Medical College, Fudan University, No 180 Fenglin Road, Shanghai 200032, China. [2]Shanghai Medical Center of Kidney, No 180 Fenglin Road, Shanghai 200032, China. [3]Shanghai Institute for Kidney and Dialysis, No 180 Fenglin Road, Shanghai 200032, China. [4]Shanghai Key Laboratory of Kidney and Blood Purification, No 180 Fenglin Road, Shanghai 200032, China. [5]Department of Critical Care Medicine, Zhongshan Hospital, Shanghai Medical College, Fudan University, No 180 Fenglin Road, Shanghai 200032, China. [6]Hemodialysis Quality of Control Center of Shanghai, No 180 Fenglin Road, Shanghai 200032, China. [7]Department of Nephrology, Xiamen Branch, Zhongshan Hospital, Fudan University, No 668 Jinhu Road, Xiamen 361015, Fujian, China. [8]Department of Cardiovascular Surgery, Zhongshan Hospital, Shanghai Medical College, Fudan University, No 180 Fenglin Road, Shanghai 200032, China.

References

1. Demir A, Yarali N, Fisgin T, Duru F, Kara A. Most reliable indices in differentiation between thalassemia trait and iron deficiency anemia. Pediatrics international : official journal of the Japan Pediatric Society. 2002; 44(6):612–6.
2. Sun XP, Chen WM, Sun ZJ, Ding XS, Gao XY, Liang SW, et al. Impact of red blood cell distribution width on long-term mortality in patients with ST-elevation myocardial infarction. Cardiology. 2014;128(4):343–8.
3. Pascual-Figal DA, Bonaque JC, Manzano-Fernandez S, Fernandez A, Garrido IP, Pastor-Perez F, et al. Red blood cell distribution width predicts new-onset anemia in heart failure patients. Int J Cardiol. 2012;160(3):196–200.
4. Liu T, Shao Q, Miao S, Liu E, Xu G, Yuan R, et al. Red cell distribution width as a novel, inexpensive marker for paroxysmal atrial fibrillation. Int J Cardiol. 2014;171(2):e52–3.
5. Zhao K, Li YJ, Gao S. Role of red blood cell distribution in predicting drug-eluting stent restenosis in patients with stable angina pectoris after coronary stenting. Coron Artery Dis. 2015;26(3):220–4.
6. Wang H, Xu H, Wang X, Wu R, Gao X, Jin Q, et al. Red blood cell distribution width to platelet ratio is related to histologic severity of primary biliary cirrhosis. Medicine. 2016;95(11):e3114.

7. Karagoz E, Tanoglu A, Ulcay A, Erdem H, Turhan V, Kara M, et al. Mean platelet volume and red cell distribution width to platelet ratio for predicting the severity of hepatic fibrosis in patients with chronic hepatitis C. Eur J Gastroenterol Hepatol. 2016;28(7):744–8.
8. Zorlu A, Bektasoglu G, Guven FM, Dogan OT, Gucuk E, Ege MR, et al. Usefulness of admission red cell distribution width as a predictor of early mortality in patients with acute pulmonary embolism. Am J Cardiol. 2012; 109(1):128–34.
9. Tertemiz KC, Ozgen Alpaydin A, Sevinc C, Ellidokuz H, Acara AC, Cimrin A. Could "red cell distribution width" predict COPD severity? Rev Port Pneumol. 2016;22(4):196–201.
10. AHRQ. KDIGO clinical practice guideline for acute kidney injury. Kidney Int Suppl. 2012;2:1–138.
11. Zou Z, Zhuang Y, Liu L, Shen B, Xu J, Luo Z, et al. Role of body mass index in acute kidney injury patients after cardiac surgery. Cardiorenal Med. 2017; 8(1):9–17.
12. Docci D, Delvecchio C, Gollini C, Turci F, Baldrati L, Gilli P. Red blood cell volume distribution width (RDW) in uraemic patients on chronic haemodialysis. The International journal of artificial organs. 1989;12(3):170–4.
13. Peng F, Li Z, Zhong Z, Luo Q, Guo Q, Huang F, et al. An increasing of red blood cell distribution width was associated with cardiovascular mortality in patients on peritoneal dialysis. Int J Cardiol. 2014;176(3):1379–81.
14. Yoon HE, Kim SJ, Hwang HS, Chung S, Yang CW, Shin SJ. Progressive rise in red blood cell distribution width predicts mortality and cardiovascular events in end-stage renal disease patients. PLoS One. 2015;10(5):e0126272.
15. Sicaja M, Pehar M, Derek L, Starcevic B, Vuletic V, Romic Z, et al. Red blood cell distribution width as a prognostic marker of mortality in patients on chronic dialysis: a single center, prospective longitudinal study. Croatian medical journal. 2013;54(1):25–32.
16. Kurtul A, Yarlioglues M, Murat SN, Demircelik MB, Acikgoz SK, Ergun G, et al. Red cell distribution width predicts contrast-induced nephropathy in patients undergoing percutaneous coronary intervention for acute coronary syndrome. Angiology. 2015;66(5):433–40.
17. Yao HM, Sun TW, Zhang XJ, Shen DL, Du YY, Wan YD, et al. Red blood cell distribution width and long-term outcome in patients undergoing percutaneous coronary intervention in the drug-eluting stenting era: a two-year cohort study. PLoS One. 2014;9(4):e94887.
18. Dabbah S, Hammerman H, Markiewicz W, Aronson D. Relation between red cell distribution width and clinical outcomes after acute myocardial infarction. Am J Cardiol. 2010;105(3):312–7.
19. Mizuno A, Ohde S, Nishizaki Y, Komatsu Y, Niwa K. Additional value of the red blood cell distribution width to the Mehran risk score for predicting contrast-induced acute kidney injury in patients with ST-elevation acute myocardial infarction. J Cardiol. 2015;66(1):41–5.
20. Akin F, Celik O, Altun I, Ayca B, Ozturk D, Satilmis S, et al. Relation of red cell distribution width to contrast-induced acute kidney injury in patients undergoing a primary percutaneous coronary intervention. Coron Artery Dis. 2015;26(4):289–95.
21. Pearson TA, Mensah GA, Alexander RW, Anderson JL, Cannon RO 3rd, Criqui M, et al. Markers of inflammation and cardiovascular disease: application to clinical and public health practice: a statement for healthcare professionals from the Centers for Disease Control and Prevention and the American Heart Association. Circulation. 2003;107(3):499–511.
22. Zakkar M, Guida G, Suleiman MS, Angelini GD. Cardiopulmonary bypass and oxidative stress. Oxidative Med Cell Longev. 2015;2015:189863.
23. Laffey JG, Boylan JF, Cheng DC. The systemic inflammatory response to cardiac surgery: implications for the anesthesiologist. Anesthesiology. 2002; 97(1):215–52.
24. Christen S, Finckh B, Lykkesfeldt J, Gessler P, Frese-Schaper M, Nielsen P, et al. Oxidative stress precedes peak systemic inflammatory response in pediatric patients undergoing cardiopulmonary bypass operation. Free Radic Biol Med. 2005;38(10):1323–32.
25. Pierce CN, Larson DF. Inflammatory cytokine inhibition of erythropoiesis in patients implanted with a mechanical circulatory assist device. Perfusion. 2005;20(2):83–90.
26. Scharte M, Fink MP. Red blood cell physiology in critical illness. Crit Care Med. 2003;31(12 Suppl):S651–7.
27. Ghali JK. Anemia and heart failure. Curr Opin Cardiol. 2009;24(2):172–8.
28. Laftah AH, Sharma N, Brookes MJ, McKie AT, Simpson RJ, Iqbal TH, et al. Tumour necrosis factor alpha causes hypoferraemia and reduced intestinal iron absorption in mice. The Biochemical journal. 2006;397(1):61–7.
29. Purtle SW, Moromizato T, McKane CK, Gibbons FK, Christopher KB. The association of red cell distribution width at hospital discharge and out-of-hospital mortality following critical illness*. Crit Care Med. 2014;42(4):918–29.
30. Patel KV, Ferrucci L, Ershler WB, Longo DL, Guralnik JM. Red blood cell distribution width and the risk of death in middle-aged and older adults. Arch Intern Med. 2009;169(5):515–23.
31. Perlstein TS, Weuve J, Pfeffer MA, Beckman JA. Red blood cell distribution width and mortality risk in a community-based prospective cohort. Arch Intern Med. 2009;169(6):588–94.
32. Weiss G, Goodnough LT. Anemia of chronic disease. N Engl J Med. 2005; 352(10):1011–23.
33. Hunziker S, Celi LA, Lee J, Howell MD. Red cell distribution width improves the simplified acute physiology score for risk prediction in unselected critically ill patients. Crit Care. 2012;16(3):R89.
34. Park TS, Zambidis ET. A role for the renin-angiotensin system in hematopoiesis. Haematologica. 2009;94(6):745–7.
35. Vlahakos DV, Marathias KP, Madias NE. The role of the renin-angiotensin system in the regulation of erythropoiesis. American journal of kidney diseases : the official journal of the National Kidney Foundation. 2010;56(3):558–65.
36. Pongstaporn W, Bunyaratavej A. Hematological parameters, ferritin and vitamin B12 in vegetarians. J Med Assoc Thail. 1999;82(3):304–11.
37. Morgan DL, Peck SD. The use of red cell distribution width in the detection of iron deficiency in chronic hemodialysis patients. Am J Clin Pathol. 1988; 89(4):513–5.
38. Kaskel FJ, Bamgbola OF. Validation of a composite scoring scheme in the diagnosis of folate deficiency in a pediatric and adolescent dialysis cohort. Journal of renal nutrition : the official journal of the Council on Renal Nutrition of the National Kidney Foundation. 2008;18(5):430–9.
39. Forhecz Z, Gombos T, Borgulya G, Pozsonyi Z, Prohaszka Z, Janoskuti L. Red cell distribution width in heart failure: prediction of clinical events and relationship with markers of ineffective erythropoiesis, inflammation, renal function, and nutritional state. Am Heart J. 2009;158(4):659–66.

18

Implantation of cardiac resynchronization therapy pacemaker via the coronary sinus in a patient with triple valve replacement

Cheng Zheng[1], Wei-Qian Lin[1], Yuan-Zheng Lin[1], Hao Lian[1], Zhi-Rui Liu[1], Jia-Hui Chen[2] and Jia-Feng Lin[1*]

Abstract

Background: In patients with triple valve replacement developing third-degree atrioventricular block (AVB), the most appropriate approach for permanent pacemaker implantation remains questionable.

Case presentation: In this case presentation, we first described the approach of implantation of the cardiac resynchronization therapy pacemaker (CRT-P) via one bipolar pacing lead in middle cardiac vein (MCV) and one quadripolar pacing lead in anterior interventricular vein (AIV) in a patient developing complete AVB, who had been previously diagnosed with rheumatic valvular heart disease with triple valve replaced. After the CRT-P implantation, the two pacing leads in coronary sinus (CS) provided a dual-site ventricular pacing from the anterior septum and posterior septum, which resulted in a narrow QRS complex and an increased ventricular synchrony. During the long-term follow-up, no deterioration of heart function was documented and pacing parameters remained good.

Conclusion: In this patient developing complete AVB with triple valve replaced, our approach of CRT-P implantation provides an effective and reliable ventricular pacing, and is an alternative option when transvenous right ventricular pacing, transseptal left ventricular pacing and transpericardial epicardium pacing are not possible. Further prospective randomized trials are required to confirm the efficiency of our approach of dual-site ventricular pacing by CRT-P in this kind patients.

Keywords: Cardiac resynchronization therapy pacemaker, Triple valve replacement, Narrow QRS duration, Ventricular synchrony

Background

In rheumatic heart disease patients with triple mechanical valve replacement and complete atrioventricular block (AVB), the most appropriate and beneficial method of pacemaker implantation remains questionable. With the tricuspid mechanical valve replaced, endocardial pacing of the right ventricle is not possible because such a manipulation may cause disastrous damage to the prosthetic valve [1]. In addition, left ventricular endocardial pacing via the atrial septum puncture was contraindicated due to the replacement of the mitral mechanical valve [2]. Epicardial pacing was also limited because of rheumatic pericardial adhesion and unsatisfying pacing parameters [3]. In this kind patients, a single lead in the coronary sinus (CS) to pace the left ventricle has been reported [3–5], however, it may lead ventricular dyssynchronization, and in the event of CS lead dislodgement or malfunction, the underlying complete AVB could be life-threatening. Here, we presented a case where we applied dual-site ventricular pacing by cardiac resynchronization therapy pacemaker (CRT-P) implantation, with one bipolar pacing lead in the middle cardiac vein (MCV) and one quadripolar pacing lead in the anterior interventricular vein (AIV)

* Correspondence: linjiafeng_wzmcfey@163.com
[1]Department of Cardiology, Second Affiliated Hospital and Yuying Children's Hospital of Wenzhou Medical University, 109 Xueyuan Road, Wenzhou, Zhejiang 325000, China
Full list of author information is available at the end of the article

to simultaneously stimulate the ventricle in a patient with triple valve replacement.

Case presentation

A 42-year-old woman with a history of rheumatic valvular heart disease and permanent atrial fibrillation underwent open triple valvotomy 14 years ago and routinely took the warfarin to anti-coagulate since then. The international normalized ratio of prothrombin time (PT-INR) was monitored every 2 weeks to keep it range between 2.5 and 3.5 s. She complained of persistent abdominal distension and repeated exertional dyspnea for 2 years at admission. Physical examination showed obvious body signs of right heart failure, including jugular vein distention, lower limb pitting edema. The 12-lead surface ECG showed atrial fibrillation rhythm with narrow QRS complex. The transthoracic echocardiography indicated a normal ventricular size of 35 mm with left ventricular ejection fraction (LVEF) of 65% and a moderate stenosis of tricuspid valve with the pressure gradient across the tricuspid valve of 8 mmHg. Laboratory examination revealed the NT-pro-BNP of 1780 ng/ml. Due to progression of heart failure from her valvular heart disease, she underwent tricuspid valve replacement again (Medtronic bileaflet prosthesis). On the second day after surgery, the patient developed sudden cardiac arrest with bedside electrocardiographic monitor recording atrial fibrillation, complete third-degree AVB with repeated episodes of torsade de point secondary to the long QT interval (0.6 s). Thus, a permanent pacemaker was required to oppose this malignant arrhythmia.

After taking full consideration of the patient's basic situations, the CRT-P implantation via two pacing leads in cardiac venous system to provide dual-site ventricular pacing was primarily planned. As the patient with triple mechanical valve replaced had a relatively higher risk for thrombosis, the oral warfarin was not interrupted before operation. The instant blood test prior to operation showed a PT-INR of 2.42 s. The intravenous unfractionated heparin was used during the procedure to keep an activated clotting time (ACT) range between 250 and 300 s. Electric surgical knives were applied to stop bleeding of the incision during the whole procedure. A guiding catheter was delivered via left subclavian vein puncture to access the coronary sinus ostium, which was located between the inferior vena cava and the mechanical tricuspid valve on the inferior aspect of the atrial septum. A retrograde occlusion venogram was then performed to evaluate the anatomy of the cardiac venous system. As the lateral cardiac vein was too thin and the posterolateral vein was too tortuous for pacing leads to access, the MCV and the AIV were selected as target vessels for pacing leads placement. A quadripolar pacing lead (Quartet LV lead model 1458Q, St Jude Medical) was introduced into the AIV, while bipolar pacing lead (Quick Flex μ model 1258 T, St Jude Medical) into the MCV, both leads were secured to the pectoral muscle fascia and attached to a CRT-P (Allure Quadra™ CRT-P, St Jude Medical), Fig. 1. For the patient was in the permanent atrial fibrillation rhythm, the atrial lead placement was abandoned due to the inability to achieve an atrioventricular synchrony. The pacing rate was initially set at 100 bpm in a VVI pacing mode (ventricle paced, ventricle sensed, pacing is inhibited if beat is sensed). By the procedure of pacing interval optimization between the two pacing leads, we obtained a relatively narrowest QRS duration of 116 ms among all bipolar and unipolar pacing configurations, using the vector from the proximal tip (P4) of quadripolar lead to the coil of bipolar lead in MCV, vector P4–MCV coil, Fig. 2 and Table 1. At the beginning of the pacemaker implantation, the quadripolar lead paced with a capture threshold of 1.75 V at 1.0 ms pulse width with an impedance

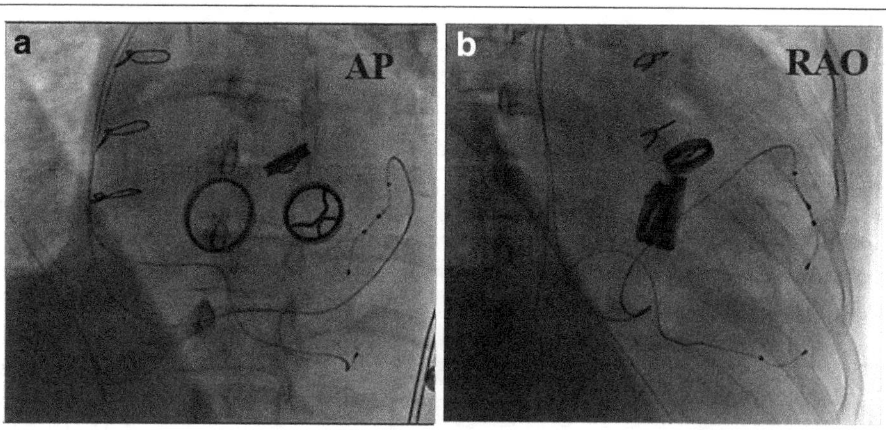

Fig. 1 A quadripolar pacing lead (Quartet LV lead model 1458Q, StJude Medical) was introduced into anterior interventricular vein (AIV), while a bipolar pacing lead (QuickFlex μ model 1258 T, St Jude Medical) into middle cardiac vein (MCV). **a**. Anteroposterior position. **b**. Right anterior oblique position

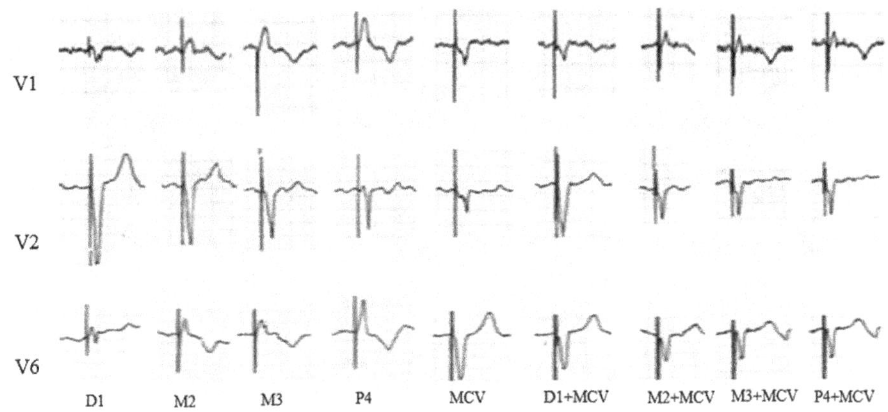

Fig. 2 The procedure of pacing interval optimization between the two pace leads

of 430 Ω, while the bipolar lead paced with a capture threshold of 1.5 V at 1.0 ms pulse width with an impedance of 600 Ω, using the vector P4–MCV coil. After the operation, the compression of pacemaker pocket with elastic bandage was immediately performed and removed after 48 h, no pocket hematoma and other bleedings was found, the PT-INR was measured of 2.28 s 24 h later. The left ventricular systolic function was evaluated with Simpsons method by transthoracic echocardiography within the first 24 h after pacemaker implantation. The ventricular dual-site pacing exhibited an obvious acute hemodynamic improvement over single-site pacing (LVEF: ventricular dual-site pacing 71.5 ± 0.96% vs ventricular single-site pacing 62.9 ± 2.38%), and the best left ventricular systolic function was obtained by ventricular dual-site pacing of P4 combined with MCV, Table 2. A remarkable decline in pacing threshold of both leads was found 2 months later, the quadripolar lead paced with a capture threshold of 0.75 V at 0.5 ms pulse width with an impedance of 490 Ω while the bipolar lead paced with a capture threshold of 1.25 V at 0.8 ms pulse width with an impedance of 550 Ω using the vector P4–MCV coil. During one-year follow-up, the patient was VVI pacing mode dependent with an intrinsic heart rhythm of atrial fibrillation with complete AVB. She did not present deteriorations of heart function in transthoracic echocardiography (LVEDD 40 mm, LVEF 75.4%, see Fig. 3) with 6-min walking test recording a walking distance more than 450 m, meanwhile, CRT programming control showed good pacing parameters all the time.

Discussion

In this case, we first described the method of implantation of CRT-P with two pacing leads in coronary venous system, which provided an effective dual-site ventricular pacing in a patient developing complete atrioventricular block after triple mechanical valves replacement.

In this patient, as the mechanical tricuspid and mitral valves implanted, placing pacing lead in right ventricular endocardium across the tricuspid valve was forbidden because of underlying risk of valve damage and failure, in addition, delivering pacing lead to left ventricular endocardium via the atrial septum puncture was also contraindicated due to the potential damage to the mitral valve [1, 2]. The method of placing an epicardial pacing lead via the thoracotomy was technically challenging, because of severe pericardial adhesion caused by the rheumatic heart disease and previous surgery in this patient, meanwhile, in such a situation, long-term epicardial pacing tended to be unreliable with high pacing thresholds [3]. The method of the coronary sinus single-site ventricular pacing was also taken into consideration [4]. Recently, a retrospective clinical study reported that in patients with tricuspid valvular replacement, coronary sinus single-site left ventricular pacing was a feasible alternative to right apical ventricular pacing. However, this study also revealed that long-term coronary sinus single-site pacing resulted in an inferior left ventricular systolic function compared with standard cardiac resynchronization therapy, in addition, in their study, a patient of long-term coronary sinus single-site ventricular pacing was found developing pacing-induced cardiomyopathy with progressive decline in LVEF [5]. Moreover, in this patient of complete AVB, if single pacing lead in coronary sinus was selected, in the event of coronary sinus lead

Table 1 QRS duration produced by pacing interval optimization

Vector	D1	M2	M3	P4	MCV	D1 + MCV	M2 + MCV	M3 + MCV	P4 + MCV	Basic
QRS (ms)	128	126	124	123	134	126	122	120	116	120

Table 2 Left ventricular systolic ejection fraction produced by different pacing sites

Pacing site	D1	M2	M3	P4	MCV	D1 + MCV	M2 + MCV	M3 + MCV	P4 + MCV	basic
Ejection (%)	64.3	58.8	64.4	64.2	62.9	72.2	70.4	71.0	72.4	55

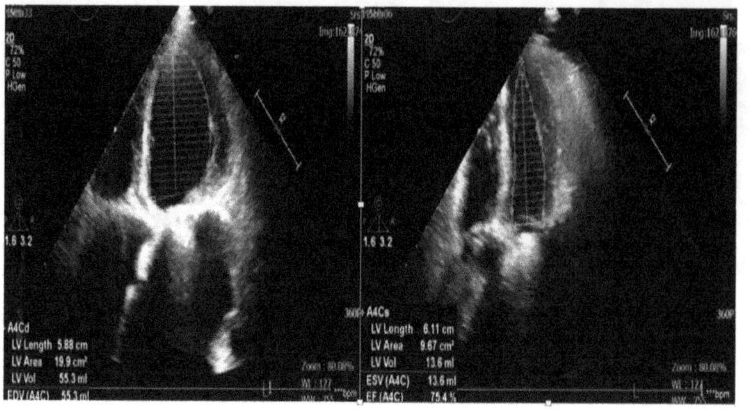

Fig. 3 Systolic heart function evaluated by Simpsons method

dislodgement or malfunction, the underlying complete AVB could be life-threatening. Based on these considerations, the idea of CS single-site pacing was abandoned. The outcomes of BLOCK-HF research indicated that the superior long-term clinical and functional benefit of dual-site ventricular pacing in patients with AV block and mild/moderate heart dysfunction compared with single-site ventricular pacing [6]. Thus, in this patient, after full consideration, the dual-site ventricular pacing via coronary sinus method was primarily chosen. Different from classical cardiac resynchronization therapy with dual-site pacing (LV free wall pacing from the coronary venous system in conjunction with RV apical pacing), in this patient, we performed dual-site ventricular pacing via coronary sinus by implantation of CRT-P with one bipolar lead in the MCV and one quadripolar lead in the AIV, which provided an anterior ventricular wall pacing in conjunction with a posterior ventricular wall pacing. By our method of ventricular dual-site pacing in coronary sinus, increased ventricular electrical and mechanical synchronization was obtained, long-term follow up also showed a good clinical outcome. However, before our approach of dual-site CS pacing can be recommended to more patients, a prospective study is needed to prove this preliminary finding.

In this patient, due to a relatively higher thrombotic risk associated with triple mechanical valve replacement, the oral anticoagulant therapy of warfarin was not interrupted and a bridging therapy with low-molecular-weight heparin (LMWH) was not initiated. Though this protocol was some different from the standard anticoagulation protocol at the time of pacemaker implantation, which required stopping oral anticoagulation therapy and initiating a bridging therapy with subcutaneous LMWH, no pocket hematoma and thromboembolic events was found in this patient. Our observation further confirmed the safety of anticoagulation protocol proposed by the POCKET study [7].

Conclusions

CRT-P implantation with two pacing leads in coronary sinus can provide an effective and reliable dual-site ventricular pacing. Further prospective randomized trials are required to confirm the efficiency of our approach of dual-site ventricular pacing by CRT-P.

Abbreviations

ACT: Activated clotting time; AIV: Anterior interventricular vein; AVB: Atrioventricular block; CRT-P: Cardiac resynchronization therapy pacemaker; CS: Coronary sinus; LMWH: Low-molecular-weight heparin; LVEDD: Left ventricular end diastolic diameter; LVEF: Left ventricular ejection fraction; MCV: Middle cardiac vein; PT-INR: International normalized ratio of prothrombin time; VVI: ventricle paced, ventricle sensed, pacing is inhibited if beat is sensed

Acknowledgements

None.

Funding

This case presentation is supported by Zhejiang Provincial Public Technology Application Research Project (Grant No. 2016C33181).

Authors' contributions

ZC, LWQ, LYZ, LH, LZR, CJH and LJF collected, analyzed and interpreted the data, ZC and LJF performed the operation and drafted the article. CJF revised written English of the article. All authors have seen and approved the final version of the manuscript being submitted. The article is the authors' original work, hasn't received prior publication and isn't under consideration for publication elsewhere.

Competing interests

The authors declare that they have no competing interests.

Author details

[1]Department of Cardiology, Second Affiliated Hospital and Yuying Children's Hospital of Wenzhou Medical University, 109 Xueyuan Road, Wenzhou, Zhejiang 325000, China. [2]Department of Cardiology, Taishun general hospital, Wenzhou 325000, China.

References

1. Lee ME. Special considerations in ventricular pacing in patients with tricuspid valve disease. Ann Thorac Surg. 1983;36(1):89–92.
2. Bracke FA, van Gelder BM, Dekker LR, Houthuizen P, Ter Woorst JF, Teijink JA. Left ventricular endocardial pacing in cardiac resynchronisation therapy: moving from bench to bedside. Neth Heart J. 2012;20(3):118–24.
3. Vijayakumar M, Kamath P, Pai PG. Permanent pacing in a patient with tricuspid prosthesis-widening therapeutic use of coronary sinus. Indian Heart J. 2013;65(5):611–3.
4. Sideris S, Drakopoulou M, Oikonomopoulos G, Gatzoulis K, Stavropoulos G, Limperiadis D, Toutouzas K, Tousoulis D, Kallikazaros I. Left ventricular pacing through coronary sinus is feasible and safe for patients with prior tricuspid valve intervention. Pacing Clin Electrophysiol. 2016;39(4):378–81.
5. Noheria A, van Zyl M, Scott LR, Srivathsan K, Madhavan M, Asirvatham SJ, McLeod CJ. Single-site ventricular pacing via the coronary sinus in patients with tricuspid valve disease. Europace. 2017. Epub ahead of print.
6. Goldschmidt H. Biventricular pacing for atrioventricular block and systolic dysfunction. N Engl J Med. 2013;369(6):578–9.
7. Malagu M, Trevisan F, Scalone A, Marcantoni L, Sammarco G, Bertini M. Frequency of "pocket" hematoma in patients receiving vitamin K antagonist and antiplatelet therapy at the time of pacemaker or cardioverter defibrillator implantation (from the POCKET study). Am J Cardiol. 2017; 119(7):1036–40.

19

Meta-analysis and systematic review of intravascular ultrasound versus angiography-guided drug eluting stent implantation in left main coronary disease in 4592 patients

Yue Wang[1], Gary S. Mintz[2], Zhichun Gu[3], Yue Qi[4], Yue Wang[1], Mengru Liu[1] and Xiaofan Wu[1*]

Abstract

Background: Although several meta-analyses have demonstrated the utility of intravascular ultrasound (IVUS) in guiding drug-eluting stent (DES) implantation compared to angiography-guidance, there has been a dearth of evidence in the left main coronary artery (LMCA) lesion subset.

Methods: We performed a meta-analysis to compare clinical outcomes of IVUS versus conventional angiography guidance during implantation of DES for patients with LMCA disease. Pubmed, Cochrane Library, Embase were searched.

Results: A total of 1002 publications were reviewed; and finally, seven clinical studies - one prospective randomized controlled trial and six observational studies with 4592 patients (1907 IVUS-guided and 2685 angiography-guided) - were included in the meta-analysis. IVUS guidance was associated with a significant reduction in major adverse cardiac events (relative ratio [RR] 95% CI 0.61; 95% confidence interval [CI] 0.53 to 0.70; $P < 0.001$), all-cause death (RR 0.55; 95% CI 0.42 to 0.71; $P < 0.001$), cardiac death (RR 0.45; 95% CI 0.32 to 0.62; $P < 0.001$), myocardial infarction (RR 0.66; 95% CI 0.55 to 0.80; $P < 0.001$), and stent thrombosis (RR 0.48; 95% CI 0.27 to 0.84; $P = 0.01$) compared with angiographic guidance. However, there was no significant difference regarding target lesion revascularization (RR 0.60; 95% CI 0.31 to 1.18; $P = 0.099$) and target vessel revascularization (RR 0.64; 95% CI 0.26 to 1.56; $P = 0.322$).

Conclusions: Compared to angiographic guidance, IVUS-guided DES implantation was associated with better clinical outcomes for patients with LMCA lesions, especially hard endpoints of death, myocardial infarction, and stent thrombosis.

Keywords: Intravascular ultrasound, Angiography, Drug eluting stent, Left main disease, Meta-analysis

Background

Intravascular ultrasound (IVUS) has played a key role in contemporary stent-based percutaneous coronary interventions (PCI) by providing more detailed coronary anatomic information, assessing plaque burden accurately, selecting proper stent sizes, and optimizing stent expansion, apposition, and geographic miss [1–5]. One meta-analysis of seven randomized trials in the bare metal stent era [6] and seven meta-analyses including both registries and randomized studies [7–13] in the drug-eluting stent (DES) era concluded that IVUS guidance improved patient outcomes compared to angiography guidance alone. However, and with one exception, these previously published meta-analyses did not address stent implantation to treat the subset of patients who present for PCI of left main coronary artery (LMCA) lesions; and there is increased interest in PCI intervention for LMCA disease since the results of two randomized DES versus bypass surgery studies – EXCEL and NOBLE – were recently presented [14, 15]. Therefore, we performed the

* Correspondence: drwuxf@163.com
[1]Department of Cardiology, Beijing Anzhen Hospital, Capital Medical University, Beijing 100029, China
Full list of author information is available at the end of the article

current meta-analysis of published studies comparing IVUS-guided versus angiography-guided DES implantation to treat LMCA lesions.

Methods

Data sources and search strategy

A computerized search was performed of Pubmed, Cochrane Library, Embase from January 1993 to October 2017. Mesh and combinations of the following terms were used in the search process: "ultrasonography, intravascular," "intravascular ultrasound," "intravascular ultrasound-guided," "IVUS," "IVUS-guided," "angiography," "angiography-guided," "left main coronary artery," "left main coronary stenosis," "left main coronary disease," "left main," "left main lesion," "LMCA," "drug-eluting stent," "sirolimus-eluting stent," "paclitaxel-eluting stent," "everolimus-eluting stent," "zotarolimus-eluting stent," "stent," and "DES." Two investigators (Yue Wang* and Yue Qi) independently screened the titles and abstracts and eventually examined the full texts of the original reports included in the study. Additional searches for potential studies were performed by reviewing the references of earlier meta-analyses concerning IVUS versus angiography-guided DES implantation. Complete data were retrieved from the studies for quantitative synthesis. In addition, studies with incomplete information - including abstracts of major meetings (Transcatheter Cardiovascular Therapeutics [TCT], Angioplasty Summit, American Heart Association [AHA], American College of Cardiology [ACC], EuroPCR, and World Congress of Cardiology [WCC]) and studies of IVUS versus angiography-guided DES implantation that included a *subgroup* of LMCA patients - were reviewed for other potentially relevant citations.

Selection criteria

Final inclusion of studies was based on the agreement of both reviewers. Randomized control trials (RCTs) and observational studies in English language were considered while studies in the non-English language literature were not included. Studies met the following pre-specified criteria: 1) clinical studies published in peer-reviewed journals with fully available data; 2) studies that included a comparison of IVUS-guided versus angiography-guided PCI with DES in LMCA lesions; and 3) follow up time of at least 12 months. Reports of mixed treatment with bare-metal stent and DES implantation without separate clinical outcomes for the DES subgroup were excluded. Within this study, [16] patients ($n = 1899$) predominantly underwent DES implantation, with BMS implanted in only a small proportion of the study population (IVUS-guided arm: 1.3%, angiography-guided arm: 3.0%). It was therefore deemed appropriate to include this study in the meta-analysis. In addition, studies with incomplete data were reviewed and later discussed, but not included in the formal meta-analysis.

Endpoints and definition

The primary endpoint in this meta-analysis was major adverse cardiac events (MACE), defined as the composite of death, MI (myocardial Infarction), and repeat revascularization. The secondary endpoint was all-cause death, cardiac death, MI, target lesion revascularization (TLR), target vessel revascularization (TVR) and stent thrombosis (ST; included definite, probable or possible ST) according to the definition of the Academic Research Consortium [17].

Data extractions

We extracted DES data exclusively, thereby excluding bare metal stent data. The study's first author's name, publication date, study design, and follow-up duration; baseline clinical, angiographic, and procedural characteristics; and clinical outcomes were systematically reviewed and recorded by the same two reviewers (Yue Wang* and Yue Qi). Disagreements were resolved by discussion between them.

Quality assessments

The methodological quality of RCTs was assessed by the Cochrane Collaboration Risk of Bias tool [18]. The methodological quality of observational studies was assessed by the Newcastle-Ottawa scale (NOS) that consists of three factors: patient selection, comparability of the study groups, and assessment of outcomes [19]. A score of 0–9 was allocated to each study except RCTs. Observational studies achieving six or more scores were considered to be of high quality [20].

Statistical analyses

Baseline characteristics between IVUS-guided versus angiography-guided groups were analyzed and compared, with mean ± SD for continuous variables using two-sample student's unpaired t-test and proportions for categorical variables using chi-square statistics. Across-study summary relative ratios (RRs) with 95% confidence interval (CI) were produced to assess the efficacy of IVUS versus angiography guidance on adverse clinical events. The statistical heterogeneity between trials was assessed with chi-square tests and I^2 statistics. When the p value of chi-square test was < 0.10 and/or the I^2 was $\geq 50\%$, significant heterogeneity was considered and a random-effects model would be selected. If not, the fixed-effects model was used instead. Egger's linear regression analysis was performed to quantitatively assess the underlying publication bias across the studies. In order to evaluate the stability and reliability of the primary endpoint result, we performed a sensitivity analysis of MACE by omitting each individual study in turn. All reported p-values were 2-sided, and $P < 0.05$ was considered to indicate statistical significance. All statistical analyses were performed using STATA 14.0 (Stata Corp, College Station, TX, USA).

Results

Studies included

A total of 1002 publications were reviewed, and 801 citations were screened by checking the title or abstract. Of these, 49 studies were reviewed in detail; and seven clinical studies (4592 patients) were included in the current formal meta-analysis, [16, 21–26] in which 1907 patients underwent IVUS-guided PCI and 2685 underwent angiography-guided PCI with DES implantation. (Fig. 1) One study was a RCT, [25] and the other six studies were observational registries [16, 21–24, 26]. Four studies performed propensity score matching [16, 22, 23, 26]. As specified in the Methods, one meeting abstract published in 2016 (Effectiveness and safety of intravascular ultrasound guidance on clinical outcomes following drug-eluting stent implantation in unprotected left main coronary artery) and one study [27] that included LMCA subgroup analysis were reviewed in the Discussion, not included in our meta-analysis.

Study characteristics

Baseline characteristics of the included studies have been shown in Table 1. The follow-up time ranged from 12 to 36 months. Of the seven studies, the follow-up time in four was 36 months. There were no statistically significant differences in the baseline characteristics between the IVUS-guided versus the angiography-guided groups, except for age, left ventricular ejection fraction and previous PCI. Table 2 demonstrating angiographic and procedural characteristics. Four studies mainly used first generation DES [21, 22, 24, 25], and both first and second-generation DES were implanted in two studies [16, 26]. However, one study did not report the type of DES [23]. Most studies were frequent use of a two-stent technique except for one study by Kim [26].

Assessment of quality

Table 3 presented quality assessment results of included observational trials. Among the six observation studies, all had a scoring of ≥6. The summary risk of bias of the RCT study was low. All studies were considered to be of high quality.

Clinical outcomes

Analyses for clinical outcomes have been presented in Fig. 2. The definition of MACE was slightly different across studies; two studies included cardiac death, [21, 25] and the other five included all-cause deaths [16, 21–24, 26]. Three studies reported TVR, [21, 22, 24] two reported TLR, [23, 25] and one study reported any revascularization not restricted to the target lesion [26] (Table 4).

MACE was reported in all seven studies (Table 5), the summary RR was 0.61 (95% CI 0.53 to 0.70; $P < 0.001$) in

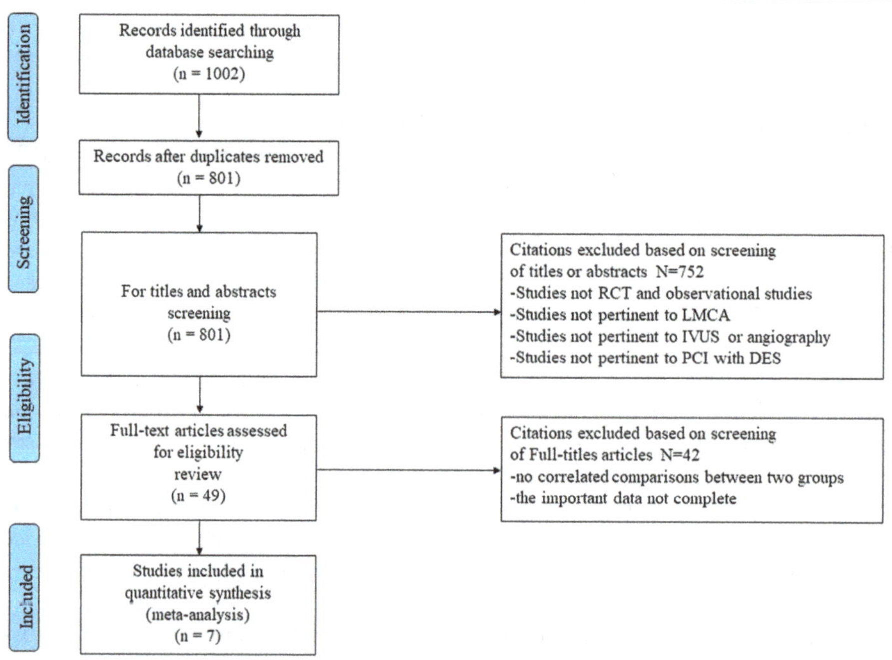

Fig. 1 Flow diagram of the process followed to identify the relevant studies that were included in the present meta-analysis

Table 1 Study design, baseline characteristics of the included studies

First author	Year	Design	Sample size	F/U (months)	Age (years)	Male	Smoker	DM	Hyperlipidemia	Hypertension	Renal failure	LVEF %	Previous PCI	Previous MI
Agostoni et al. [21]	2005	Observational Unadjusted	24/34	14	62/64	15/25	4/7	9/10	15/23	14/20	–	52/44[a]	12/17[a]	9/17
Park et al. [22]	2009	Observational Adjusted	145/145	36	64/65[a]	102/102	28/30	49/49	42/44	86/85	110/112	60/61	–	10/11
De La Torre Hernandez et al. [23]	2014	Observational Adjusted	505/505	36	66/67	404/397	148/161	183/175	314/284	342/325	35/31	55/55	111/107	122/130
Gao et al. [24]	2014	Observational Unadjusted	337/679	12	66/67	274/526	111/230	109/232	228/487	244/489	88/214	59/57[a]	60/119	60/123
Tan et al. [25]	2015	RCT	61/62	24	77/76	38/43	27/29	21/18	–	25/29	–	55/53	–	10/13
Kim et al. [26]	2017	Observational Adjusted	122/74	36	62/65[a]	95/53	60/37	47/33	28/17	75/54	10/7[b]	55/49[a]	9/14[a]	4/5
Tian et al. [16]	2017	Observational Adjusted	713/1186	36	60/60	576/920	256/316	173/314	387/597	400/654	–	63.2/62.9	165/270	163/293

Data are presented as IVUS-guided/angiography-guided PCI with DES for left main lesions

DM diabetes mellitus, *F/U* follow-up, *LVEF* left ventricular ejection fraction, *MI* myocardial infarction, *PCI* percutaneous coronary intervention, *RCT* randomized controlled trial

[a] $p < 0.05$

[b] Chronic kidney disease

Table 2 Angiographic and procedural characteristics

First author	Lesion number	Ostial lesion	Midshaft lesion	Distal lesion	LM only	LM plus 1 Vessel disease	LM plus 2 vessel disease	LM plus 3 vessel disease	Types of Stent	Stent number	Stent diameter (mm)	Stent Length (mm)	Two-stent technique	Final kissing balloon	Post-dilation
Agostoni et al. [21]	–	7/3	7/9	10/22	–	–	11/25	–	SES/PES	1.5/1.4	3.2/3.2	27/23	7/11	4/10	22/26
Park et al. [22]	–	61/62[a]		84/83	6/8	35/32	48/48	56/57	SES/PES	1.23/1.24	–	35.16/35.63	39/42	–	–
De La Torre Hernandez et al. [23]	1.47/1.5	151/145	133/134	221/226	–	160/168	161/149	–	–	–	3.8/3.65	16.0/16.8	63/62	–	–
Gao et al. [24]	1.2/1.3	32/59	16/30	191/359	–	–	–	–	SES	1.5/1.4	3.5/3.4	35.4/33.3	154/280	–	321/543
Tan et al. [25]	–	29/28[a]		32/34	7/10	14/13	24/22	16/17	SES	1.39/1.42	3.43/3.44	21.48/18.24	24/26	–	23/9
Kim et al. [26]	–	–	–	–	–	–	–	–	First and second-generation	–	–	25/28	0/0	26/12	–
Tian et al. [16]	1.7/1.68	81/148	45/82	587/956	59/66	141/240	258/416	255/464	First and second-generation	–	3.54/3.39	21.7/24.3	266/236	399/395	551/638

Data are presented as IVUS-guided /angiography-guided PCI with DES for left main coronary artery lesions
***SES* sirolimus eluting stent, *PES* paclitaxel eluting stent**
[a]Ostial or midshaft LM lesions

Table 3 Quality assessment results of included observational trials

First author	Year	Selection				Comparability	Outcomes			NOS score
		Representativeness of the exposed cohort	Selection of the unexposed cohort	Ascertainment of exposure	No interest outcomes at start of the study	Comparability of cohorts on the basis of design and analysis	Assessment of outcomes	Was follow-up sufficient for the outcome	Adequacy of follow-up	
Agostoni et al. [21]	2005	*	*	*	*			*	*	6
Park et al. [22]	2009	*	*	*	*	**		*	*	8
De La Torre Hernandez et al. [23]	2014	*	*	*	*	**	*	*		8
Gao et al. [24]	2014	*	*	*	*	**	*	*		6
Kim et al. [26]	2017	*	*	*	*		*	*		6
Tian et al. [16]	2017	*	*	*	*	*	*	*	*	8

Footnote: Each asterisk represents one star in the Newcastle-Ottawa Scale system. The maximum number of stars is 2 for comparability and 1 for each of the other categories, for a total of up to 9 stars. *NOS* Newcastle-Ottawa scale

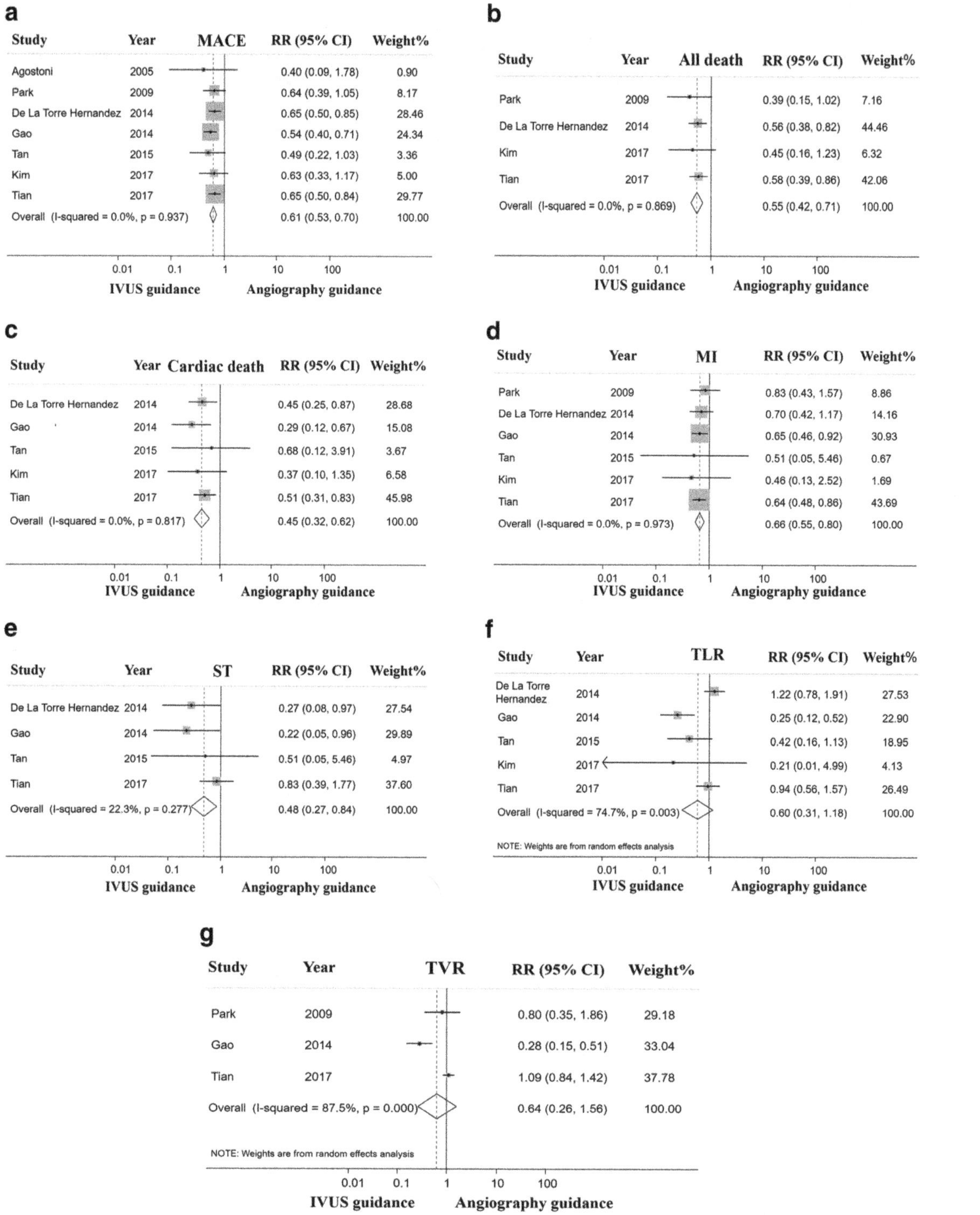

Fig. 2 Forest plot of RR for MACE (**a**), all cause death (**b**), cardiac death (**c**), MI (**d**), ST (**e**), TLR (**f**) and TVR (**g**) associated with IVUS guided vs angiography guided DES implantation to treat LMCA disease. Squares is the effect size of the individual studies; diamonds, the summarized effect size; horizontal lines, upper and lower border of 95% confidence interval. DES = drug eluting stent; LMCA = left main coronary artery; IVUS = intravascular ultrasound; MACE = major adverse cardiac event; MI = myocardial infarction; relative ratio = RR; ST = stent thrombosis; TLR = target lesion revascularization; TVR = target vessel revascularization

Table 4 The endpoint events and definitions

First author	MACE	Repeat revascularization	Stent thrombosis
Agostoni et al. [21]	Cardiac death, MI, TVR	–	–
Park et al. 22]	All cause death, MI, TVR	TVR	–
De La Torre Hernandez et al. [23]	All cause death, MI, TLR	TLR	Definite, probable
Gao et al. [24]	All cause death, MI, TVR	TLR, TVR	Definite, probable, possible
Tan et al. [25]	Cardiac death, MI, TLR	TLR	Definite, probable
Kim et al. [26]	All cause death, MI, TVR, TLR	TLR, TVR	–
Tian et al. [16]	All cause death, MI	TLR, TVR	Definite, probable

MACE major adverse cardiovascular event, *MI* myocardial infarction, *TLR* target lesion revascularization, *TVR* target vessel revascularization

favor of IVUS-guided DES implantation. No evidence of statistical heterogeneity was noted among the included studies ($I^2 = 0\%$; $P = 0.937$) (Fig. 2a).

Four studies reported all-cause death and indicated that IVUS-guided DES implantation was associated with a significant reduction of all-cause mortality (RR 0.55; 95% CI 0.42 to 0.71; $P < 0.001$) with no statistical heterogeneity across the studies ($I^2 = 0\%$; $P = 0.869$) (Fig. 2b).

Of the seven studies, five were included in the analysis of cardiac death; the risk of cardiac death was significantly lower with IVUS guidance (RR 0.45; 95% CI 0.32 to 0.62; $P < 0.001$) with no statistically significant heterogeneity ($I^2 = 0\%$; $P = 0.817$) (Fig. 2c).

Six studies were applied to the analysis of MI. The result was significantly in favor of IVUS-guided DES implantation (RR 0.66; 95% CI 0.55 to 0.80; $P < 0.001$) with no heterogeneity ($I^2 = 0\%$; $P = 0.973$) (Fig. 2d).

Data on ST was reported in four studies. In PCI with DES implantation, IVUS-guidance markedly lowered the risk of definite/probable ST compared with the angiography guidance group (RR 0.48; 95% CI 0.27 to 0.84; $P = 0.01$), again with no statistical heterogeneity ($I^2 = 22.3\%$; $P = 0.277$) (Fig. 2e).

Six studies reported data regarding TLR and three reported TVR. Due to significant heterogeneities (TLR $I^2 = 74.7\%$; $P = 0.003$, and TVR $I^2 = 87.5\%$; $P < 0.001$), random effects models were used to estimate the summary effect of all studies. There were no significant statistical differences regarding TLR (RR 0.60; 95% CI 0.31 to 1.18; $P = 0.099$) and TVR (RR 0.64; 95% CI 0.26 to 1.56; $P = 0.\ 322$) between the two groups (Fig. 2f and Fig. 2g).

Sensitivity analysis

Sensitivity analysis regarding the primary endpoint MACE has been presented in Fig. 3. After removing each study in sequence, the results were not statistically different from the summary RR across the seven studies, further indicating that IVUS-guided DES implantation was associated with a significant reduction in MACE.

Publication bias

Because only seven clinical studies were included the current meta-analysis, we assessed the asymmetry of publication using quantitative tools. No significant evidence of publication bias ($P = 0.401$ for MACE, $P = 0.058$ for all death, $P = 0.709$ for cardiac death, $P = 0.842$ for MI, $P = 0.338$ for ST and $P = 0.75$ for TLR) were observed on the basis of Egger's test (Fig. 4).

Discussion

This meta-analysis of seven studies consisting of 4592 patients demonstrated that IVUS-guided DES implantation when treating LMCA lesions was associated with a significantly reduced risk of MACE, all-cause death,

Table 5 Clinical outcomes for MACE in the IVUS-guided and angiography-guided groups

First author	Year	Sample size	IVUS guidance[a]	Angiography guidance[a]	RR	95% CI	*P*-value
Agostoni et al. [21]	2005	24/34	8%	20%	0.4	0.09–1.78	0.18
Park et al. [22]	2009	145/145	–	–	0.64	0.39–1.05	0.074
De La Torre Hernandez et al. [23]	2014	505/505	14.4%	22.2%	0.65	0.5–0.85	0.006
Gao et al. [24]	2014	337/679	14.8%	27.7%	0.54	0.4–0.71	< 0.001
Tan et al. [25]	2015	61/62	13.1%	27.4%	0.49	0.22–1.03	0.031
Kim et al. [26]	2017	122/74	21%	43%	0.63	0.33–1.17	0.149
Tian et al. [16]	2017	713/1186	5.3%	8.1%	0.65	0.5–0.84	0.001

CI confidence interval, *MACE* major adverse cardiac events, *RR* relative ratio
[a]Percentage of total population

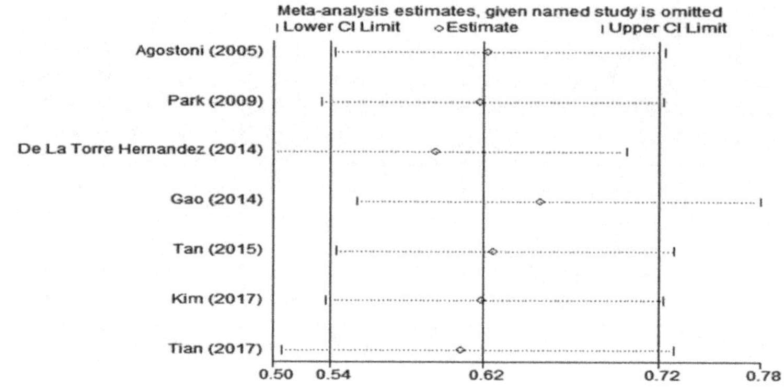

Fig. 3 Sensitivity analysis of MACE by omitting each individual study in turn. Cycle is relative ratio; horizontal lines, upper and lower border of 95% confidence interval. MACE = major adverse cardiac event

cardiac death, MI, and ST, when compared with angiography-guidance.

Using coronary angiography, LMCA lesions may be obscured by overlapping vessels, streaming of injected contrast, and lack of a normal reference segment that limits the utility of angiography in determining lesion severity and selecting treatment strategy [28]. A study by Chakrabarti demonstrated that 11.2% (17 of 152) patients with LMCA disease by core laboratory assessment were deemed normal by clinical assessment in the National Cardiovascular Data Registry (NCDR), whereas 56.7% (177 of 312) patients having significant LMCA disease by clinical assessment in the NCDR had no LMCA lesions by core laboratory analysis [29]. In addition, visual inspection of the angiogram may result in an incorrect diagnosis of LMCA disease severity. In one study including 213 patients with LMCA stenosis, 23% of patients had a diameter stenosis < 50% on the angiogram while the FFR was < 0.80, who actually had hemodynamically significant stenosis and needed revascularization [30].

Conversely, IVUS can detect significant narrowing and assess angiographically ambiguous LMCA lesions; [31] and IVUS correlates with FFR [32]. IVUS has been used to guide decision-making with regards to PCI or bypass surgery in patients with LMCA disease [33]. IVUS also has the ability to assess LMCA plaque distribution and predict hemodynamically significant jailing of the left circumflex after single stent cross-over in a manner not possible using coronary angiography [34, 35]. More

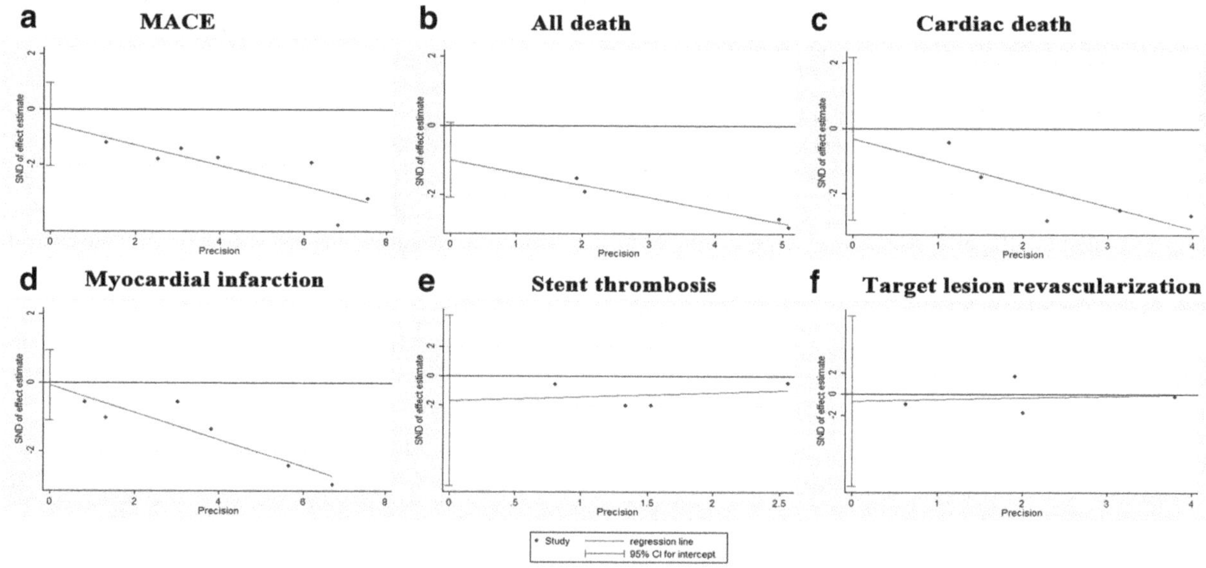

Fig. 4 Assessment of publication bias using the Egger's linear regression analysis for MACE (**a**), all cause death (**b**), cardiac death (**c**), MI (**d**), ST (**e**), TLR (**f**). MACE = major adverse cardiac event; MI = myocardial infarction; ST = stent thrombosis. TLR = target lesion revascularization; TVR = target vessel revascularization

importantly, IVUS can assess stent underexpansion, incomplete lesion coverage (ie, large residual stent edge plaque burden), and malapposition in both LMCA and non-LMCA lesions after DES implantation [36, 37]. Optimal DES implantation is the key to improved patient outcomes. A multivariable logistic regression model of PCI treatment of LMCA lesions showed that IVUS-determined stent underexpansion was an independent predictor for MACE (adjusted hazard ratio [HR] = 5.56; $P < 0.001$); and the two-year MACE-free survival rate was significantly lower in patients with underexpansion of at least one segment versus lesions with no underexpansion (90% vs 98%; $P < 0.001$) [37].

The current meta-analysis demonstrating that IVUS-guided DES implantation led to a significant reduction in the incidence of MACE compared with angiography guidance. This has also been seen in several abstracts at major meetings, and in LMCA subset analyses of larger IVUS versus angiography-guided DES implantation studies. For example, a recently published summary in WCC_2016 concluded that the risk of MACE was significantly lower in LMCA lesions stented with IVUS guidance (15%) vs angiography guidance (24%) ($X^2 = 42.76$; $P = 0.009$). In addition, the subset analyses of LMCA patients in the ADAPT-DES study also showed a trend toward a reduction in MACE (HR 0.54; 95% CI 0.23–1.26; $P = 0.15$) [30].

The beneficial results of IVUS-guidance demonstrated in the current meta-analysis were mainly related to the lower risk of death and MI. In addition, the use of IVUS was associated with a lower ST risk than reliance on angiography. Considering that ST within LMCA stents may present as sudden death, the incidence of this complication may have been underestimated, but was likely captured in the assessment of patient mortality and/or MI [22].

However, we found that IVUS guidance did not reduce TLR or TVR. This may be attributed to the fact that underpowered study population, low incidence of events and the discretion of the operator who might prefer IVUS guidance for lesions with more complex coronary anatomy.

Limitations

This meta-analysis had the following limitations. Firstly, only seven studies were included in our meta-analysis; and only one was an (admittedly relatively small) RCT. Indeed, observational studies have significant limitations with selection and ascertainment bias, which influenced the quality of the evidence across studies. In the present meta-analysis, four of six observational studies included propensity score matching to reduce selection biases. Moreover, IVUS-guided DES implantation was still associated with a significant reduction in MACE after sensitivity analysis was performed. The result indicated that IVUS was worthy of being recommended while performing DES placement for LMCA. However, adequately powered, large-scale RCT studies are needed. Secondly, the location of LMCA lesions, the numbers of other diseased vessels, DES type, and specific treatment strategies may also have impacted the clinical outcomes; but most studies did not provide this detailed data so that subgroup analyses could not be conducted. Thirdly, this meta-analysis lacked the power to detect meaningful differences in TLR and TVR due to little sample size and significant heterogeneities.

Conclusions

The current meta-analysis and systematic review of the literature demonstrate potential clinical value of IVUS in guiding DES implantation for LMCA patients by a significantly reduced risk of MACE, all-cause death, cardiac death, MI, and ST compared with angiography guidance alone. Future studies are warranted as more data becoming available.

Abbreviations

ACC: American College of Cardiology; AHA: Angioplasty Summit, American Heart Association; CI: Confidence interval; DES: Drug eluting stent; FFR: Fractional flow reserve; HR: Hazard ratio; IVUS: Intravascular ultrasound; MACE: Major adverse cardiac event; MI: Myocardial infarction; NCDR: National Cardiovascular Data Registry; NOS: Newcastle-Ottawa scale; PCI: Percutaneous coronary interventions; PES: Paclitaxel eluting stent; RCTs: Randomized control trials; RRs: Relative ratios; SES: Sirolimus eluting stent; ST: Stent thrombosis; TCT: Transcatheter Cardiovascular Therapeutics; TLR: Target lesion revascularization; TVR: Target vessel revascularization; WCC: World Congress of Cardiology

Funding

This study was supported by grants for National Natural Science Foundations of China (NSFC, Grant No. 81470492 and 81670317) and Beijing Administration of Foreign Experts Affairs (GDJ-20171100001).

Authors' contributions

YW, XFW and ZCG designed the study; YW, ZCG and YQ acquired, analyzed, and interpreted data; YW and MRL drafted the manuscript; YW and YQ did the literature search and study selection procedures; MSG and XFW did critical revisions for important; All authors read and approved the final manuscript.

Authors' information

Yue Wang (first author) is a postgraduate student of grade 2016; Yue Wang (fifth author) is a postgraduate student of grade 2017.

Competing interests

Dr. Mintz receives grant support and/or honoraria from Boston Scientific, Volcano, and ACIST. The other authors have no potential conflicts of interest.

Author details
[1]Department of Cardiology, Beijing Anzhen Hospital, Capital Medical University, Beijing 100029, China. [2]Cardiovascular Research Foundation, New York, NY, USA. [3]Department of Pharmacy, Renji Hospital, School of Medicine, Shanghai Jiao Tong University, Shanghai 200127, China. [4]Department of Epidemiology, The Key Laboratory of Remodeling-Related Cardiovascular Diseases, Ministry of Education, Beijing Institute of Heart, Lung and Blood Vessel Diseases, Beijing Anzhen Hospital, Capital Medical University, Beijing, China.

References

1. McDaniel MC, Eshtehardi P, Sawaya FJ, Douglas Jr JS, Samady H. Contemporary clinical applications of coronary intravascular ultrasound. JACC Cardiovasc Interv. 2011;4:1155–67.
2. Park SJ, Hong MK, Lee CW, et al. Elective stenting of unprotected left main coronary artery stenosis: effect of debulking before stenting and intravascular ultrasound guidance. J Am Coll Cardiol. 2001;38:1054–60.
3. Kang SJ, Yang DH, Kweon J, et al. Better diagnosis of functionally significant intermediate sized narrowings using intravascular ultrasound-minimal lumen area and coronary computed tomographic angiography-based myocardial segmentation. Am J Cardiol. 2016;117:1282–8.
4. Saito S, Maehara A, Yakushiji T, et al. Serial intravascular ultrasound findings after treatment of chronic total occlusions using drug-eluting stents. Am J Cardiol. 2016;117:727–34.
5. Kang SJ, Ahn JM, Kim WJ, et al. Intravascular ultrasound assessment of drug-eluting stent coverage of the coronary ostium and effect on outcomes. Am J Cardiol. 2013;111:1401–7.
6. Parise H, Maehara A, Stone GW, Leon MB, Mintz GS. Meta-analysis of randomized studies comparing intravascular ultrasound versus angiographic guidance of percutaneous coronary intervention in pre-drug-eluting stent era. Am J Cardiol. 2011;107:374–82.
7. Ahn JM, Kang SJ, Yoon SH, et al. Meta-analysis of outcomes after intravascular ultrasound-guided versus angiography-guided drug-eluting stent implantation in 26,503 patients enrolled in three randomized trials and 14 observational studies. Am J Cardiol. 2014;113:1338–47.
8. Zhang YJ, Farooq V, García-García HM, et al. Comparison of intravascular ultrasound versus angiography-guided drug-eluting stent implantation: a meta-analysis of one randomised trial and ten observational studies involving 19,619 patients. Eur Secur. 2012;8:55–65.
9. Zhang YJ, Pang S, Chen XY, et al. Comparison of intravascular ultrasound guided versus angiography guided drug eluting stent implantation: a systematic review and meta-analysis. BMC Cardiovasc Disord. 2015;15:153.
10. Klersy C, Ferlini M, Raisaro A, et al. Use of IVUS guided coronary stenting with drug eluting stent. A systematic reviewandmeta-analysis of randomized controlled clinical trials and high quality observational studies. Int J Cardiol. 2013;170:54–63.
11. Steinvil A, Zhang YJ, Lee SY, et al. Intravascular ultrasound-guided drug-eluting stent implantation: an updated meta-analysis of randomized control trials and observational studies. Int J Cardiol. 2016;216:133–9.
12. Jang JS, Song YJ, Kang W, et al. Intravascular ultrasound-guided implantation of drug-eluting stents to improve outcome a meta-analysis. JACC Cardiovasc Interv. 2014;7:233–43.
13. Elgendy IY, Mahmoud AN, Elgendy AY, Bavry AA. Outcomes with intravascular ultrasound-guided stent implantation a meta-analysis of randomized trials in the era of drug-eluting stents. Circ Cardiovasc Interv. 2016;9:e003700.
14. Stone GW, Sabik JF, Serruys PW, et al. Everolimus-eluting stents or bypass surgery for left main coronary artery disease. N Engl J Med. 2016;375:2223–5.
15. Mäkikallio T, Holm NR, Lindsay M, et al. Percutaneous coronary angioplasty versus coronary artery bypass grafting in treatment of unprotected left main stenosis (NOBLE): a prospective, randomised, open-label, non-inferiority trial. Lancet. 2016;388:2743–52.
16. Tian J, Guan C, Wang W, et al. Intravascular ultrasound guidance improves the long-term prognosis in patients with unprotected left main coronary artery disease undergoing percutaneous coronary intervention. Sci Rep. 2017;7:2377.
17. Laskey WK, Yancy CW, Maisel WH. Thrombosis in coronary drug eluting stents: report from the meeting of the circulatory system medical devices advisory panel of the Food and Drug Administration Center for devices and radiologic health, December 7-8, 2006. Circulation. 2007;115:2352–7.
18. Higgins JP, Altman DG, Gotzsche PC, et al. The Cochrane Collaboration's tool for assessing risk of bias in randomised trials. BMJ. 2011;343:d5928.
19. Wells GA, Shea B, O'Connell D, Tugwell P. The Newcastle-Ottawa Scale (NOS) for assessing the quality if nonrandomized studies in meta-analyses Available at: http://www.ohri.ca/programs/clinical_epidemiology/oxford.htm. Accessed 19, Oct 2009.
20. Cheng J, Gao J, Shuai X, Wang G, Tao K. Two-dimensional versus three-dimensional laparoscopy in surgical efficacy: a systematic review and meta-analysis. Oncotarget. 2016;7:70979–90.
21. Agostoni P, Valgimigli M, Van Mieghem CA, et al. Comparison of early outcome of percutaneous coronary intervention for unprotected left main coronary artery disease in the drug-eluting stent era with versus without intravascular ultrasonic guidance. Am J Cardiol. 2005;95:644–7.
22. Park SJ, Kim YH, Park DW, et al. Impact of intravascular ultrasound guidance on long-term mortality in stenting for unprotected left main coronary artery stenosis. Circ Cardiovasc Interv. 2009;2:167–77.
23. De La Torre Hernandez JM, Baz Alonso JA, Gomez Hospital JA, et al. Clinical impact of intravascular ultrasound guidance in drug-eluting stent implantation for unprotected left main coronary disease pooled analysis at the patient-level of 4 registries. JACC Cardiovasc Interv. 2014;7:244–54.
24. Gao XF, Kan J, Zhang YJ, et al. Comparison of one-year clinical outcomes between intravascular ultrasound-guided versus angiography-guided implantation of drug-eluting stents for left main lesions: a single-center analysis of a 1,016-patient cohort. Patient Prefer Adherence. 2014;8:1299–309.
25. Tan Q, Wang Q, Liu D, Zhang S, Zhang Y, Li Y. Intravascular ultrasound-guided unprotected left main coronary artery stenting in the elderly. Saudi Med J. 2015;36:549–53.
26. Kim YH, Her AY, Rha SW, et al. Three-year major clinical outcomes of angiography-guided single stenting technique in non-complex left main coronary artery diseases. Int Heart J. 2017;58:704–13.
27. Witzenbichler B, Maehara A, Weisz G, et al. Relationship between intravascular ultrasound guidance and clinical outcomes after drug-eluting stents the assessment of dual antiplatelet therapy with drug-eluting stents (ADAPT-DES) study. Circulation. 2014;129:463–70.
28. Ragosta M. Left main coronary artery disease: importance, diagnosis, assessment, and management. Curr Prob Cardiol. 2015;40:93–126.
29. Chakrabarti AK, Grau-Sepulveda MV, O'Brien S, et al. Angiographic validation of the american college of cardiology foundation-the society of thoracic surgeons collaboration on the comparative effectiveness of revascularization strategies study. Circ Cardiovasc Interv. 2014;7:11–8.
30. Hamilos M, Muller O, Cuisset T, et al. Long-term clinical outcome after fractional flow reserve-guided treatment in patients with angiographically equivocal left main coronary artery stenosis. Circulation. 2009;120:1505–12.
31. Sano K, Mintz GS, Carlier SG, et al. Assessing intermediate left main coronary lesions using intravascular ultrasound. Am Heart J. 2007;154:983–8.
32. Jasti V, Ivan E, Yalamanchili V, Wongpraparut N, Leesar MA. Correlations between fractional flow reserve and intravascular ultrasound in patients with an ambiguous left main coronary artery stenosis. Circulation. 2004;110:2831–6.
33. De la Torre Hernandez JM, Hernandez Hernandez F, Alfonso F, et al. Prospective application of pre-defined intravascular ultrasound criteria for assessment of intermediate left main coronary artery lesions results from the multicenter LITRO study. J Am Coll Cardiol. 2011;58:351–8.
34. Oviedo C, Maehara A, Mintz GS, et al. Intravascular ultrasound classification of plaque distribution in left main coronary artery bifurcations where is the plaque really located? Circ Cardiovasc Interv. 2010;3:105–12.
35. Kang SJ, Ahn JM, Kim WJ, et al. Functional and morphological assessment of side branch after left main coronary artery bifurcation stenting with cross-over technique. Catheter Cardiovasc Interv. 2014;83:545–52.
36. Fujii K, Carlier SG, Mintz GS, et al. Stent underexpansion and residual reference segment stenosis are related to stent thrombosis after sirolimus-eluting stent implantation: an intravascular ultrasound study. J Am Coll Cardiol. 2005;45:995–8.
37. Kang SJ, Ahn JM, Song H, et al. Comprehensive intravascular ultrasound assessment of stent area and its impact on restenosis and adverse cardiac events in 403 patients with unprotected left main disease. Circ Cardiovasc Interv. 2011;4:562–9.

Heart rate in patients with reduced ejection fraction: relationship between single time point measurement and mean heart rate on prolonged implantable cardioverter defibrillator monitoring

Marlena V. Habal[1], Kumaraswamy Nanthakumar[1,2], Peter C. Austin[1,3], Cassandra Freitas[2,4], Christopher Labos[3] and Douglas S. Lee[1,2,3,4,5*]

Abstract

Background: Heart rate (HR) is a prognostic marker that is increasingly used as a therapeutic target in patients with cardiovascular disease. The association between resting and mean HR remains unclear. We therefore set out to determine the relationship between resting HR on the electrocardiogram (ECG) obtained at a single time point, and mean HR on implantable cardioverter defibrillator (ICD) interrogation amongst patients with a reduced left ventricular ejection fraction (LVEF).

Methods: Prospective ICD data were obtained from 54 patients with LVEF < 40%. Mean HR determined using the ICD HR histograms was compared with resting HR measured on the ECG performed in the clinic.

Results: Average resting and ICD mean HRs were 67.9 ± 10.1 and 67.8 ± 9.6 bpm respectively. There was good correlation in the overall cohort ($r = 0.79$), in those with resting ECG HRs ≤ 70 bpm ($r = 0.62$), and amongst the 27 patients on intermediate-to-high dose beta-blockers ($r = 0.91$). However, Bland-Altman analysis demonstrated wide limits of agreement in the overall cohort (– 12.5, 12.7 bpm), at resting HRs ≤ 70 bpm (– 12.7, 9.8 bpm), and on intermediate-to-high dose beta-blockers (– 8.9, 7.4 bpm). Moreover, resting HR did not predict the 10-bpm interval where the most time was spent.

Conclusions: While resting HR correlated with mean HR in patients with reduced LVEF, and in important subgroups, the limits of agreement were unacceptably wide raising concern over the use of single time point resting HR as a therapeutic target.

Keywords: Mean heart rate, Resting heart rate, Beta-blockers

Background

Elevated heart rate (HR) has been associated with higher mortality in otherwise healthy individuals [1–3] and in those with coronary artery disease [4, 5]. In the Framingham cohort, higher HR was associated with an increased risk of cardiovascular disease, heart failure, and death [6]. Our group and others have previously shown that an elevated HR is associated with increased all-cause and cardiovascular mortality as well as with 30-day re-hospitalization in chronic heart failure [7–9]. The negative effect of elevated HR on the myocardial supply-demand balance is implicated in this process and clinically, elevated HR has been associated with progression of atherosclerosis in patients with an MI at a young age [10] and plaque disruption [11].

Ivabradine, an I_f current inhibitor that selectively lowers HR was initially shown to improve time to ST-segment depression in patients with stable angina [12].

* Correspondence: dlee@ices.on.ca
[1]University of Toronto, Toronto, ON, Canada
[2]Peter Munk Cardiac Centre, University Health Network, Toronto, ON, Canada
Full list of author information is available at the end of the article

More recently, ivabradine was studied in the heart failure (HF) population where it reduced HF hospitalizations (SHIFT) [13] resulting in its inclusion as part of guideline recommended therapy for HF patients with HR ≥ 70 bpm despite optimal medical therapy [14, 15]. However, despite the growing interest in heart rate modulation as a target for therapeutic intervention, there is a paucity of literature on the optimal method of HR assessment.

While resting HR is commonly used in the clinical setting due to its simplicity, it has been shown that single time-point HR measurement reproducibility is poor with only modest correlation between resting HR and mean HR obtained on extended monitoring [16–18]. Moreover a recent study examining ambulatory monitoring suggested that continuous HR was an independent predictor of all-cause mortality after adjusting for resting HR while adjusted resting HR was not [19]. This has implications not only from a therapeutic perspective but also merits investigation to inform clinical trial design. Indeed, the ivabradine trials have shown mixed results both in the setting of ischemic heart disease [12, 20], and chronic HF [13, 21]. Therefore we sought to examine the relationship between resting and mean HR on prolonged monitoring in patients with reduced LVEF. However, because correlation does not necessarily imply agreement, we further sought to investigate the level of agreement between these measures in order to ascertain the safety and validity of these methods of HR determination.

Methods

Study population and study design

We prospectively recruited a convenience sample of patients with systolic dysfunction between April 2015 and March 2016 who were followed in the device clinic at Toronto General Hospital, a large tertiary care centre in the University Health Network, Toronto, Canada. Patients were eligible for inclusion if they were older than 18 years old, had an LVEF less than 40%, had an ICD in situ, and were paced in the atrium or ventricle less than 20% of the time. Patients with an LVEF greater than or equal to 40%, who were paced more than 20% of the time, who had a HR less than 40 bpm, or a paced rhythm on resting rhythm strip during their clinic visit were excluded. Patients with a left ventricular assist device or complex congenital heart disease were also excluded.

Baseline characteristics and device indication were obtained from the electronic patient record (EPR). Medication lists were obtained directly from the patient, or if not available, from the chart or EPR. Analyses were limited to those patients whose medication lists were documented within 13 weeks of HR assessment. Beta-adrenoreceptor blockers were stratified into low and intermediate-high dose categories. Carvedilol ≥12.5 mg twice daily, bisoprolol ≥5 mg daily, and metoprolol ≥ 50 mg twice daily were considered to be intermediate-high doses. The intermediate-high dose category which we analyzed together, is consistent with high dose group in the recent OBTAIN study [22].

Ascertainment of heart rate

Resting HR was defined as that obtained from the device interrogation at the end of the clinic visit in the seated or recumbent position after the patient had been resting both prior to and during the clinic visit. Mean HR was obtained from the HR histogram available upon device interrogation. The HR histogram is divided into 10 bpm heart rate intervals, (for example 60–69 bpm, 70–79 bpm, etc.) and provides the relative amount of time spent in each heart rate interval as a percentage of the total time since last device interrogation. Mean HR was calculated by taking the median of each 10-bpm heart rate interval and multiplying it by the percentage of time spent in that interval. The mean HR was the sum of the products calculated in each interval. The highest % HR interval was defined as the 10-bpm interval that the patient spent the most time in. If multiple 10-bpm intervals had equal frequencies, the one closest to the resting HR was used. An illustrative example of our calculation of mean heart rate can be seen in Additional file 1: Figure S1.

Outcomes

The primary goal was to determine the agreement between resting HR on the ECG at a single time point and mean HR from the ICD interrogation. Secondary analyses included the correlation between resting HR and the highest % HR interval. We also conducted a sensitivity analysis to examine the relationship in important subgroups including HR ≤ 70 bpm, diabetics, patients with arrhythmias on interrogation (atrial fibrillation and ventricular tachycardia), those taking intermediate-high doses of beta-blockers, the subgroups with and without pacing on interrogation, and those with cardiac resychronization therapy (CRT).

Statistical analysis

Continuous variables are reported as mean ± standard deviation and categorical variables as numbers (percentages). The correlation coefficient (r) was determined for the association between resting HR and mean HR, as well as the association between resting HR and the highest % HR interval. Percent agreement between the two HR measurements was assessed using Bland-Altman plots with 95% limits of agreement. Statistical analysis was performed using STATA version 12, StataCorp, College Station, Texas.

Results

Patient characteristics

A total of 54 patients were included in the present study of which 41 (76%) were male. The average age was 63.6 ± 12.6 years. The baseline characteristics are shown in Table 1. Twenty-four patients (44%) had an LVEF between 20 and 29% and 32 (59%) had an ischemic etiology for their cardiomyopathy. With regards to the ICD indication, 41 devices (76%) were for primary prevention. Nineteen patients (35%) were paced > 1% in the chamber used to quantify heart rate (ie. excluding CRT) with an overall mean percentage time paced of 6.6%.

Table 1 Baseline Characteristics

Age (years)	63.6 ± 12.6
Male, n (%)	41 (76)
Indication for ICD, n (%)	
1°	41 (76)
2°	13 (24)
Ischemic HF, n (%)	32 (59)
LVEF, n (%)	
30–39	16 (30)
20–29	24 (44)
< 20%	14 (26)
Comorbidities, n (%)	
Hypertension	29 (54)
Dyslipidemia	30 (56)
Diabetes	20 (37)
Device, n (%)	
Medtronic	15 (28)
St. Jude	34 (63)
Boston	4 (7)
Biotronik	1 (2)
Dual chamber, n (%)	36 (67)
CRT, n (%)	22 (41)
Paced> 1%, n (%)	19 (35)
Mean time paced	6.6%
Atrial fibrillation history, n (%)	16 (30)
Atrial fibrillation on interrogation, n (%)	15 (28)
History of VT/VF, n (%)	30 (56)
VT on interrogation, n (%)	6 (11)
NSVT on interrogation, n (%)	13 (24)
Medications, n(%)[a]	
Beta-blockers	39 (100%)
Amiodarone	7 (18%)
Digoxin	12 (31%)
ACEI or ARB	37 (95%)
Mineralocorticoid antagonist	29 (74%)
Furosemide	24 (62%)

ICD Implantable Cardioverter Defibrillator, *HF* heart failure, *LVEF* left ventricular systolic function, *CRT* cardiac resynchronization therapy, *VT* ventricular tachycardia, *VF* ventricular fibrillation, *NSVT* nonsustained ventricular tachycardia
[a]medication data were known and available for 39 patients

Association between resting and mean heart rate

For the total study population, the mean resting HR was 67.9 ± 10.1 bpm and the ICD derived mean HR was 67.8 ± 9.6 bpm. There was good linear correlation ($r = 0.79$; $p < .001$) between these two measurements (Fig. 1a). Using Bland-Altman analysis, the mean difference was minimal (0.1). However the limits of agreement were wide (− 12.5, 12.7 bpm) (Fig. 1b). When the limits of agreement were set to ±5 bpm, 20 (37%) of the values fell outside of this range (Additional file 2: Figure S2).

Association between resting heart rate ≤ 70 bpm and mean heart rate

The association between resting and mean HR in the subgroup with resting HR ≤ 70-bpm is presented in Fig. 2a. Moderate correlation ($r = 0.62$; $p < .001$) was found in this subgroup of patients. Bland-Altman analysis demonstrated a slight difference between resting and mean HR (−1.4 bpm) (Fig. 2b). Similar to the overall cohort, the limits of agreement were wide (−12.7, 9.8 bpm). When the limits of agreement were set to ±5 bpm, 11 (30.6%) of the values fell outside of this range.

Association between resting heart rate and mean heart rate in patients prescribed beta-blockers

We performed a sensitivity analysis for the 39 patients for whom beta-blocker dose was recorded. There was excellent correlation ($r = 0.91$, $p < .001$) between the resting and mean HR amongst patients taking intermediate-to-high dose beta-blockers (Fig. 3a). Bland-Altman analysis demonstrated minimal mean difference (−0.74 bpm) with narrower limits of agreement than for the overall cohort (− 8.9, 7.4 bpm) (Fig. 3b). When the limits of agreement were set to ±5 bpm, 7 (25.9%) of the values fell outside of this range.

Association between resting heart rate and mean heart rate in subgroup analysis

Since HR and HR variability are influenced by diabetic neuropathy, we performed a sensitivity analysis for the 20 patients with documented diabetes. Amongst this subgroup, the average ECG HR and ICD HR was 69.5 ± 7.6 and 70.2 ± 8.7, respectively. Correlation between resting and ICD HR was moderate ($r = 0.61$, limits of agreement − 15.0, 13.5). We also performed sensitivity analysis for the 16 patients with ventricular tachycardia or nonsustained ventricular tachycardia on interrogation. Correlation was strong with persistently wide limits of

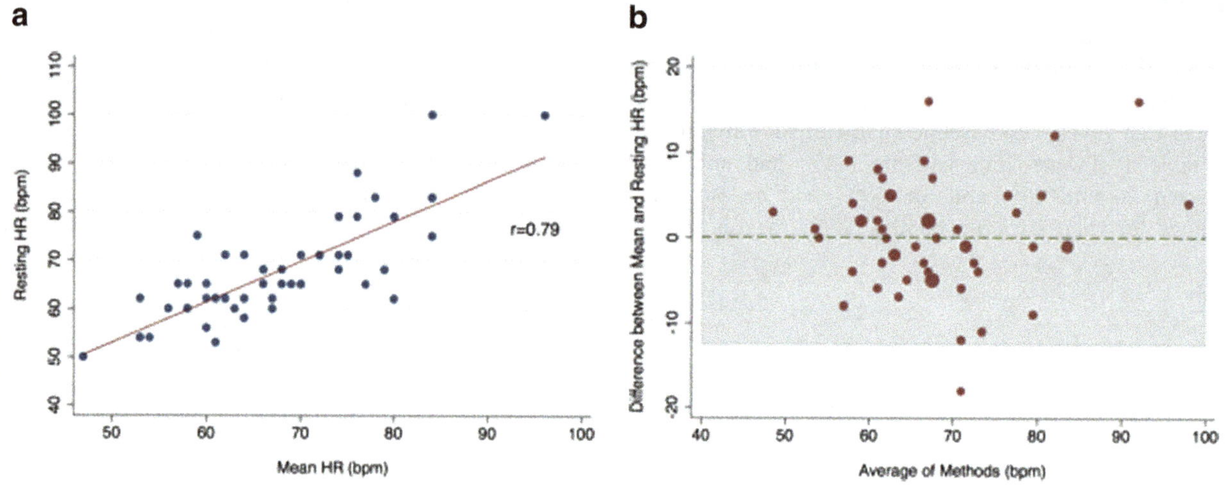

Fig. 1 **a** Resting HR/mean HR. **b** Bland-Altman Plot of resting HR/mean HR. HR, heart rate

agreement ($r = 0.93$, limits of agreement − 8.0, 8.8 bpm). Given that pacing could affect the ICD HR, we performed a sensitivity analysis of the patients paced < 1% in the cardiac chamber from which the mean HR was determined, those paced > 1%, and those with a CRT device in situ (Additional file 3: Table S1). In all three groups the mean difference remained low (0.3, − 0.2, and − 0.7 respectively), the correlation was moderate to strong (0.80, 0.60, and 0.61 respectively), and the limits of agreement were wide (− 13.6, 14.1; − 9.8, 9.4; − 14.2, 12.7 respectively).

Association between resting heart rate and heart rate interval

To further validate our findings, we sought to determine whether resting HR could predict the HR interval in which a patient spent the most time. Data were categorized by 10-bpm intervals on the histogram and compared with the resting HR. In the overall cohort, 28% ($n = 15$) had a resting HR above the highest % HR interval, 50% ($n = 27$) had a resting HR within this interval, and 22% ($n = 12$) had a resting HR below the highest % interval (Table 2). In the subgroup with HR ≤ 70 bpm ($n = 36$), 22% ($n = 8$) had a resting HR above the highest % HR interval, 47% ($n = 17$) had a HR within this interval, and 31% ($n = 11$) had a resting HR below the highest % HR interval (Table 2).

Discussion

In the present, hypothesis generating study, we examined a novel method of mean HR determination from prolonged ICD monitoring. Although our data demonstrated good correlation between resting and mean HR with minimal systematic bias between the 2 methods,

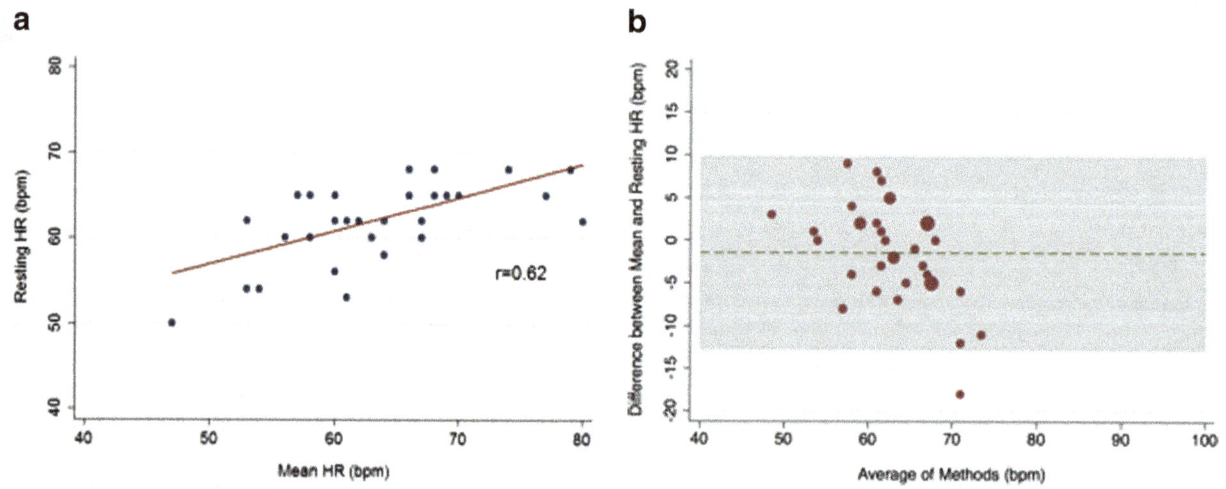

Fig. 2 **a** Resting HR/mean HR amongst the subgroup with resting HR ≤ 70 bpm. **b** Bland-Altman Plot of resting HR/mean HR amongst the subgroup with resting HR ≤ 70 bpm

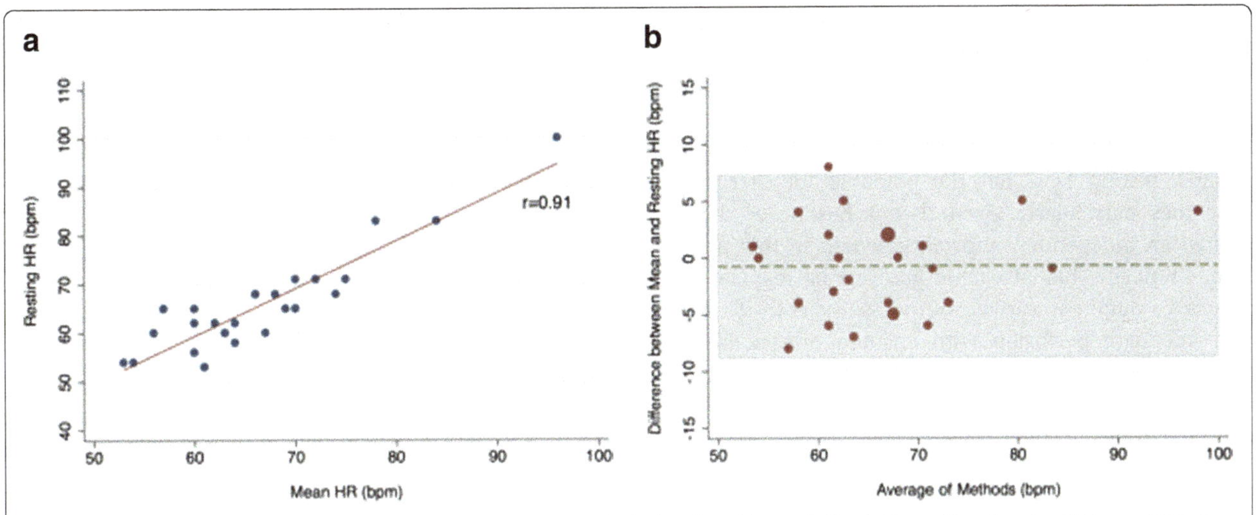

Fig. 3 a Resting HR/mean HR in the subgroup on an intermediate-to-high dose beta-blocker. **b** Bland-Altman Plot of resting HR/mean HR in the subgroup on an intermediate-to-high dose beta-blocker

the limits of agreement were unacceptably wide. Since there is no gold standard for HR determination we further assessed whether resting HR obtained at a single time point could predict the highest frequency HR interval over the duration of ICD monitoring. Our findings demonstrated that resting HR only reflected the highest frequency HR interval half of the time as determined from the HR histogram. Importantly, resting HR more frequently overestimated the HR interval than underestimated it. From a clinical perspective, this suggests that single time point resting HR is an imperfect surrogate for mean HR when titrating pharmacotherapies.

Our findings of correlation between methods are consistent with other small studies comparing resting and HRs obtained by Holter monitoring. Carlson et al., found partial correlation between resting ECG HR and both mean daytime HR as well as resting HR determined by Holter monitoring in a cohort of otherwise healthy participants [17]. The strength of correlation was weaker than in the present study, which may be explained by the lower activity levels of the patients in our study as well as lower heart rate variability. Moreover, the routine use of beta-blockers in this population would be expected to further contribute as evidenced by the strong correlation between methods in the subgroup on an intermediate-to-high dose beta-blocker. Furthermore, in a telemonitoring study of ICD patients with NYHA class III heart failure, resting HR correlated with mean 24-h HR [18]. More recently Jolly et al., showed a positive correlation between ambulatory Holter mean HR and ECG resting HR in patients with atrial fibrillation [23].

Table 2 Agreement between resting HR and 10-bpm HR interval

	Overall cohort ($n = 54$)		Resting HR ≤ 70 bpm ($n = 36$)	
	N	%	*N*	%
Resting HR higher than highest% HR interval	15	28%	8	22%
Resting HR within highest% HR interval	27	50%	17	47%
Resting HR below highest% HR interval	12	22%	11	31%

HR heart rate

Our study extends the literature by demonstrating that correlation between methods for determining HR does not necessarily imply that the two different approaches yield the same measurements. After confirming correlation, we determined that the limits of agreement between resting single time point HR and mean HR on prolonged monitoring were wide. While there is no consensus on how wide a limit of agreement is acceptable, from a clinical perspective, a 10-bpm difference would be likely to alter clinical decision-making. When the limits of agreement were set to a clinically meaningful interval of ±5 bpm, 37% of patients fell outside of this range. Furthermore, we demonstrated that resting HR was frequently above the mean HR, which is consistent with the findings of Pastor-Perez et al., who identified a subgroup of patients with HF in whom resting HR was above the mean with 7 day ambulatory HR monitoring [24].

The present findings, both using Bland-Altman analysis and comparing resting HR to the highest frequency heart rate interval, raise concern for iatrogenic bradycardia when resting ECG heart rate is used to titrate therapies. This issue was clinically highlighted in both the SHIFT [13] (Systolic Heart failure treatment with the I_f inhibitor ivabradine Trial) and SIGNIFY [20] (Study Assessing the Morbidity-Mortality Benefits of the

I_f Inhibitor Ivabradine in Patients with Coronary Artery Disease) trials where resting ECG was used to measure heart rate. In these trials, the rate of bradycardia in the treatment arm was 10.3% and 18.9% respectively. Thus, uptitrating HR lowering therapies, such as ivabradine, using a resting ECG has the potential for detrimental outcomes particularly given that it has never demonstrated an independent mortality benefit in this population. Clinically this iatrogenic bradycardia may result in failure to augment cardiac output sufficiently to maintain adequate perfusion with ensuing presyncope and falls. Moreover, while there is no consensus on the lower HR limit for a mortality benefit, our group found a non-significant trend towards increased 30-day mortality in a cohort of community-based HF patients with HR < 60 bpm [7]. Furthermore, in the MESA cohort, there was a U-shaped mortality distribution amongst individuals taking HR-modifying therapies with increased mortality at HR < 50 bpm on resting ECG [25]. Finally, in a heart failure population such as ours, who frequently are recipients of an ICD or pacemaker, over titration of medications may result in increased RV pacing which also carries negative prognostic implications [26]. In the context of these concerns, our findings suggest that an alternative method of HR assessment to supplement single time point measurements, should be considered by clinicians. Since many of these patients will have an ICD, either the mean HR or highest frequency HR interval could be used in order to reduce the risk of iatrogenic bradycardia. Long-term studies are then required to assess whether this method will also have prognostic implications.

Our study has several limitations. Firstly, mean HR could not be directly assessed from the ICD, as most commercially available devices do not offer this function. However, we developed a novel method of mean HR determination using the HR histogram which demonstrated strong correlation with resting HR, confirming its validity as a tool to measure HR. Secondly, the presence of tachyarrhythmias such atrial fibrillation or ventricular tachycardia could have influenced the results. With respect to atrial fibrillation, the documented burden was low and only three of these patients had single lead device in which case it would have been difficult to assess the atrial fibrillation burden. The episodes of NSVT/VT were also brief and unlikely to have affected the overall results. Our sensitivity analyses of these subgroups demonstrated results similar to the overall cohort, with moderate to good correlation but wide limits of agreement.

Thirdly, resting HR was taken at a single time point near the end of the clinic visit after the patient had been seated or recumbent and thus, in some instances the patient may have moved or become anxious, thus transiently raising their resting HR. However, this would have been expected to weaken the correlation between the two methods of measurement, which nonetheless remained robust. Fourthly, it is possible that the beta-blocker dose was adjusted during the time between device interrogations. However, it is equally likely that the doses would be increased or decreased. Given that this would result in non-differential misclassification, it would bias the results toward the null and thus is unlikely to affect the finding of the present study.

Conclusion

In conclusion, while there is good correlation between single time point resting HR and mean HR as determined from the ICD histogram, the limits of agreement are unacceptably wide and resting HR is frequently above the mean. These findings raise concern for the current clinical strategy of using a single time point method of heart rate assessment to titrate negative chronotropic therapies, which may result in iatrogenic bradycardia. Further studies are warranted to address the prognostic implications of these findings and the relative safety of these two methods when titrating chronotropic therapies.

Abbreviations

ECG: Electrocardiogram; HR: Heart rate; ICD: Implantable cardioverter defibrillator; LVEF: Left ventricular ejection fraction

Acknowledgements

Not applicable.

Funding

The Institute for Clinical Evaluative Sciences (ICES) is supported in part by a grant from the Ontario Ministry of Health and Long-Term Care. The opinions, results and conclusions are those of the authors and no endorsement by the Ministry of Health and Long-Term Care or by the Institute for Clinical Evaluative Sciences is intended or should be inferred.

This study was supported by a Foundation Grant from the Canadian Institutes of Health Research (grant # FDN 148446). Dr. Lee is supported by a mid-career investigator award from the Heart and Stroke Foundation and the Ted Rogers Chair in Heart Function Outcomes, a joint Hospital-University Chair of the University Health Network and the University of Toronto. Dr. Austin is supported by a Career Investigator Award from the Heart and Stroke Foundation of Ontario.

Authors' contributions

MVH and DSL conceived the idea for the study. MVH, DSL and KN designed the study. MVH drafted the manuscript. MVH, PCA and CL analyzed the data. DSL and KN provided supervision. DSL,CF and CL critically revised the manuscript. KN, CL and CF prepared the manuscript for submission. DSL provided the funding for the study. All authors read and approved the final manuscript.

Competing interests

The authors declare that they have no competing interests.

Author details
[1]University of Toronto, Toronto, ON, Canada. [2]Peter Munk Cardiac Centre, University Health Network, Toronto, ON, Canada. [3]Institute for Clinical Evaluative Sciences, Toronto, ON, Canada. [4]Ted Rogers Centre for Heart Research, Toronto, ON, Canada. [5]University Health Network, Toronto General Hospital, 200 Elizabeth Street, 4NU-482, Toronto, ON M5G 2C4, Canada.

References

1. Jensen MT, Marott JL, Allin KH, Nordestgaard BG, Jensen GB. Resting heart rate is associated with cardiovascular and all-cause mortality after adjusting for inflammatory markers: the Copenhagen City heart study. Eur J Prev Cardiol. 2012;19(1):102–8.
2. Dyer AR, Persky V, Stamler J, Paul O, Shekelle RB, Berkson DM, et al. Heart rate as a prognostic factor for coronary heart disease and mortality: findings in three Chicago epidemiologic studies. Am J Epidemiol. 1980;112:736–49.
3. Jouven X, Empana JP, Schwartz PJ, Desnos M, Courbon D, Ducimetiere P. Heart-rate profile during exercise as a predictor of sudden death. N Engl J Med. 2005;352:1951–8.
4. Hjalmarson A, Gilpin EA, Kjekshus J, Schieman G, Nicod P, et al. Influence of heart rate on mortality after acute myocardial infarction. Am J Cardiol. 1990;65:547–53.
5. Diaz A, Bourassa MG, Guertin MC, Tardif JC. Long-term prognostic value of resting heart rate in patients with suspected or proven coronary artery disease. Eur Heart J. 2005;26:967–74.
6. Ho JE, Bittner V, Demicco DA, Breazna A, Deedwania PC, Waters DD. Usefulness of heart rate at rest as a predictor of mortality, hospitalization for heart failure, myocardial infarction, and stroke in patients with stable coronary heart disease. Am J Cardiol. 2010;105:905–11.
7. Habal MV, Liu PP, Austin PC, Ross HJ, Newton GE, Wang X, et al. Association of Heart Rate at hospital discharge with mortality and hospitalizations in patients with heart failure. Circ Heart Fail. 2014;7:12–20.
8. Laskey WK, Alomari I, Cox M, Schulte P, Zhao X, Hernandez AF, et al. Heart rate at hospital discharge in patients with heart failure is associated with mortality and Rehospitalization. J Am Heart Assoc. 2015;4:e001626. https://doi.org/10.1161/JAHA.114.001626.
9. Castagno D, Skali H, Takeuchi M, Swedberg K, Yusuf S, Michelson EL, et al. Association of Heart Rate and Outcomes in a broad Spectrum of patients with chronic heart failure. J Am Coll Cardiol. 2012;59:1785–95.
10. Perski A, Olsson G, Landou C, de Faire U, Theorell T, et al. Minimum heart rate and coronary atherosclerosis: independent relations to global severity and rate of progression of angiographic lesions in men with myocardial infarction at a young age. Am Heart J. 1992;123:609–16.
11. Heidland UE, Stauer BE. Left ventricular muscle mass and elevated heart rate are associated with coronary plaque disruption. Circulation. 2001;104:1477–82.
12. Borer JS, Fox K, Jaillon P, Lerebours G. Antianginal and antiischemic effects of ivabradine, an I_f inhibitor, in stable angina. A randomized, double-blind, multicentered, placebo-controlled trial. Circulation. 2003;107:817–23.
13. Swedberg K, Komajda M, Bohm M, Borer JS, Ford I, Dubost-Brama A, et al. SHIFT investigators. Heart rate as a risk factor in chronic heart failure (SHIFT): the association between heart rate and outcomes in a randomized placebo-controlled trial. Lancet. 2010;376:886–94.
14. Howlett J, Chan M, Ezekowitz J, Harkness K, Heckman G, Kouz S, et al. The Canadian cardiovascular society heart failure companion: bridging guidelines to your practice. Can J Cardiol. 2016;32:296–310.
15. Ponikowski P, Voors AA, Anker SD, Bueno H, Cleland JG, Coats AJ et al. 2016 ESC Guidelines for the diagnosis and treatment of acute and chronic heart failure: The Task Force for the diagnosis and treatment of acute and chronic heart failure of the European Society of Cardiology (ESC) Developed with the special contribution of the Heart Failure Association (HFA) of the ESC. Eur Heart J. 2016;37:2129-200.
16. Palatini P, Winnicki M, Santonastaso M, De Venuto G, Zanata G, Bertolo O, et al. Reproducibility of heart rate measured in the clinic and with 24-hour intermittent recorders. Am J Hypertens. 2000;13:92–8.
17. Carlson N, Dixen U, Marott JL, Jensen MT, Jensen GB. Predictive value of casual ECG-based resting heart rate compared with resting heart rate obtained from Holter recording. Scand J Clin Lab Invest. 2014;74:163–9.
18. Lieback A, Proff J, Weeel K, Fleck E, Gotze S. Remote monitoring of heart failure patients using implantable cardiac pacing devices and external sensors: results of the insight-HF study. Clin Res Cardiol. 2012;101:101–7.
19. Korshoj M, Lidegaard M, Kittel F, Van Herck K, De Backer G et al. The Relation of Ambulatory Heart Rate with All-Cause Mortality among Middle-Aged Men: A prospective Cohort Study. PLoS One. 2015. https://doi.org/10.1371/journal.pone.0121729.
20. Fox K, Ford I, Steg PG, Tardif M, Ferrari R, et al. Ivabradine in stable coronary artery disease without clinical heart failure. NEJM. 2014;371:1091–9.
21. Fox K, Ford I, Steg PG, Tendera M, Ferrari R, et al. Ivabradine for patients with stable coronary artery disease and left-ventricular systolic dysfunction (BEAUTIFUL): a randomized, double-blind, placebo-controlled trial. Lancet. 2008;372:807–16.
22. Goldberger JJ, Bonow RO, Cuffe M, Liu L, Rosenberg Y, et al. Effect of Beta-blocker dose on survival after acute myocardial infarction. J Am Coll Cardiol. 2015;66:1431–41.
23. Jolly US, Klein G. Utility of ambulatory Holter monitoring in patients with permanent Atrial fibrillation. Can J Cardiol. 2015;31:S246.
24. Pastor-Perez FJ, Manzano-Fernandez S, Goya-Esteban R, Pascual-Figal DA, Bravo IP, Barquero-Perez O, et al. Heart rate control in chronic heart failure: resting versus mean heart rate with prolonged ambulatory ECG recording. Int J Cardiol. 2013;170:e45–7.
25. Dharod A, Soliman EZ, Dawood F, Chen H, Shea S, et al. Association of Asymptomatic Bradycardia with Incident Cardiovascular Disease and Mortality: the multi-ethnic study of atherosclerosis. JAMA Intern Med. 2016;176:219–27.
26. Wilkoff B, Cook J, Epstein A, Greene HL, Hallstrom AP, Hsia H, et al. Dual chamber pacing or ventricular backup pacing in patients with an implantable defibrillator. The dual chamber and VVI implantable defibrillator (DAVID) trial. JAMA. 2002;288(24):2123–3115.

Endovascular treatment of transplant renal artery stenosis based on hemodynamic assessment using a pressure wire

Yoshito Kadoya*, Kan Zen and Satoaki Matoba

Abstract

Background: Transplant renal artery stenosis (TRAS) is a serious complication after renal transplantation, leading to hypertension, deterioration in renal function, and/or graft loss. The incidence of TRAS reportedly varies from 1 to 23%, depending on its definition or diagnostic tools. The hemodynamic definition or therapeutic indication of TRAS is unclear.

Case presentation: A 66-year-old man with a history of diabetes, chronic kidney disease, and angina presented with a 2-week history of dyspnea and leg edema. He had undergone living-donor kidney transplantation for end-stage renal disease secondary to diabetic nephropathy 7 years earlier. He developed acute deterioration in renal function after the administration of an angiotensin II receptor blocker and required emergency hospitalization owing to acute congestive heart failure with pulmonary edema. A vasodilator and loop diuretics were administered following his admission, and the patient's symptoms resolved quickly. Further investigation, including magnetic resonance angiography and ultrasonography, revealed severe stenosis of the transplant renal artery. Renal arteriography and pressure gradient measurement using a 0.014-inch pressure wire were performed. The systolic pressure gradient was 40 mmHg, and the resting Pd/Pa ratio (ratio of mean distal to lesion and mean proximal pressures) was 0.90 without hyperemia. Hemodynamically significant stenosis was suspected. Intravascular ultrasonography revealed vessel shrinkage in the stenotic area, suggestive of the end-to-end anastomosis site. Pre-dilation using a 4-mm balloon, implantation of a 6-mm self-expandable stent, and post-dilatation using a 5-mm balloon were performed. Although the moderate stenosis persisted angiographically, the systolic pressure gradient dropped to 20 mmHg with the mean systolic pressure ratio increased to 0.95, which was considered an acceptable result. One month after the procedure, the patient's renal function and blood pressure control had significantly improved.

Conclusions: Hemodynamic assessment using a pressure wire is useful in determining the appropriate therapeutic indication and endpoint of endovascular treatment of TRAS.

Keywords: Endovascular treatment, Transplant renal artery stenosis, Case report

* Correspondence: m03020kdy@gmail.com
Department of Cardiovascular Medicine, Graduate School of Medical Science, Kyoto Prefectural University of Medicine, 465 Kajii-cho, Kawaramachi-Hirokoji, Kamigyo-ku, Kyoto 602-8566, Japan

Background

Transplant renal artery stenosis (TRAS) is a serious complication after renal transplantation, and is an important cause of hypertension, renal function deterioration, and/or graft loss [1]. The reported incidence of TRAS is in the range of 1–23%, depending on its definition or on the diagnostic tools [2]. Endovascular treatment (EVT), including percutaneous transluminal angioplasty and stent implantation, is considered the first-line therapy for TRAS [3]. However, the hemodynamic definition or therapeutic indication of TRAS remains unclear. Herein, we report a case of TRAS that was successfully treated via EVT based on hemodynamic assessment using a 0.014-inch pressure wire.

Case presentation

A 66-year-old Japanese man with a history of diabetes, chronic kidney disease, and angina was admitted to our hospital with a 2-week history of dyspnea and leg edema. He also had a history of end-stage renal failure secondary to diabetic nephropathy and had been undergoing peritoneal dialysis. He had received living-donor kidney transplantation from his wife 7 years earlier, in which an end-to-end anastomosis of the donor renal artery to the patient's left internal iliac artery was performed. After the transplantation, he was able to discontinue dialysis and his renal function was stable with an estimated glomerular filtration rate (eGFR) of approximately 40 mL/min/1.73 m^2. A few months before admission to our hospital, his blood pressure control gradually deteriorated, and he experienced acute deterioration in renal function after the administration of an angiotensin II receptor blocker (ARB). Antihypertensive medication on admission included 2.5 mg of carvedilol, 80 mg of nifedipine, and 2 mg of benidipine. On physical examination, he exhibited wheezing in the chest and pitting edema in the bilateral limbs. His body temperature was 36.8 °C; blood pressure, 166/71 mmHg; regular pulse rate, 91 beats/min; and oxygen saturation, 93% (without oxygen administration). Laboratory findings showed acute exacerbation of renal function with an eGFR of 24 mL/min/1.73 m^2 and an elevation of the brain natriuretic peptide level (483.3 pg/mL; normal range: < 18.4 pg/mL). Electrocardiography showed the strain pattern. Echocardiography revealed concentric left ventricular hypertrophy as well as moderate aortic stenosis with an aortic mean gradient of 11 mmHg, a valve area of 1.12 cm^2, and an ejection fraction of 68%. The severity of aortic stenosis had been followed up echocardiographically once yearly, showing no significant progression at this hospitalization. Plain chest radiography and computed tomography of the chest showed a bilateral infiltrative shadow, suggestive of pulmonary edema (Fig. 1). The patient's diagnosis was acute congestive heart failure with pulmonary edema. A vasodilator and loop diuretics were administered following admission, and the patient's symptoms resolved quickly. Because of the worsened blood pressure control and renal function deterioration caused by ARB, transplant renal artery stenosis was suspected. Magnetic resonance angiography was performed and it revealed the bending and narrowing of the transplant renal artery (Fig. 2). On ultrasound examination, the peak systolic velocity of the narrowing part was observed to be above 2 m/sec. The peak systolic velocity ratio could not be determined owing to poor echographic imaging of the proximal non-stenosed part. A 5-French guiding catheter (Destination®, Terumo, Japan) was inserted into the left common iliac artery via the right femoral artery and an angiography revealed significant stenosis in the transplant renal artery (Fig. 3).

In addition, pressure gradient measurement was conducted using a 0.014-inch pressure wire (Aeris®, Abbott, USA). The mean pressure was 96 mmHg proximally and 87 mmHg distally with a resting Pd/Pa ratio (ratio of mean distal to lesion and mean proximal pressures) of 0.90, and the peak-to-peak systolic pressure gradient was 40 mmHg without hyperemia. Based on these findings in addition to

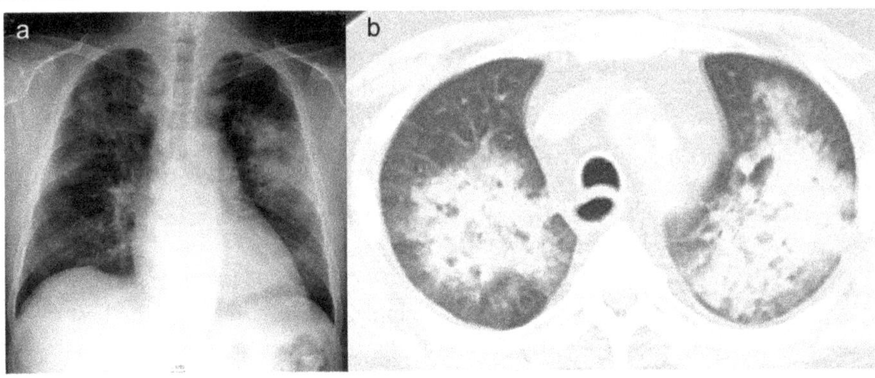

Fig. 1 **a** Plain chest radiography showing a bilateral infiltrative shadow. **b** Computed tomography of the chest showing a bilateral infiltrative shadow in the hilar region dominant

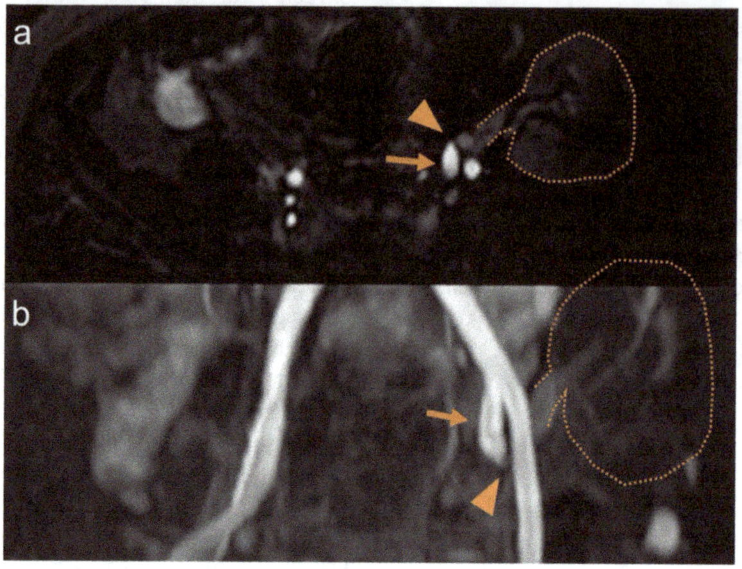

Fig. 2 Magnetic resonance angiography showing the bending and narrowing of the transplant renal artery (**a** axial view; **b** three-dimensional image) (arrow: the left internal iliac artery; arrowhead, the narrowing part; dash line: the transplanted kidney)

the clinical course, such as worsening of blood pressure control and acute renal function deterioration after the administration of an ARB, we assessed that the stenosis was hemodynamically significant. Therefore, we did not perform hyperemic evaluation of the stenosis. Intravascular ultrasonography (IVUS) revealed shrinkage of the vessel in the stenotic area, with a diameter of 5 mm, suggestive of the anastomosis site (Fig. 4). Pre-dilation using a

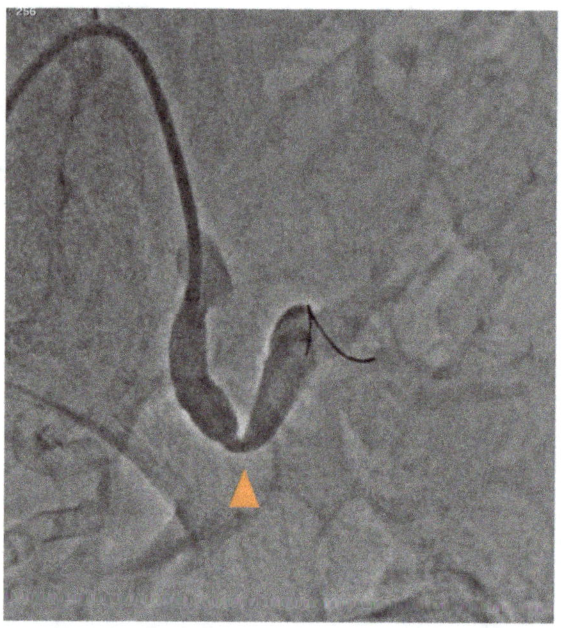

Fig. 3 Angiography showing significant stenosis in the transplant renal artery (arrowhead: the narrowing part)

4-mm balloon, implantation of a 6-mm self-expandable stent, and post-dilatation using a 5-mm balloon were sequentially performed (Fig. 5). Thereafter, moderate stenosis persisted angiographically (Fig. 6). However, we had concerns that too much dilatation would increase the risk of vessel dissection or perforation because the lesion might be at the anastomosis site. We repeated the resting pressure gradient measurement. The mean pressure proximally was 101 mmHg and the pressure distally was 96 mmHg, with a resting Pd/Pa ratio of 0.95, and the peak-to-peak systolic pressure gradient was 20 mmHg. This was thought to be acceptable as the endpoint of TRAS-EVT. Moreover, the self-expandable stent was expected to further expand in the remote phase. Therefore, we concluded the procedure. After the procedure, the peak systolic velocity in the stenosed part based on an ultrasound examination had dropped to 1.45 m/sec. Renal function and blood pressure control improved, which resulted in the preservation of graft function. Moreover, antihypertensive medication could be significantly reduced; carvedilol 1.25 mg and nifedipine 40 mg. Four months later, a follow-up angiography demonstrated no restenosis and the pressure gradient had dropped to 15 mmHg.

Discussion and conclusions

We present a case of TRAS, which was successfully treated via EVT based on a hemodynamic assessment using a pressure wire. To the best of our knowledge, this is the first reported case of pressure wire-guided EVT of TRAS. Hemodynamic assessment should be conducted to determine the therapeutic indication and endpoint of EVT for TRAS.

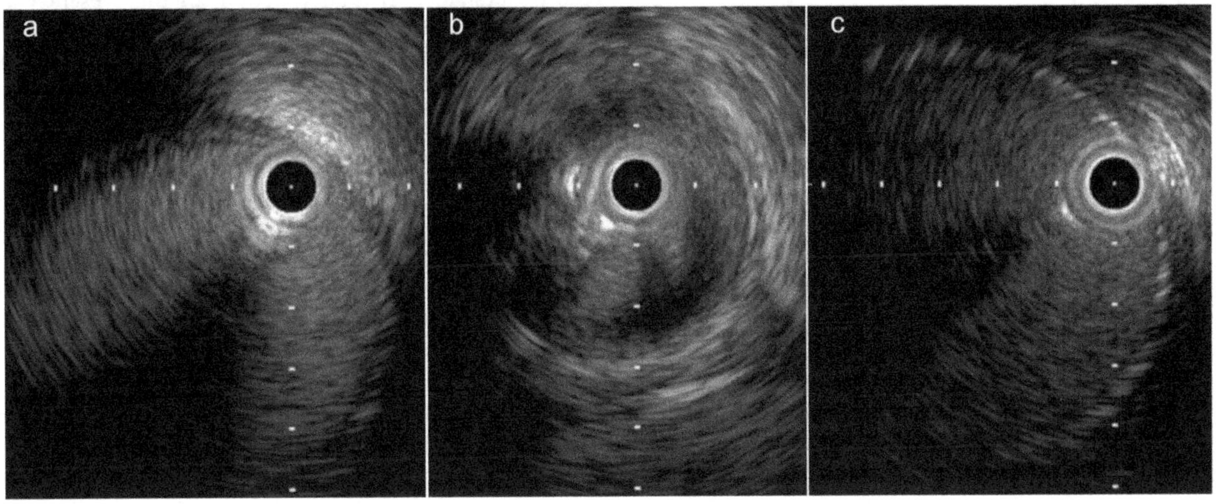

Fig. 4 Intravascular ultrasonography showing vessel shrinkage at the narrowing part, with a diameter of 5 mm (**a** proximal part; **b** the narrowing part; **c** distal part)

The reported incidence of TRAS in the literature varies from 1 to 23%, being an important cause of hypertension, renal function deterioration, and/or graft loss (1). The wide range of TRAS incidence may be influenced by the non-standard definition of the hemodynamic significance of TRAS [2, 3]. Marini et al. defined hemodynamically significant TRAS as > 75% narrowing of the lumen diameter [2]. On the other hand, Nasserala et al. defined it as > 50% narrowing of the arterial lumen [4]. Although the gold standard for the diagnosis of TRAS remains renal arteriography, angiographic stenosis was reported to have a poor correlation with hemodynamic parameters [5]. Doppler ultrasonography might provide hemodynamic information; however, such data cannot be obtained accurately owing to patients' anatomical factors, such as obesity or vessel angulation. Invasive pressure measurement using 4- or 5-French catheters during angiography also seems inappropriate because it can overestimate the true pressure gradient due to the flow obstruction [6, 7]. Thus, we thought pressure gradient measurement using a 0.014-inch pressure wire might be a more useful and appropriate method for the assessment of hemodynamic function in TRAS.

In recent years, the concept of renal fractional flow reserve (FFR) using a pressure wire has been developed. Renal FFR is calculated as the ratio of the mean distal renal pressure to the mean aortic pressure during hyperemia. Intrarenal papaverine is commonly used for eliciting maximal renal hyperemia. Although renal FFR threshold still remains controversial regarding the clinical

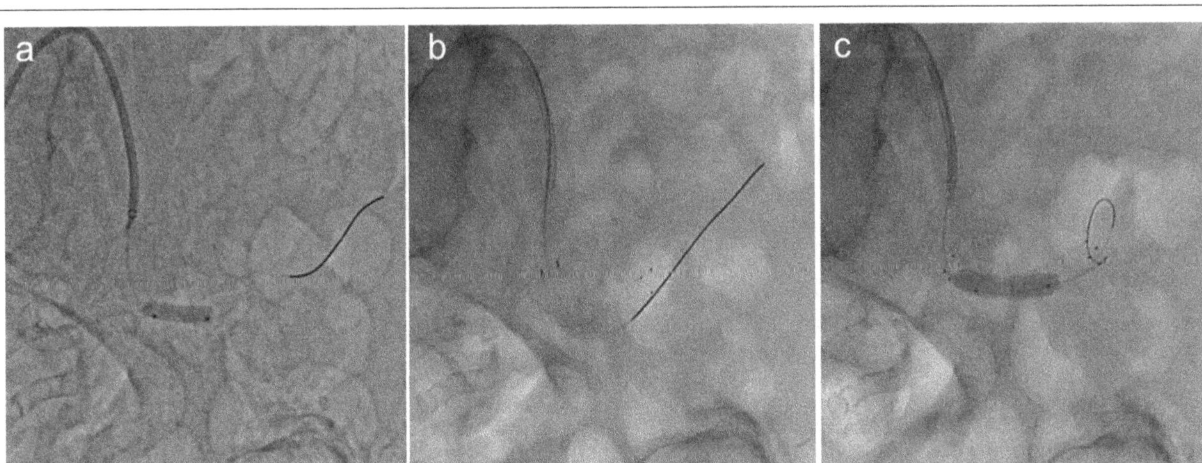

Fig. 5 Procedure of endovascular treatment. **a** Pre-dilation using a 4-mm balloon. **b** Implantation of a 6-mm self-expandable stent. **c** Post-dilatation using a 5-mm balloon

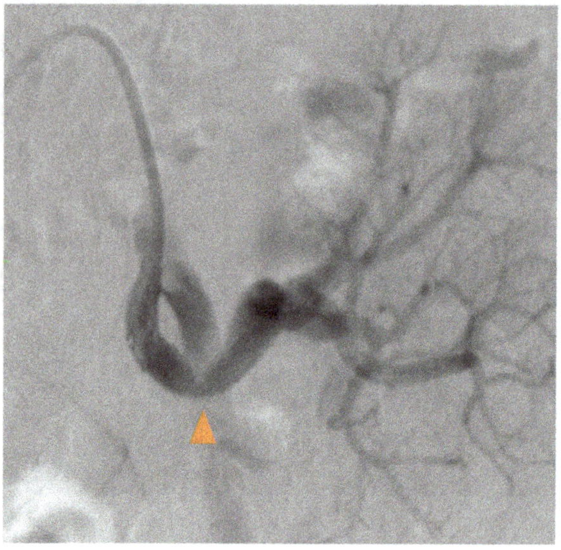

Fig. 6 Final angiography showing persistent moderate stenosis (arrowhead)

benefit of revascularization in a patient with renovascular hypertension [8, 9], Leesar MA et al. showed that a hyperemic systolic gradient ≥21 mmHg is the predictor of hypertension improvement after stenting of renal artery stenosis [10]. Kapoor N et al. suggested that a hyperemic systolic gradient ≥21 mmHg or a renal FFR of 0.90 can be considered a hemodynamically significant stenosis, and resting systolic gradient would underestimate the significance of stenosis [11]. In the present case, resting pressure measurement using 0.014-inch wire revealed a systolic pressure gradient of 40 mmHg and a Pd/Pa ratio of 0.90; therefore, we assessed the lesion as a hemodynamically significant stenosis. We considered that hyperemic evaluation would not be mandatory when it was clear that the lesion was a significant stenosis based on resting hemodynamic evaluation. To evaluate the indication of TRAS treatment, the patients' clinical course, such as worsening of blood pressure control and acute renal function deterioration, is undoubtedly important. In addition, we believe the hemodynamic evaluation with or without hyperemia adds useful information to confirm the indication of TRAS treatment.

Using a 0.014-in. wire during renal arteriography offers some technical advantages to TRAS-EVT. Regarding the treatment strategy, EVT is recognized as the first-line therapy for TRAS; its technical success is reported in 89–100% of cases [12]. After pressure measurement using a 0.014-in. wire, the subsequent EVT procedure can be performed and completed using the same wire. Moreover, pressure measurement seems to be useful to determine the endpoint of EVT. We thought that angiographically complete dilation may increase the risk of vessel dissection or perforation; and is not required for the maintenance of graft function. In the present case, the patients' renal function and blood pressure control sufficiently improved despite the persistent moderate stenosis. Therefore, it is important to identify the appropriate endpoints and avoid serious complications induced by excessive dilatation.

Recently, hemodynamic evaluation using a pressure wire has become quite popular in cardiac catheterization. This technology should be used more widely in various peripheral artery interventions, including lower limb arteries or renal arteries. It is essential to clarify the correct therapeutic indication and endpoint of EVT in non-coronary locations based on the hemodynamic evaluation with or without hyperemia. Although the possible limitation of hyperemia achievement in chronic kidney disease patients was reported [13], coronary circulation and other peripheral circulations should not be considered in the same way, and we think further studies are necessary.

In conclusion, we described a case of TRAS that was successfully treated via EVT based on pressure gradient measurement using a pressure wire. Hemodynamic evaluation using a pressure wire is useful in determining the therapeutic indication and endpoint of EVT in TRAS treatment.

Abbreviations

ARB: Angiotensin II receptor blocker; eGFR: Estimated glomerular filtration rate; EVT: Endovascular treatment; FFR: Fractional flow reserve; IVUS: Intravascular ultrasound; TRAS: Transplant renal artery stenosis

Authors' contributions

YK managed the patient, wrote and revised the manuscript. KZ and SM revised the manuscript and figures. All the authors read and approved the final manuscript.

Competing interests

The authors declare that they have no competing interests.

References

1. Fervenza FC, Lafayette RA, Alfrey EJ, Petersen J. Renal artery stenosis in kidney transplants. Am J Kidney Dis. 1998;31:142–8.
2. Marini M, Fernandez-Rivera C, Cao I, Gulias D, Alonso A, Lopez-Muniz A, et al. Treatment of transplant renal artery stenosis by percutaneous transluminal angioplasty and/or stenting: study in 63 patients in a single institution. Transplant Proc. 2011;3:2205–7.
3. Bruno S, Remuzzi G, Ruggenenti P. Transplant renal artery sltenosis. J Am Soc Nephrol. 2004;15:134–41.
4. Nasserala JC, Oliveira CM, Cerqueira JB, Souza S, Silva SL, Santos LC, et al. Artery stenosis of the renal graft: experience of a center of Northeastern Brazil. Transplant Proc. 2016;48:74–80.
5. Subramanian R, White CJ, Rosenfield K, Bashir R, Almagor Y, Meerkin D, et al. Renal fractional flow reserve: a hemodynamic evaluation of moderate renal artery stenoses. Catheter Cardiovasc Interv. 2005;64:480–6.
6. Parham W, Shafei A, Rajjoub H, Ziaee A, Kern M. Retrograde left ventricular hemodynamic assessment across bileaflet prosthetic aortic valves: the use

of a high-fidelity pressure sensor angioplasty guidewire. Catheter Cardiovasc Interv. 2003;59:509–13.
7. Colyer WR Jr, Cooper CJ, Burket MW, Thomas WJ. Utility of a 0.014" pressure-sensing guidewire to assess renal artery translesional systolic pressure gradients. Catheter Cardiovasc Interv. 2003;59:372–7.
8. Mitchell JA, Subramanian R, White CJ, Soukas PA, Almagor Y, Stewart RE, et al. Predicting blood pressure improvement in hypertensive patients after renal artery stent placement: renal fractional flow reserve. Catheter Cardiovasc Interv. 2007;69:685–9.
9. Kadziela J, Januszewicz A, Prejbisz A, Michałowska I, Januszewicz M, Florczak E, et al. Prognostic value of renal fractional flow reserve in blood pressure response after renal artery stenting (PREFER study). Cardiol J. 2013;20:418–22.
10. Leesar MA, Varma J, Shapira A, Fahsah I, Raza ST, Elghoul Z, et al. Prediction of hypertension improvement after stenting of renal artery stenosis: comparative accuracy of translesional pressure gradients, intravascular ultrasound, and angiography. J Am Coll Cardiol. 2009;53:2363–71.
11. Kapoor N, Fahsah I, Karim R, Jevans AJ, Leesar MA. Physiological assessment of renal artery stenosis: comparisons of resting with hyperemic renal pressure measurements. Catheter Cardiovasc Interv. 2010;76:726–32.
12. Touma J, Costanzo A, Boura B, Alomran F, Combes M. Endovascular management of transplant renal artery stenosis. J Vasc Surg. 2014;59:1058–65.
13. Tebaldi M, Biscaglia S, Fineschi M, Manari A, Menozzi M, Secco GG, et al. Fractional flow reserve evaluation and chronic kidney disease: analysis from a multicenter Italian registry (the FREAK study). Catheter Cardiovasc Interv. 2016;88:555–62.

22

Relationship between high platelet reactivity on clopidogrel and long-term clinical outcomes after drug-eluting stents implantation (PAINT-DES)

Xiao-Fei Gao[1†], Shu Lu[2†], Zhen Ge[3], Guang-Feng Zuo[3], Zhi-Mei Wang[1], Feng Wang[1], Xiang-Quan Kong[3], Da-Yang Chai[2], Shao-Liang Chen[1,3] and Jun-Jie Zhang[1,3*]

Abstract

Background: The relationship between platelet reactivity and long-term clinical outcomes remains controversial. The present prospective study was designed to explore the association between high platelet reactivity (HPR) on clopidogrel and long-term clinical outcomes following implantation of drug eluting stents (DES).

Methods: A total of 1769 consecutive patients assessed by Aggrestar (PL-11) were enrolled at our center from February 2011 to December 2017. The primary end point was major adverse cardiovascular and cerebrovascular events (MACCE), defined as definite or probable stent thrombosis, spontaneous myocardial infarction, all cause death, clinically driven target vessel revascularization (TVR), or ischemic stroke. Bleeding served as the safety endpoint. Propensity score matching (PSM) analysis was performed to adjust for baseline differences in the overall cohort.

Results: Finally, 409 patients (23.1%) were identified with HPR on clopidogrel. At a median follow-up of 4.1 years (interquartile range, 1.8 years), the occurrence of MACCE was significantly higher in HPR on clopidogrel group than normal platelet reactivity (NPR) on clopidogrel group (15.6% vs. 5.4%, $p < 0.001$). After PSM, 395 paired patients were matched, and the difference in MACCE between HPR (15.7%) versus NPR (9.4%) on clopidogrel groups remained significant ($P < 0.001$), mainly driven by increased all cause death (5.3% vs. 1.8%, $p < 0.001$), and clinically driven TVR (8.1% vs. 6.3%, $p = 0.019$) in the HPR group. The risk of bleeding between two groups was similar.

Conclusions: This prospective study confirms the relationship between HPR on clopidogrel and long-term adverse cardiovascular events after coronary stenting.

Keywords: Platelet function testing, Clopidogrel, High platelet reactivity, Drug eluting stent

Background

Dual antiplatelet therapy with aspirin and clopidogrel, an adenosine diphosphate (ADP)-receptor inhibitor, is widely prescribed for patients with percutaneous coronary intervention (PCI) to prevent stent thrombosis, which has a high risk of myocardial infarction (MI) and cardiac death [1, 2]. However, patients treated with protocolized aspirin and clopidogrel may still develop adverse cardiovascular events, and high platelet reactivity (HPR) on clopidogrel (clopidogrel no-response or clopidogrel resistance) has been thought to play a critical role in their occurrence [3].

In platelet function testing studies [4, 5], the rate of HPR on clopidogrel was 4–46% in patients on conventional dose of clopidogrel. Randomized clinical trials (RCTs) [6–9] failed to show benefit of antiplatelet

* Correspondence: jameszll@163.com
†Xiao-Fei Gao and Shu Lu contributed equally to this work.
1Department of Cardiology, Nanjing First Hospital, Nanjing Medical University, No. 68 Changle Road, Nanjing 210006, China
3Department of Cardiology, Nanjing Heart Center, Nanjing, China
Full list of author information is available at the end of the article

regimen adjustment according to platelet function testing for coronary stenting, which might partly be due to exclusion of high-risk patients, and randomization performed a few hours after PCI. The current consensus [10] from large observational studies [3, 11–14] is that HPR on clopidogrel is associated with increased short-term risk of cardiac events following drug-eluting stents (DES) implantation. However, there is scarce evidence on the relationship between HPR on clopidogrel and long-term cardiovascular events in PCI patients. Therefore, the present prospective, propensity score-matched (PSM) cohort study explored the long-term impact of HPR on clopidogrel in patients with DES implantation.

Methods

Study design and population

The PAINT-DES is a prospective, single-center cohort study designed to assess the association between HPR on clopidogrel and long-term cardiovascular events in patients with DES implantation. From February 2011 to December 2017, a total of 6200 consecutive real-word PCI patients at our center with loading dose of aspirin and clopidogrel were candidates for this study. Finally, 1769 patients with platelet function testing were enrolled in the present study if they met the following inclusion criteria: age > 18 years, and at least one successful DES implantation. The major exclusion criteria were: patients on ticagrelor or oral anticoagulation (warfarin, dabigatran, rivaroxaban, etc.); platelet count $< 10 \times 10^9$ /L; acute myocardial infarction < 24 h; suspected intolerance to study drugs; major complication during PCI; and an estimated life expectancy < 12 months (Additional file 1: Figure S1). Cases missing > 10% of baseline variables also were excluded. The study protocol and informed consent were reviewed and approved by the Institutional Review Board of Nanjing First Hospital. Written informed consent for participation was obtained from all enrolled patients.

Procedure and medication

All coronary interventions were performed according to current standards. Use of coronary imaging tools, type of DES, low molecular weight heparin, glycoprotein IIb/IIIa inhibitors, and intra-aortic balloon pump counterpulsation were at operator's discretion. Patients not on aspirin 100 mg daily for more than 7 days were loaded with 300 mg at least 6 h prior to index procedure. A loading dose of clopidogrel of 300 mg or 600 mg was prescribed at least 6 h before the procedure, followed by a daily maintenance dose of 75 mg. Total creatine kinase (CK), CK-myocardial-band isoenzyme (MB), and troponin T/I were dynamically measured before the procedure and until 72 h post-procedure. After the procedure, all patients were prescribed aspirin 100 mg daily indefinitely and clopidogrel 75 mg daily for at least 12 months.

Platelet function testing

Platelet function testing with Aggrestar (PL-11) analyzer (SINNOWA Co., Nanjing, China) was performed before heparin or antithrombotic agent administration during the index procedure in the cardiac catheterization lab. Blood samples were stored at room temperature and tested within 2 h after collection. Information on the Aggrestar analyzer has been provided in detail before [12, 15]. Briefly, platelet function was tested using sequentially platelet counting method, with automatically and sequentially counting platelet numbers in the citrated whole blood sample before and after adding agonists at fixed time intervals. Aggrestar analyzer provides more stable and accurate platelet maximum aggregation ratio (MAR%) than standardized test method. HPR on clopidogrel was defined as MAR% ≥ 55% according to a previous study [12]. It was not recommended to adjust antiplatelet strategy based on the results of platelet function testing.

Endpoints and definitions

The primary endpoint was rate of major adverse cardiovascular and cerebrovascular events (MACCE), defined as definite or probable stent thrombosis, spontaneous MI, all cause death, clinically driven target vessel revascularization (TVR), or ischemic stroke. The secondary endpoints included stent thrombosis, cardiac death, clinically driven target lesion revascularization (TLR), and individual components of the primary endpoint. Spontaneous MI was diagnosed based on Third Universal Definition of Myocardial Infarction [16]. Cardiac death was defined as any death without a clear non-cardiac cause. Clinically driven TLR or TVR was defined as angina or ischemia referable to the target lesion or target vessel requiring repeated PCI or bypass surgery. Ischemic stroke was defined as neurological deficit of cerebrovascular cause according to the related symptoms and physical examination and brain imaging. Bleeding served as the safety endpoint, defined in accordance to the Bleeding Academic Research Consortium (BARC) classification [17]. Stent thrombosis was defined based on the Academic Research Consortium (ARC) classification [18]. Lesion specificities were defined based on American Heart Association/American College of Cardiology criteria [19]. Complex coronary lesions in this study were defined as one of the following: multi-vessel lesions, moderate to severe calcification, chronic total occlusion, coronary bifurcations treated with two-stent techniques, and unprotected left main lesions.

Follow up

Clinical follow-up was conducted with visits (preferred) or telephone contact at 1, 6, 12 months, and yearly thereafter. Angiographic follow-up was scheduled for all patients at 13 months after PCI, unless clinically indicated earlier. An independent committee that was blinded to the study assessed all adverse clinical events.

Statistical analysis

Continuous baseline variables are expressed as means ± standard deviation (SD) or median (interquartile range) and were compared using Students' *t*-test for normal data and Wilcoxon rank sum scores for non-normally distributed data. Categorical variables are expressed as counts and percentages and were compared by Chi-square test or Fisher's exact test. Time-to-first event curves between two groups were generated by Kaplan-Meier analysis and compared by a log-rank test. For significant differences ($p < 0.10$) in baseline clinical characteristics (age, male, body mass index [BMI], hypertension, hyperlipidemia, current smoker, prior stroke, prior MI, and prior PCI), and procedural characteristics (chronic total occlusion, and complete revascularization) between two groups, propensity score matching at a ratio of 1:1 was performed to minimize any selection bias using logistic regression according to the nearest rule, with matching tolerance of 0.01. Potential interactions between the subgroups and platelet reactivity were examined for the primary outcome. Multivariable Cox proportional hazards forward stepwise regression was performed to determine independent predictors of the primary endpoint with purposeful selection of covariates. The variables showing possible statistical significance ($P < 0.10$) in univariable model and those judged to be of clinical importance from previous studies (age, male, body mass index, hypertension, diabetes, current smoker, complex lesions, stent number, intravascular ultrasound used, and complete revascularization) were entered into the Cox multivariable model. All statistical tests were two-sided, and a *p*-value of < 0.05 was considered statistically significant. All statistical analyses were performed with SPSS version 24.0 (SPSS Institute Inc., Chicago, Illinois, USA).

Results

Baseline clinical characteristics

Of 1769 patients with DES implantation, 409 (23.1%) were in the HPR on clopidogrel group, and the remainder was in the normal platelet reactivity (NPR) on clopidogrel group. The baseline clinical characteristics are summarized in Table 1. Notably, patients in the HPR on clopidogrel group were older (66.9 ± 10.2), and with higher BMI (25.1 ± 3.6 kg/mm^2), and more frequent hypertension (76.0%), hyperlipidemia (49.9%), and prior stroke (3.7%) when compared with the NPR on clopidogrel group (64.6 ± 10.2, $p < 0.001$; 24.6 ± 2.9 kg/mm2, $p = 0.003$; 69.8%, $p = 0.014$; 38.3%, $p < 0.001$; 1.3%, $p = 0.005$, respectively). They also were less often men (70.7% versus 75.6%, $p = 0.045$). All the other baseline variables were similarly distributed.

Lesion and procedural characteristics

Table 2 shows that patients in the HPR on clopidogrel group had more frequent chronic total occlusion (15.4%) compared with the NPR on clopidogrel group (10.0%, $p = 0.003$). Moreover, there was a numerically lower rate of complete revascularization for all diseased coronary segments (defined as ≥2.5 mm in diameter by visual estimation) in the HPR on clopidogrel group than that in the NPR on clopidogrel group (59.6% vs. 64.8%, $p = 0.054$). All the other angiographic and procedural characteristics were comparable between two groups.

Unadjusted clinical outcomes

Clinical follow-up was available in 94.7% of all patients, and angiographic follow-up was conducted in 70.1% of patients. Unadjusted clinical outcomes are listed in Table 3. After a median follow-up of 4.1 years (interquartile range, 1.8 years), the incidence of definite and probable stent thrombosis, all cause death, clinically driven TVR, and ischemic stroke in the HPR on clopidogrel group was 1.5, 5.1, 7.8, and 2.2%, respectively, which was significantly higher than 0.3% ($p = 0.003$), 1.3% ($p < 0.001$), 3.2% ($p < 0.001$), and 0.5% ($p < 0.001$), respectively, in the NPR on clopidogrel group, resulting in more frequent MACCE in the HPR on clopidogrel group (15.6% vs. 5.4%, $p < 0.001$). The occurrence of bleeding (BARC classification ≥2) was 2.9% in the HPR on clopidogrel group, which was comparable with 2.6% in the NPR on clopidogrel group ($p = 0.754$).

Propensity score matched analysis

After PSM, 395 pairs of patients were matched. The baseline characteristics became comparable between two groups (Tables 1 and 2). There was still a significant difference in MACCE between the NPR on clopidogrel group and the HPR on clopidogrel group (9.4% vs. 15.7%, $p < 0.001$; Table 3, Fig. 1), mainly driven by increased all cause death (1.8% vs. 5.3%, $p < 0.001$), and clinically driven TVR (6.3% vs. 8.1%, $p = 0.019$) in the latter group. The risk of bleeding (BARC classification≥2) between these two groups remained similar. There were no significant interactions between any of the subgroups and platelet reactivity for MACCE (Fig. 2). In Cox regression multivariable analysis, diabetes (hazard ratio [HR]: 1.566, 95% confidence interval [CI]: 1.028–2.385, $p = 0.037$), HPR on clopidogrel (HR: 2.146, 95% CI: 1.387–3.320, $p = 0.001$), and complex coronary lesions (HR: 2.510, 95% CI: 1.522–4.140, $p < 0.001$) were

Table 1 Baseline clinical characteristics

	Before propensity score matching			After propensity score matching		
	NPR on clopidogrel (n = 1360)	HPR on clopidogrel (n = 409)	P Value	NPR on clopidogrel (n = 395)	HPR on clopidogrel (n = 395)	P Value
Age, year	64.6 ± 10.2	66.9 ± 10.2	< 0.001	66.5 ± 9.8	66.7 ± 10.2	0.765
Male, n (%)	1028 (75.6)	289 (70.7)	0.045	264 (66.8)	278 (70.4)	0.283
BMI, kg/mm^2	24.6 ± 2.9	25.1 ± 3.6	0.003	25.3 ± 3.1	25.0 ± 3.1	0.169
Hypertension, n (%)	949 (69.8)	311 (76.0)	0.014	298 (75.4)	305 (77.2)	0.558
Hyperlipidemia, n (%)	521 (38.3)	204 (49.9)	< 0.001	198 (50.1)	200 (50.6)	0.887
Diabetes, n (%)	372 (27.4)	127 (31.1)	0.145	118 (29.9)	125 (31.6)	0.589
Current smoker, n (%)	511 (37.6)	132 (32.3)	0.051	137 (34.7)	131 (33.2)	0.652
ACS, n (%)	1226 (90.1)	361 (88.3)	0.272	359 (90.9)	349 (88.4)	0.243
eGFR ≥60 ml/min/1.73m^2, n(%)	1205 (88.9)	359 (88.0)	0.625	339 (86.5)	347 (88.1)	0.503
Prior stroke, n (%)	18 (1.3)	15 (3.7)	0.005	5 (1.3)	12 (3.0)	0.086
Prior MI, n (%)	124 (9.1)	49 (12.0)	0.088	42 (10.6)	48 (12.2)	0.502
Prior PCI, n (%)	267 (19.6)	96 (23.5)	0.092	76 (19.2)	96 (24.3)	0.085
Prior CABG, n (%)	12 (0.9)	6 (1.5)	0.397	3 (0.8)	6 (1.5)	0.505
LVEF, %	59.7 ± 9.0	58.4 ± 8.2	0.488	58.5 ± 9.4	58.4 ± 8.2	0.952
Symptomatic HF, n (%)	222 (16.5)	79 (19.6)	0.155	97 (24.6)	79 (20.0)	0.124
Treatment at discharge						
Aspirin maintenance dose, n (%)	1360 (100)	408 (99.8)	0.231	395 (100)	394 (99.7)	0.317
Clopidogrel maintenance dose of 75 mg, n (%)	1331 (97.9)	395 (96.6)	0.137	381 (96.5)	381 (96.5)	NS
Clopidogrel maintenance dose of 150 mg, n (%)	29 (2.1)	14 (3.4)	0.137	14 (3.5)	14 (3.5)	NS
Treatment at last follow-up visit						
Aspirin maintenance dose, n (%)	1292 (95)	386 (94.4)	0.617	376 (95.2)	372 (94.2)	0.526
Clopidogrel maintenance dose, n (%)	494 (36.3)	140 (34.2)	0.439	132 (33.4)	127 (32.2)	0.705
Ticagrelor maintenance dose, n (%)	11 (0.8)	5 (1.2)	0.388	6 (1.5)	4 (1.0)	0.524
Laboratory						
Red blood cell, × 10^{12}/L	4.4 ± 0.6	4.6 ± 6.5	0.314	4.3 ± 0.6	4.6 ± 6.5	0.596
Hemoglobin, g/L	133.7 ± 17.2	132.1 ± 55.3	0.436	132.0 ± 17.9	132.2 ± 55.8	0.973
Platelet count, × 10^9/L	190.6 ± 66.9	190.3 ± 51.5	0.937	186.1 ± 55.5	189.9 ± 51.1	0.431
hsCRP, ug/ml	32.1 ± 8.9	31.9 ± 8.8	0.858	31.8 ± 8.6	31.9 ± 8.9	0.883

NPR normal platelet reactivity, *HPR* high platelet reactivity, *BMI* body mass index, *ACS* acute coronary syndrome, *eGFR* estimated glomerular filtration rate, *MI* myocardial infarction, *PCI* percutaneous coronary intervention, *CABG* coronary artery bypass grafting, *LVEF* left ventricular ejection fraction, *HF* heart failure, *hsCRP* high sensitivity C reactive protein

independent predictors of MACCE at a median follow-up of 4.1 years.

Discussion

The present prospective, propensity score-matched cohort study for the first time evaluated the relationship between HPR on clopidogrel and long-term outcomes following DES implantation. The major findings were: 1) 23.1% of patients with DES implantation were identified with HPR on clopidogrel despite having received loading dose of clopidogrel; 2) HPR on clopidogrel was associated with dramatic increment in unadjusted and adjusted long-term MACCE, mainly driven by increased all cause death and clinically driven TVR; and 3) there was no significant association between platelet reactivity and unadjusted and adjusted risk of bleeding.

Antiplatelet agents, aspirin and clopidogrel, have a critical role in the treatment of coronary heart disease, ischemic stroke and peripheral artery disease. However, stented patients suffer from recurrent thrombotic events despite being on regular aspirin and clopidogrel, which might be due to HPR on clopidogrel. Several factors [20–22] might underlie HPR on clopidogrel including patient noncompliance, intestinal absorption (ABCB1

Table 2 Angiographic and procedural characteristics

	Before propensity score matching[a]			After propensity score matching		
	NPR on clopidogrel (*n* = 1360)	HPR on clopidogrel (*n* = 409)	*P* Value	NPR on clopidogrel (*n* = 395)	HPR on clopidogrel (*n* = 395)	*P* Value
Radial access, n (%)	1249 (92.9)	372 (92.1)	0.596	355 (89.9)	367 (92.9)	0.128
Multi-vessel disease, n (%)	605 (46.4)	200 (49.5)	0.280	188 (50.4)	196 (51.0)	0.860
Bifurcation lesion, n (%)	410 (30.5)	135 (33.4)	0.268	129 (32.7)	133 (33.7)	0.762
Chronic total occlusion, n (%)	133 (10.0)	63 (15.4)	0.003	64 (16.2)	62 (15.7)	0.846
Unprotected Left main lesions, n (%)	146 (10.9)	46 (11.4)	0.765	51 (12.9)	45 (11.4)	0.514
Second-generation DES used, n (%)	1360 (100)	409 (100)	NS	395 (100)	395 (100)	NS
IABP used, n (%)	23 (1.8)	6 (1.6)	0.753	13 (3.5)	6 (1.6)	0.108
IVUS used, n (%)	291 (22.9)	100 (26.1)	0.189	79 (21.2)	97 (26.2)	0.106
Stent number	1.9 ± 1.1	1.9 ± 1.1	0.328	1.9 ± 1.1	1.9 ± 1.1	0.946
Mean stent diameter, mm	3.0 ± 0.7	2.9 ± 0.7	0.770	3.0 ± 0.6	2.9 ± 0.7	0.166
Stent length, mm	49.1 ± 31.2	51.0 ± 30.4	0.299	49.6 ± 31.1	50.6 ± 30.2	0.650
Complete revascularization, n (%)	852 (64.8)	240 (59.6)	0.054	252 (63.8)	237 (60.0)	0.272
Final TIMI grade 3, n (%)	1301 (98.3)	393 (97.5)	0.339	387 (98.5)	384 (97.5)	0.315

[a] There is some data loss in dozens of patients
NPR normal platelet reactivity, *HPR* high platelet reactivity, *DES* drug-eluting stent, *IABP* intra-aortic balloon pump, *IVUS* intravascular ultrasound, *TIMI* thrombolysis in myocardial infarction

gene polymorphism), polymorphisms in CYP2C19, drug-drug interactions (e.g. omeprazole, β-Blockers [23]), and other clinical factors (age, BMI, diabetes, chronic renal insufficiency, heart failure). More potent ADP-receptor inhibitors, such as ticagrelor and prasugrel, were expected to overcome HPR on clopidogrel because they showed better clinical outcomes than clopidogrel in patients with acute coronary syndrome (ACS) [24, 25]. However, ticagrelor and prasugrel were associated with higher risk of major bleeding [24–26]. Furthermore, recent studies [27, 28] demonstrated that clopidogrel was superior to ticagrelor to prevent bleeding complications without increased risk of ischemic events in low-to-moderate risk of ACS, especially among those treated with newer-generation DES. Overall, clopidogrel, with low cost and low bleeding risk, is still widely used in clinical practice, and platelet reactivity is worth exploring further.

The optimal method for platelet function testing is still a key and controversial issue. Although various methods

Table 3 Clinical outcomes

	Before propensity score matching			After propensity score matching		
	NPR on clopidogrel (*n* = 1360)	HPR on clopidogrel (*n* = 409)	*P* Value	NPR on clopidogrel (*n* = 395)	HPR on clopidogrel (*n* = 395)	*P* Value
Stent thrombosis	7 (0.5)	13 (3.2)	< 0.001	3 (0.8)	13 (3.3)	0.003
Definite/ probable Stent thrombosis	4 (0.3)	6 (1.5)	0.003	2 (0.5)	6 (1.5)	0.110
All cause death	18 (1.3)	21 (5.1)	< 0.001	7 (1.8)	21 (5.3)	< 0.001
Cardiac death	6 (0.4)	10 (2.4)	0.001	2 (0.5)	10 (2.5)	0.004
MI	12 (0.9)	7 (1.7)	0.085	6 (1.5)	7 (1.8)	0.526
STEMI	4 (0.3)	5 (1.2)	0.015	2 (0.5)	5 (1.3)	0.215
NSTEMI	10 (0.7)	3 (0.7)	NS	5 (1.3)	3 (0.8)	0.734
Clinically driven TLR	40 (2.9)	26 (6.4)	< 0.001	24 (6.1)	26 (6.6)	0.111
Clinically driven TVR	43 (3.2)	32 (7.8)	< 0.001	25 (6.3)	32 (8.1)	0.019
Ischemic stroke	7 (0.5)	9 (2.2)	< 0.001	4 (1.0)	7 (1.8)	0.093
Bleeding (BARC≥2)	36 (2.6)	12 (2.9)	0.754	11 (2.8)	11 (2.8)	NS
MACCE	74 (5.1)	64 (15.6)	< 0.001	37 (9.4)	62 (15.7)	< 0.001

Data are number of events (Kaplan-Meier estimated event rate), compared by the log-rank test
NPR normal platelet reactivity, *HPR* high platelet reactivity, *MI* myocardial infarction, *TLR* target lesion revascularization, *TVR* target vessel revascularization, *MACCE* major adverse cardiovascular and cerebrovascular events

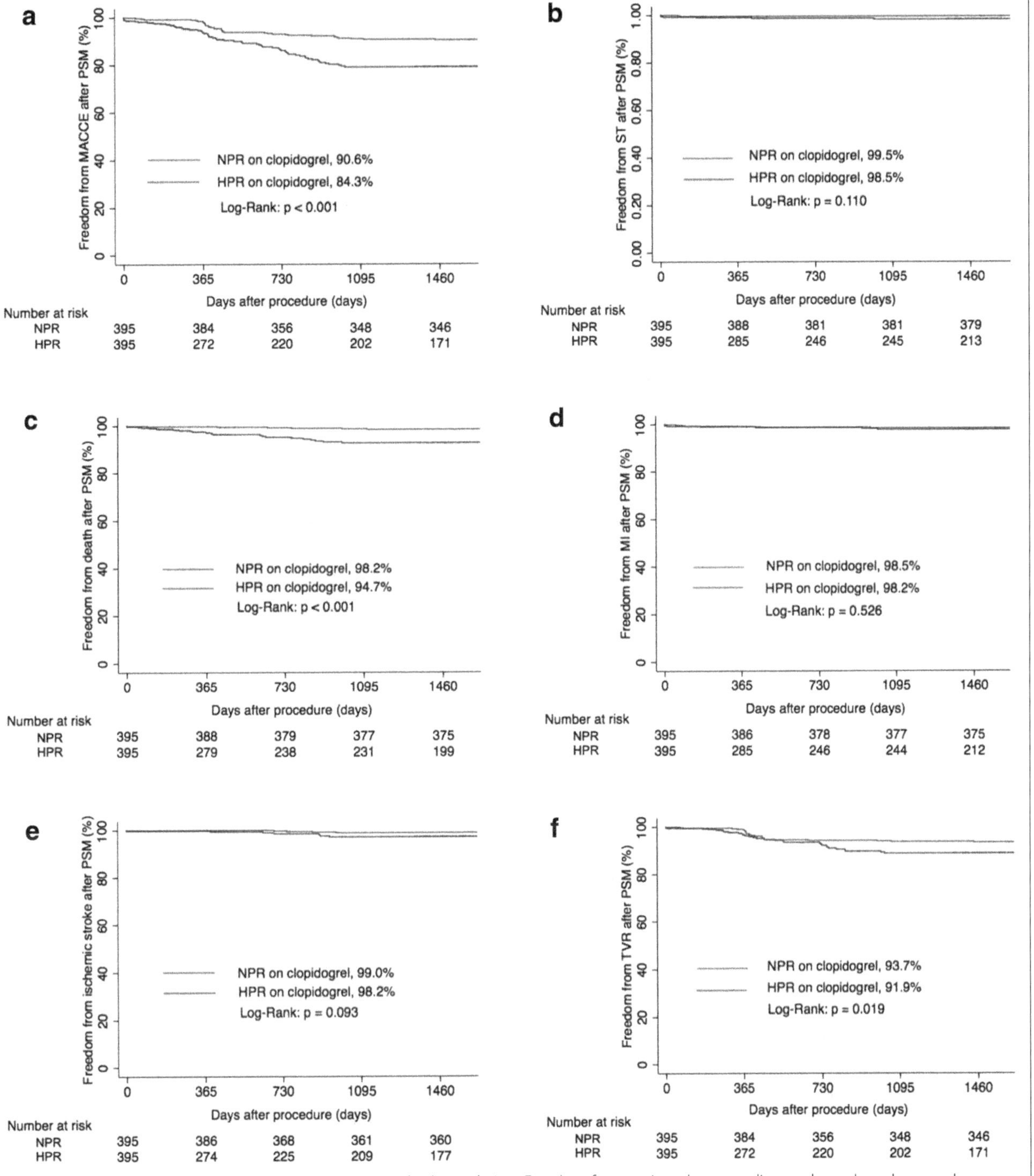

Fig. 1 Freedom from events in the propensity score-matched population. Freedom from major adverse cardiovascular and cerebrovascular events (MACCE) (**a**), definite/ probable stent thrombosis (ST) (**b**), all cause death (**c**), myocardial infarction (MI) (**d**), ischemic stroke (**e**), and clinically driven target vessel revascularization (TVR) (**f**) between high platelet reactivity (HPR) on clopidogrel and normal platelet reactivity (NPR) on clopidogrel in the propensity score-matched (PSM) population

have been developed, their results correlate poorly with each other [29, 30]. Light transmittance aggregation (LTA) is considered the gold standard, but it is time and labor consuming. VerifyNow system has been widely used in clinical trials, but it is very expensive and nonflexible [31, 32]. As described in the methods section, Aggrestar analyzer provides more stable and accurate platelet numbers, with good correlation with VerifyNow [15], which renders it a reliable alternative for platelet function testing.

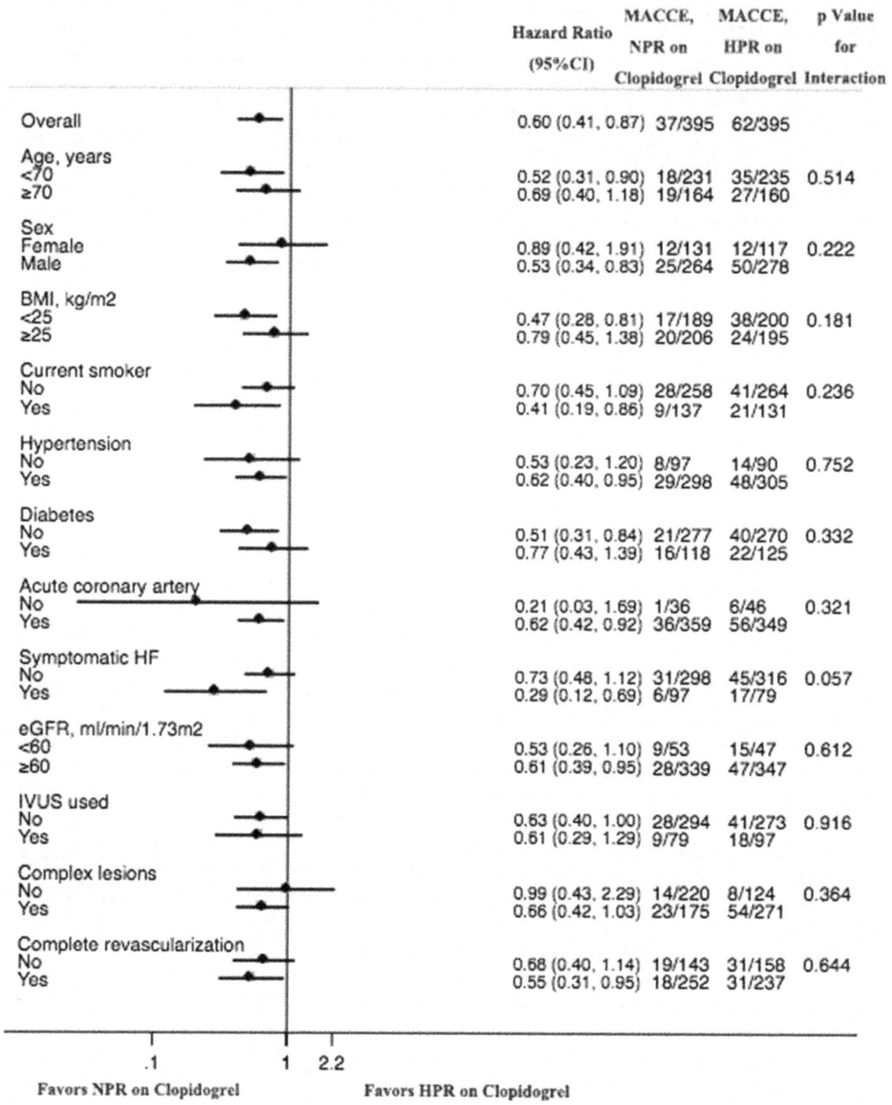

Fig. 2 Subgroup analysis. The increment in major adverse cardiovascular and cerebrovascular events (MACCE) with high platelet reactivity (HPR) on clopidogrel compared with normal platelet reactivity (NPR) on clopidogrel was consistent across pre-specified subgroups. BMI: body mass index; HF: heart failure; eGFR: estimated glomerular filtration rate; IVUS: intravascular ultrasound

Individualized treatment based on platelet function testing was expected to inform choice of more suitable antiplatelet agents and dosage for stenting patients, balancing the risk of ischemia and bleeding. In line with our previous study [12], HPR on clopidogrel was associated with increased risk for stent thrombosis in a prospective multicenter study [14]. The present prospective study with propensity-matched population is the first to confirm the relationship between HPR on clopidogrel and long-term thrombotic events in patients with DES implantation. In contrast to these findings, ARCTIC study (Bedside Monitoring to Adjust Antiplatelet Therapy for Coronary Stenting), including 2440 patients scheduled for coronary stenting, showed no significant improvements in clinical outcomes with platelet function testing and treatment adjustment for coronary stenting [7]. The latter difference might be due to the higher proportion of patients at higher risk in our study, with higher frequency of diabetes, ACS, prior MI, prior PCI, symptomatic heart failure, and complex coronary lesions. However, TROPICAL-ACS trial (The Testing Responsiveness To Platelet Inhibition On Chronic Antiplatelet Treatment For ACS) demonstrated that platelet function testing guided de-escalation of antiplatelet treatment (from prasugrel to clopidogrel) was non-inferior to standard treatment with prasugrel at 1 year after PCI, providing important evidence for ACS patients with coronary stenting in whom early de-escalation is considered as an alternative strategy [33]. Notably, the recent CREATIVE trial [34] (Clopidogrel Response

Evaluation and AnTi-platelet InterVEntion in High Thrombotic Risk PCI Patients) also showed that intensified antiplatelet strategies with adjunctive use of cilostazol significantly improved clinical outcomes without increasing the risk of major bleeding in patients with HPR on clopidogrel. Consequently, the relationship between clopidogrel hyporesponsiveness and thrombotic events has been probably established, especially in high-risk patients, and a well-designed large-scale RCT with optimal testing method is waarranted to evaluate the real benefit of platelet function testing.

Several questions remain unanswered. First, previous studies [12, 35] showed that HPR on aspirin was also associated with incremental thrombotic events after DES implantation. However, mounting evidence [36–38] supports that HPR on aspirin is either a very rare phenomenon or does not exist, and might due to patient noncompliance, delayed and reduced drug absorption of enteric coating, or drug-drug interactions (e.g. ibuprofen). Second, it was reported [3] that platelet function testing predicts bleeding in patients with bypass surgery. Nevertheless, other studies [12, 39] failed to show that platelet function testing reliably predicted future bleeding risk in stenting patients, in line with the present study, which might be due to the low bleeding risk of clopidogrel and coronary intervention. Therefore, the value of platelet function testing in PCI patients should be explored in further studies. Our ongoing PL-PLATELET (Ticagrelor Versus High-dose Clopidogrel in Patients With High Platelet Reactivity on Clopidogrel After PCI, NCT03078465) trial may offer further insight into the effect of platelet function testing on PCI patients.

Our study has several limitations. First, we did not assess the effect of platelet function testing guided therapy adjustment on cardiac events. Second, platelet function testing was performed at index procedure, and enrolled patients did not undergo repeated testing at later time periods. Third, Aggrestar, not VerifyNow, was used in this study due to the high cost of VerifyNow; however, Aggrestar has been shown to correlate well with VerifyNow [15]. Fourth, the study median follow-up of 4.1 years with interquartile range of 1.8 years (skewed distribution) indicates that more patients were enrolled at the early stage of this study, but the duration of follow-up was similar between two groups. Additionally, it was a real-world cohort study, and some patients changed the antiplatelet drugs themselves, although no differences were found between two groups.

Conclusion

This prospective, propensity score-matched cohort study showed that HPR on clopidogrel was associated with incremental long-term risk of MACCE after DES implantation, mainly driven by increased all cause death and clinically driven TVR. The present study suggests potential benefits for platelet function testing, and a well-designed RCT with optimal testing method is needed to further address the real advantages of platelet function testing.

Abbreviations

ACS: Acute coronary syndrome; ADP: Adenosine diphosphate; BMI: Body mass index; CABG: Coronary artery bypass grafting; DES: Drug-eluting stent; eGFR: Estimated glomerular filtration rate; HF: Heart failure; HPR: High platelet reactivity; hsCRP: High sensitivity C reactive protein; IABP: Intra-aortic balloon pump; IVUS: Intravascular ultrasound; LTA: Light transmittance aggregation; LVEF: Left ventricular ejection fraction; MACCE: Major adverse cardiovascular and cerebrovascular events; MAR: Maximal aggregation ratio; MI: Myocardial infarction; NPR: Normal platelet reactivity; PCI: Percutaneous coronary intervention; PSM: Propensity score matching; RCT: Randomized clinical trial; TIMI: Thrombolysis in myocardial infarction; TLR: Target lesion revascularization; TVR: Target vessel revascularization

Acknowledgements

We deeply appreciate Ms. Hai-Mei Xu, Ms. Jing Kan, and Ms. Ling Lin for remote monitoring and data collection throughout the study.

Funding

The present study was supported by National Science Foundation of China (NSFC 81770342), Nanjing Health and Family Planning Commission (YKK16124), Nanjing Health Youth Talent Training project (QRX17017), and Nanjing Municipal Commission of Science & Technology (201715026).

Authors' contributions

ZJJ designed the statistical analysis, lead the interpretation of research findings, and revised the manuscript. GXF and LS participated in design, data collection, dataset generation, statistical analysis, and drafting of the manuscript. GZ, ZGF, WZM, WF, KXQ, CDY, and CSL participated in the conception and design and data collection. All of the authors read and approved the final manuscript.

Competing interests

The authors declare that they have no competing interests.

Author details

[1]Department of Cardiology, Nanjing First Hospital, Nanjing Medical University, No. 68 Changle Road, Nanjing 210006, China. [2]Department of Cardiology, The First People's Hospital of Taicang, Suzhou, China. [3]Department of Cardiology, Nanjing Heart Center, Nanjing, China.

References

1. Iakovou I, Schmidt T, Bonizzoni E, Ge L, Sangiorgi GM, Stankovic G, Airoldi F, Chieffo A, Montorfano M, Carlino M, et al. Incidence, predictors, and outcome of thrombosis after successful implantation of drug-eluting stents. JAMA. 2005;293(17):2126–30.
2. Kimura T, Morimoto T, Kozuma K, Honda Y, Kume T, Aizawa T, Mitsudo K, Miyazaki S, Yamaguchi T, Hiyoshi E, et al. Comparisons of baseline demographics, clinical presentation, and long-term outcome among patients with early, late, and very late stent thrombosis of sirolimus-eluting stents: observations from the registry of stent thrombosis for review and reevaluation (RESTART). Circulation. 2010;122(1):52–61.

3. Stone GW, Witzenbichler B, Weisz G, Rinaldi MJ, Neumann FJ, Metzger DC, Henry TD, Cox DA, Duffy PL, Mazzaferri E, et al. Platelet reactivity and clinical outcomes after coronary artery implantation of drug-eluting stents (ADAPT-DES): a prospective multicentre registry study. Lancet. 2013;382(9892):614–23.
4. Capodanno D, Angiolillo DJ. Platelet monitoring for PCI: which test is the one to choose? Hamostaseologie. 2009;29(4):376–80.
5. Gurbel PA, Becker RC, Mann KG, Steinhubl SR, Michelson AD. Platelet function monitoring in patients with coronary artery disease. J Am Coll Cardiol. 2007;50(19):1822–34.
6. Cayla G, Cuisset T, Silvain J, Leclercq F, Manzo-Silberman S, Saint-Etienne C, Delarche N, Bellemain-Appaix A, Range G, El Mahmoud R, et al. Platelet function monitoring to adjust antiplatelet therapy in elderly patients stented for an acute coronary syndrome (ANTARCTIC): an open-label, blinded-endpoint, randomised controlled superiority trial. Lancet. 2016; 388(10055):2015–22.
7. Collet JP, Cuisset T, Range G, Cayla G, Elhadad S, Pouillot C, Henry P, Motreff P, Carrie D, Boueri Z, et al. Bedside monitoring to adjust antiplatelet therapy for coronary stenting. N Engl J Med. 2012;367(22):2100–9.
8. Price MJ, Angiolillo DJ, Teirstein PS, Lillie E, Manoukian SV, Berger PB, Tanguay JF, Cannon CP, Topol EJ. Platelet reactivity and cardiovascular outcomes after percutaneous coronary intervention: a time-dependent analysis of the gauging responsiveness with a VerifyNow P2Y12 assay: impact on thrombosis and safety (GRAVITAS) trial. Circulation. 2011; 124(10):1132–7.
9. Trenk D, Stone GW, Gawaz M, Kastrati A, Angiolillo DJ, Muller U, Richardt G, Jakubowski JA, Neumann FJA. Randomized trial of prasugrel versus clopidogrel in patients with high platelet reactivity on clopidogrel after elective percutaneous coronary intervention with implantation of drug-eluting stents: results of the TRIGGER-PCI (testing platelet reactivity in patients undergoing elective stent placement on Clopidogrel to guide alternative therapy with Prasugrel) study. J Am Coll Cardiol. 2012;59(24):2159–64.
10. Aradi D, Storey RF, Komocsi A, Trenk D, Gulba D, Kiss RG, Husted S, Bonello L, Sibbing D, Collet JP, et al. Expert position paper on the role of platelet function testing in patients undergoing percutaneous coronary intervention. Eur Heart J. 2014;35(4):209–15.
11. Viviani Anselmi C, Briguori C, Roncarati R, Papa L, Visconti G, Focaccio A, De Micco F, Latronico MV, Pagnotta P, Condorelli G. Routine assessment of on-clopidogrel platelet reactivity and gene polymorphisms in predicting clinical outcome following drug-eluting stent implantation in patients with stable coronary artery disease. JACC Cardiovasc Interv. 2013;6(11):1166–75.
12. Zhang JJ, Gao XF, Ge Z, Tian NL, Liu ZZ, Lin S, Ye F, Chen SL. High platelet reactivity affects the clinical outcomes of patients undergoing percutaneous coronary intervention. BMC Cardiovasc Disord. 2016;16(1):240.
13. Redfors B, Genereux P, Witzenbichler B, Kirtane AJ, Maehara A, Weisz G, Madhavan MV, McAndrew T, Mehran R, Stone GW. Percutaneous coronary intervention of bifurcation lesions and platelet reactivity. Int J Cardiol. 2018; 250:92–7.
14. Stuckey TD, Kirtane AJ, Brodie BR, Witzenbichler B, Litherland C, Weisz G, Rinaldi MJ, Neumann FJ, Metzger DC, Henry TD, et al. Impact of aspirin and Clopidogrel Hyporesponsiveness in patients treated with drug-eluting stents: 2-year results of a prospective, Multicenter Registry Study. JACC Cardiovasc Interv. 2017;10(16):1607–17.
15. Guan J, Cong Y, Ren J, Zhu Y, Li L, Deng X, Bai J. Comparison between a new platelet count drop method PL-11, light transmission aggregometry, VerifyNow aspirin system and thromboelastography for monitoring short-term aspirin effects in healthy individuals. Platelets. 2015;26(1):25–30.
16. Thygesen K, Alpert JS, White HD. Joint ESCAAHAWHFTFftRoMI. Universal definition of myocardial infarction. Eur Heart J. 2007;28(20):2525–38.
17. Mehran R, Rao SV, Bhatt DL, Gibson CM, Caixeta A, Eikelboom J, Kaul S, Wiviott SD, Menon V, Nikolsky E, et al. Standardized bleeding definitions for cardiovascular clinical trials: a consensus report from the bleeding academic research consortium. Circulation. 2011;123(23):2736–47.
18. Cutlip DE, Windecker S, Mehran R, Boam A, Cohen DJ, van Es GA, Steg PG, Morel MA, Mauri L, Vranckx P, et al. Clinical end points in coronary stent trials: a case for standardized definitions. Circulation. 2007;115(17): 2344–51.
19. Ryan TJ, Bauman WB, Kennedy JW, Kereiakes DJ, King SB 3rd, McCallister BD, Smith SC Jr, Ullyot DJ. Guidelines for percutaneous transluminal coronary angioplasty. A report of the American Heart Association/American College of Cardiology Task Force on assessment of diagnostic and therapeutic cardiovascular procedures (committee on percutaneous transluminal coronary angioplasty). Circulation. 1993;88(6):2987–3007.
20. Michelson AD, Bhatt DL. How I use laboratory monitoring of antiplatelet therapy. Blood. 2017;130(6):713–21.
21. Tantry US, Gesheff M, Liu F, Bliden KP, Gurbel PA. Resistance to antiplatelet drugs: what progress has been made? Expert Opin Pharmacother. 2014; 15(17):2553–64.
22. Dezsi DA, Merkely B, Skopal J, Barabas E, Varnai K, Falukozy J, Veress G, Alotti N, Aradi D. Impact of test conditions on ADP-induced platelet function results with the multiplate assay: is further standardization required? J Cardiovasc Pharmacol Ther. 2018;23(2):149–54.
23. Ignjatovic V, Pavlovic S, Miloradovic V, Andjelkovic N, Davidovic G, Djurdjevic P, Stolic R, Iric-Cupic V, Simic I, Ignjatovic VD, et al. Influence of different beta-blockers on platelet aggregation in patients with coronary artery disease on dual antiplatelet therapy. J Cardiovasc Pharmacol Ther. 2016;21(1):44–52.
24. Wallentin L, Becker RC, Budaj A, Cannon CP, Emanuelsson H, Held C, Horrow J, Husted S, James S, Katus H, et al. Ticagrelor versus clopidogrel in patients with acute coronary syndromes. N Engl J Med. 2009;361(11):1045–57.
25. Wiviott SD, Braunwald E, McCabe CH, Montalescot G, Ruzyllo W, Gottlieb S, Neumann FJ, Ardissino D, De Servi S, Murphy SA, et al. Prasugrel versus clopidogrel in patients with acute coronary syndromes. N Engl J Med. 2007; 357(20):2001–15.
26. Becker RC, Bassand JP, Budaj A, Wojdyla DM, James SK, Cornel JH, French J, Held C, Horrow J, Husted S, et al. Bleeding complications with the P2Y12 receptor antagonists clopidogrel and ticagrelor in the PLATelet inhibition and patient Outcomes (PLATO) trial. Eur Heart J. 2011;32(23):2933–44.
27. Cuisset T, Deharo P, Quilici J, Johnson TW, Deffarges S, Bassez C, Bonnet G, Fourcade L, Mouret JP, Lambert M, et al. Benefit of switching dual antiplatelet therapy after acute coronary syndrome: the TOPIC (timing of platelet inhibition after acute coronary syndrome) randomized study. Eur Heart J. 2017;38(41):3070–8.
28. Zocca P, van der Heijden LC, Kok MM, Lowik MM, Hartmann M, Stoel MG, Louwerenburg JW, de Man F, Linssen GCM, Knottnerus IL, et al. Clopidogrel or ticagrelor in acute coronary syndrome patients treated with newer-generation drug-eluting stents: CHANGE DAPT. EuroIntervention. 2017; 13(10):1168–76.
29. Lordkipanidze M, Pharand C, Nguyen TA, Schampaert E, Palisaitis DA, Diodati JG. Comparison of four tests to assess inhibition of platelet function by clopidogrel in stable coronary artery disease patients. Eur Heart J. 2008; 29(23):2877–85.
30. Lemesle G, Landel JB, Bauters A, Delhaye C, Bonello L, Sudre A, Susen S, Bauters C, Lablanche JM. Poor agreement between light transmission aggregometry, verify now P2Y(1)(2) and vasodilatator-stimulated phosphoprotein for clopidogrel low-response assessment: a potential explanation of negative results of recent randomized trials. Platelets. 2014; 25(7):499–505.
31. Franchi F, Rollini F, Cho JR, Ferrante E, Angiolillo DJ. Platelet function testing in contemporary clinical and interventional practice. Curr Treat Options Cardiovasc Med. 2014;16(5):300.
32. Paniccia R, Priora R, Liotta AA, Abbate R. Platelet function tests: a comparative review. Vasc Health Risk Manag. 2015;11:133–48.
33. Sibbing D, Aradi D, Jacobshagen C, Gross L, Trenk D, Geisler T, Orban M, Hadamitzky M, Merkely B, Kiss RG, et al. Guided de-escalation of antiplatelet treatment in patients with acute coronary syndrome undergoing percutaneous coronary intervention (TROPICAL-ACS): a randomised, open-label, multicentre trial. Lancet. 2017;390(10104):1747–57.
34. Tang Y-D, Wang W, Yang M, Zhang K, Chen J, Qiao S, Yan H, Wu Y, Huang X, Xu B, et al. Randomized comparisons of double-dose Clopidogrel or adjunctive Cilostazol versus standard dual Anti-platelet in patients with high post-treatment platelet reactivity: results of the CREATIVE trial (Clopidogrel response evaluation and AnTi-platelet InterVEntion in high thrombotic risk PCI patients). Circulation. 2018. PMID:29420189. https://doi.org/10.1161/CIRCULATIONAHA.117.030190.
35. Snoep JD, Hovens MM, Eikenboom JC, van der Bom JG, Huisman MV. Association of laboratory-defined aspirin resistance with a higher risk of recurrent cardiovascular events: a systematic review and meta-analysis. Arch Intern Med. 2007;167(15):1593–9.
36. Bhatt DL, Grosser T, Dong JF, Logan D, Jeske W, Angiolillo DJ, Frelinger AL 3rd, Lei L, Liang J, Moore JE, et al. Enteric coating and aspirin

nonresponsiveness in patients with type 2 diabetes mellitus. J Am Coll Cardiol. 2017;69(6):603–12.

37. Grosser T, Fries S, Lawson JA, Kapoor SC, Grant GR, FitzGerald GA. Drug resistance and pseudoresistance: an unintended consequence of enteric coating aspirin. Circulation. 2013;127(3):377–85.
38. Patrono C. The multifaceted clinical readouts of platelet inhibition by low-dose aspirin. J Am Coll Cardiol. 2015;66(1):74–85.
39. Kim MH, Choi SY, An SY, Serebruany V. Validation of three platelet function tests for bleeding risk stratification during dual antiplatelet therapy following coronary interventions. Clin Cardiol. 2016;39(7):385–90.

23

Incomplete intestinal obstruction as the possible main complaint in Behcet's disease after surgery for recurrent abdominal aortic pseudoaneurysms

Fang Jiang[†], Hui Xiang[†] and Zhi-Yong Peng[*]

Abstract

Background: Behcet's disease (BD) is a systemic vasculitis characterized by oral and genital aphthosis, and ocular and skin lesions. The disease is involved in vascular, gastrointestinal, and central nervous systems. Vasculitis may exacerbate fatal problems, such as anastomotic pseudoaneurysms. If the mesenteric vessels are involved, severe abdominal symptoms such as intestinal obstruction may occur.

Case presentation: This case report describes a young female patient who suffered from BD with recurrent abdominal aortic pseudoaneurysms, as well as deep venous thrombosis and subsequent complications of incomplete intestinal obstruction. This patient first underwent stent grafting, which was followed by rupture of two newly formed anastomotic pseudoaneurysms within six months. Emergency open surgical repair (OSR) was then performed on the ruptured pseudoaneurysms. Thrombosis and incomplete ileus occurred five months after surgery. This case was unique due to the presence of incomplete intestinal obstruction being the possible main complaint for a patient with Behcet's disease, and it is the first ever case to be reported.

Conclusion: Intestinal obstruction may present as the possible main complaint in BD. Careful and attentive strategy should be carried out to prevent fatal outcomes.

Keywords: Behcet's disease, Recurrent abdominal aortic pseudoaneurysm, Incomplete intestinal obstruction

Background

Behcet's disease (BD) is a disease that involves complex multisystem disorders. However, the exact physiopathologic mechanism of BD remains unclear. Evidence shows that arterial and venous systems are involved in BD. Involvement of the venous systems results in the occurrence of thrombosis and superficial phlebitis. Involvement of the arterial systems result in aneurysm or pseudoaneurysm, stenosis, and occlusion [1]. The pseudoaneurysm, which evolves quickly, is prone to rupture and can become life-threatening. Therefore, it is crucial to diagnose and manipulate this fatal condition early. If the mesenteric vessels are involved, severe abdominal symptoms such as intestinal obstruction may occur [2]. However, such symptoms, especially those presenting as the main complaint, are easily misdiagnosed. Here, we report a rare case of a patient who presented with incomplete intestinal obstruction as the possible main complaint after a second surgery. We believe that an examination of this case will help the field make progress toward developing a common procedural strategy for treating such rare conditions.

Case presentation

A 28-year-old female Chinese patient presented with the onset of acute continuous right abdomen pain, nausea

* Correspondence: pengzy5@hotmail.com
[†]Fang Jiang and Hui Xiang contributed equally to this work.
Department of Critical Care Medicine, Zhongnan Hospital of Wuhan University, 169 Dong'hu Road, Wuhan 430071, Hubei, People's Republic of China

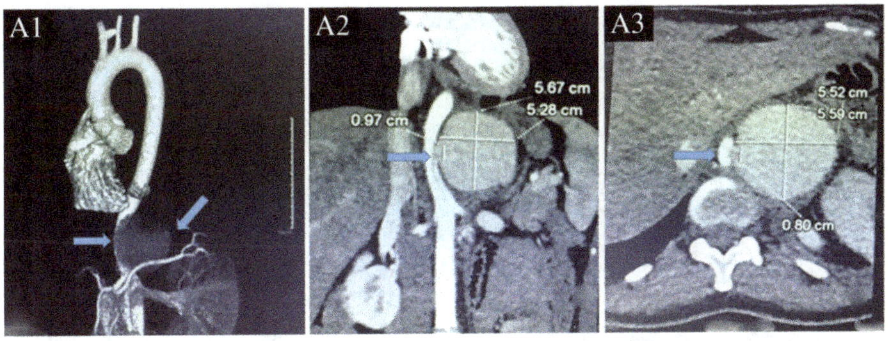

Fig. 1 The aneurysm prior to intervention. A1:The aneurysm was located in the left junction of the thoracic and abdominal aorta. A2: The size of aneurysm was 5.67 cm*5.28 cm*0.97 cm. A3: The segmental block of the starting part of the celiac trunk was approximately 0.8 cm. Arrow pointed to the aneurysm

and vomiting at the emergency department. On admission, abdominal dynamic computed tomography (CT) with a multislice detector row CT scanner showed several air-fluid levels in the enteric cavity, and the diagnosis was considered to be ileus.

The patient was diagnosed with BD four years ago. She had received medications regularly, including immunosuppressive therapy with oral prednisone (60 mg/day) and cyclophosphamide (100 mg/day).

The patient first presented with abdominal pain at the hospital. A computed tomographic angiography (CTA) was performed, which (Fig. 1) indicated an aneurysm of 5.67 cm*5.28 cm*0.97 cm located in the left junction of the thoracic aorta and abdominal aorta. An approximately 0.8 cm segment was found to block the starting part of the celiac trunk. Subsequently, a graft stent was implanted. Follow-up CTA (Fig. 2) showed no residual aneurysm. However, six months after the intervention, a rapidly growing mass was found in the lower abdomen, and the patient presented with nausea, vomiting, progressive and intermittent pain in the abdomen which radiated to her back. Before being admitted to the intensive care unit (ICU), the patient underwent CTA, which showed that there was a haematoma of approximately 6.0 × 4.8 cm in the abdomen. The extravasation of contrast agent was located in the opening of the renal artery, with a mixed soft tissue mass of 3.7 cm (Fig. 3) in the haemoperitoneum. The haemoglobin concentration decreased to 4.36 g/dL with abrupt hypotension (60/43 mmHg). The critical condition of the patient prompted the cardiac surgeons to perform open surgical repair (OSR) rather than a more conservative treatment. The patient was transferred to the ICU after the operation. Three days later, after her vital signs were stable, she was transferred back to the general ward. No recurrence of pseudoaneurysm was found during a follow-up of 15 days (Fig. 4). She continued receiving immunosuppressive therapy as usual. This course of treatment was decided based on previous studies showing that use of immunosuppressive therapy with cyclophosphamide and corticosteroids before and after surgical intervention could help prevent BD activation [3, 4].

Ten months later, after the implantation of artificial vascularization in the thoracic and abdominal aorta,

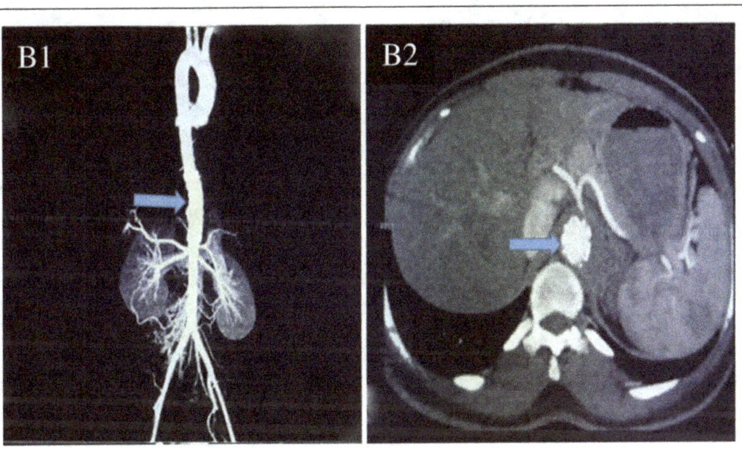

Fig. 2 The aneurysm after intervention (B1, B2). The upper end was located in the cardia level, and the lower end in the upper edge of the superior mesenteric artery opening. Arrow pointed to the stent implantation site

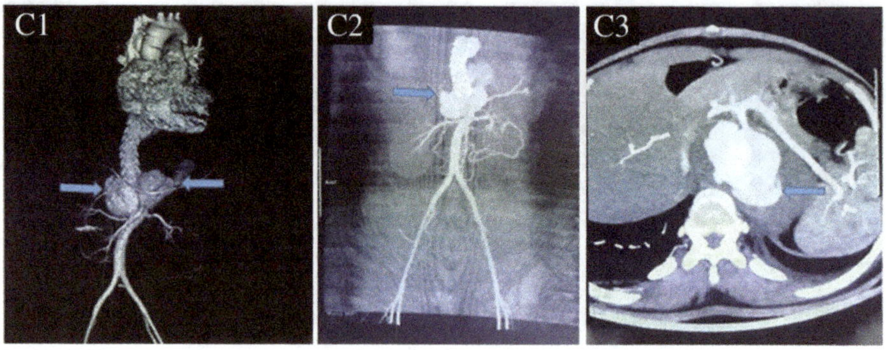

Fig. 3 The hematoncus occured at 6 months after intervention. The size was 6.0*4.8 cm. The extravasation of contrast agent located in the opening of the renal artery, and the thickness of this mixed soft tissue mass was 3.7 cm

doppler-ultrasound indicated deep venous thrombosis in the left popliteal vein (Fig. 5). Therefore, the patient was treated with anticoagulant therapy using hypodermic injections of low-molecular-weight heparin at a daily dose of 4100 U.

One month later, the patient suffered from persistent right abdominal pain with nausea and vomiting accompanied by oral aphtha and genital ulcer. Abdominal CT showed the occurrence of an air-fluid level in part of the ileum and colon (Fig. 6). The diagnosis was determined to be an incomplete intestinal obstruction, which may have been caused by the previous aneurysms. Mesenteric artery angiography showed that the root of the celiac trunk and superior mesenteric artery were stenosed (Fig. 7). Then, conservative treatment was administered, such as fasting, gastrointestinal decompression and

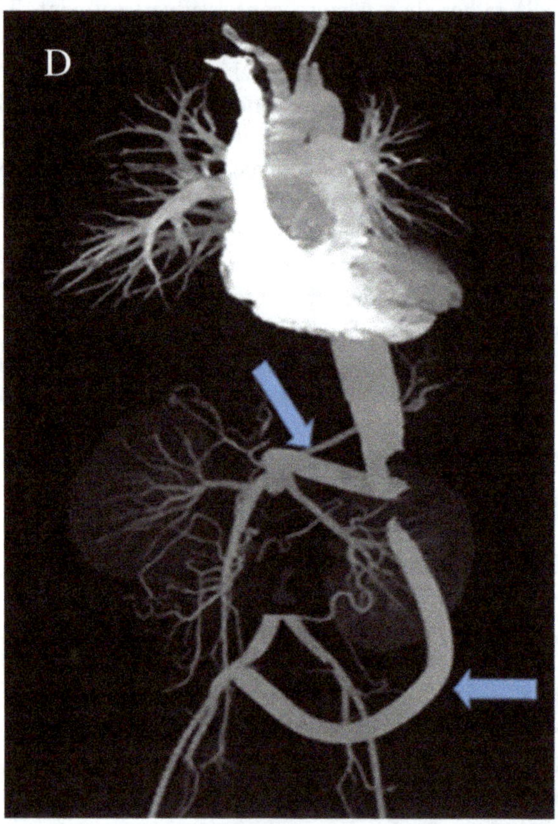

Fig. 4 Implantation of artificial vascular in the thoracic and abdominal aorta. Two transplanted vessels were seen in picture D, one of which was connected to abdominal aorta, the other connected to right common iliac artery

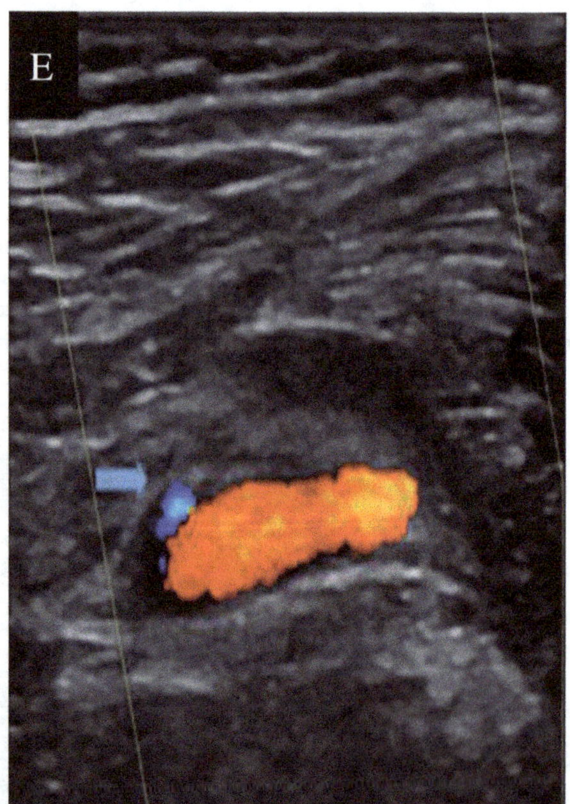

Fig. 5 The deep venous thrombosis in the left popliteal vein. It was detected by doppler-ultrasound. Arrow pointed to the thrombosis

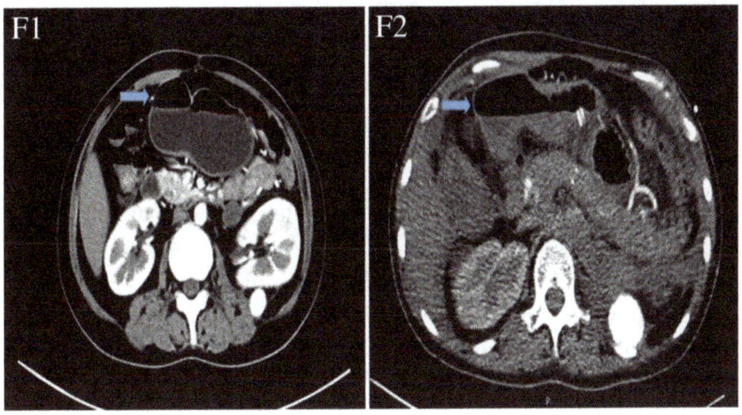

Fig. 6 Air-fluid level (arrows). Detected by abdominal computed tomography

enema. Approximately 20 days later, the patient recovered well and was discharged from the hospital.

Discussion and conclusions

Here we demonstrated a case of a patient with a diagnosis of BD who presented with incomplete intestinal obstruction as the possible main complaint. To the best of our knowledge, this is the first report of the presence of incomplete intestinal obstruction after a second surgery for BD.

Recent studies have reported that HLA-B51 is associated with a more severe disease and is related to familial BD [5]. Other studies have shown that polymorphism in the IL-21, IL-10, and IL-8 genes and in the tumour necrosis factor-(TNF-)alpha-1031C allele are correlated with the pathogenesis of BD [6–11]. The role of the IL-23/IL-17 axis has been found to be associated with the onset of BD [12, 13]. Meanwhile, delayed-type hypersensitivity to infections such as streptococcus species (especially sanguis) has also been proposed to be an important factor in inducing BD [14]. Hematological diseases such as coagulation abnormalities and platelet overactivity may play additional roles in the development of BD [15–17]. Nitric oxide (NO) accumulation after induction by interferon-gamma is also related to the activation of BD [18].

BD can be divided into two categories according to the pathological mechanism: occlusive and lesion. Although venous involvement is the most common vasculo-BD complication, Ketari et al. has been reported that arterial involvement is more common than venous involvement [19]. The most severe complication is aneurysm formation and rupture. Approximately 60% of reported arterial lesions associated with BD are aneurysms [20]. The aorta is the most commonly affected artery followed by the pulmonary artery. Aneurysms occur more frequently in the abdominal aorta than in the thoracic aorta [21–23].

Surgical repair is the standard treatment for aneurysms with dilatation, stenosis, or obstruction, while alternative treatments involve minimally invasive endovascular therapy for aneurysm repair [22, 24, 25].

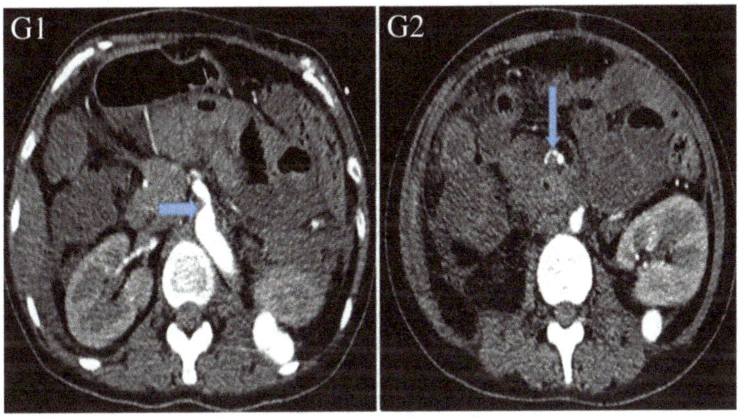

Fig. 7 The root stenosis of celiac trunk and superior mesenteric artery. Detected by mesenteric artery angiography

Table 1 Characteristics of lesion, treatment and outcome for patients complicated with intestinal obstruction from literature review

Patient	Location	symptom	Treatment (graft size: mm & type)	Complication	Immuno-suppresant	Recurrence	Follow up	Result
38 yrs. male	Infrarenal	C. Rupture	Interposition (Polytetrafluoroethylene) 16 × 8, bifurcated	Incomplete Intestinal Obstruction	Prednisolone + Colchicines	None	98 M	Alive
31 yrs. male	Suprarenal	Rupture	Patch (Polytetrafluoroethylene)	Incomplete Intestinal Obstruction	Colchicines + Azathioprine	18 M	43 M	Alive
50 yrs. male	Suprarenal	vascular thrombosis	Stent graft	Complete Intestinal Obstruction	Not clear	72 M	5 M	Alive

Shen et al. reported that both open surgery and endovascular repair were safe and effective for treating aortic pseudoaneurysm in BD [26]. Furthermore, Naganuma et al. reported that ulcer lesions in the ileum and colon, which could lead to intestinal obstruction, were found in surgical patients with intestinal BD [27].

In our report, it was challenging to diagnose the patient who presented with initial symptoms of abdominal pain and vomiting. The differential diagnoses included pseudoaneurysm, ileus, new recurrent arterial aneurysm, mesenteric arterial embolism and so on. To obtain an accurate diagnosis, abdominal computed tomography and angiography were performed. CT/CTA results showed that the patient suffered from intestinal obstruction. The cause may be related to chronic vascular lesions, which could finally lead to an insufficient blood supply in the mesenteric artery. Literature review demonstrated that intestinal obstruction presented with BD in three cases. Of them, two cases of BD that presented with abdominal aortic aneurysm were diagnosed with ileus after stent graft interposition [28]. One patient with BD suffered from complete obstruction 6 years after several operations. The operations included an aortobifemoral bypass grafting for an abdominal aortic aneurysm [2] (Table 1). However, incomplete intestine obstruction was not reported as the main complaint for these patients. Our case report is the first to present incomplete intestinal obstruction as the possible main complaint of BD. Unfortunately, there are no certain guidelines for how to prevent and treat intestinal obstruction caused by BD. Thus, prompt differential diagnosis and management are essential for future treatment.

Considering the paucity of data available, the management of patients with intestinal obstruction should be individualized, and a multidisciplinary approach should be taken. Differential diagnosis and management are essential when addressing this fatal problem.

Technologies such as abdominal computed tomography and angiography are recommended resources when determining differential diagnosis. Finally, if intestinal obstruction is confirmed with the diagnosis, appropriate measures (surgical or nonsurgical treatment) to treat this disease should be taken.

Abbreviations

BD: Behcet's disease; CT: Computed tomography; CTA: Computed tomographic angiogram; ICU: Intensive care unit; NO: Nitric oxide; OSR: Open surgical repair

Acknowledgements

We would like to express our sincere appreciation to Dr. Jinping Zhao and Dr. Ming Xu of the Department of Cardiothoracic Surgery for their valuable comments.

Funding

This study was supported by the National Natural Science Foundation of China (Z.P. 81560131) and Hubei Province Key Projects (Z.P. WJ2017Z008).

Authors' contributions

ZP designed this study and revised the manuscript. FJ & HX analyzed and interpreted the patient data regarding Behcet's disease. FJ & ZP conducted the manuscript writing. ZP, FJ & HX treated the patient in the ICU. All authors read and approved the final manuscript.

Competing interests

The authors declare that they have no competing interests.

References

1. Nair JR, Moots RJ. Behcet's disease. Clin Med (Lond). 2017;17(1):71–7.
2. Bayar S, Unal E, Esen S, Kurt T, Ensari C, Alacayir I. Aortobifemoral graft causing complete intestinal obstruction in a patient with Behcet's disease: report of a case. Surg Today. 2004;34(2):185–7.
3. Tuzun H, Seyahi E, Arslan C, Hamuryudan V, Besirli K, Yazici H. Management and prognosis of nonpulmonary large arterial disease in patients with Behcet disease. J Vasc Surg. 2012;55(1):157–63.
4. Barnes CG. Treatment of Behcet's syndrome. Rheumatology (Oxford). 2006; 45(3):245–7.
5. Fresko I, Soy M, Hamuryudan V, Yurdakul S, Yavuz S, Tumer Z, Yazici H. Genetic anticipation in Behcet's syndrome. Ann Rheum Dis. 1998;57(1):45–8.
6. Geri G, Terrier B, Rosenzwajg M, Wechsler B, Touzot M, Seilhean D, Tran TA, Bodaghi B, Musset L, Soumelis V, et al. Critical role of IL-21 in modulating TH17 and regulatory T cells in Behcet disease. J Allergy Clin Immunol. 2011; 128(3):655–64.
7. Touma Z, Farra C, Hamdan A, Shamseddeen W, Uthman I, Hourani H, Arayssi T. TNF polymorphisms in patients with Behcet disease: a meta-analysis. Arch Med Res. 2010;41(2):142–6.
8. Bonyadi M, Jahanafrooz Z, Esmaeili M, Kolahi S, Khabazi A, Ebrahimi AA, Hajialilo M, Dastgiri S. TNF-alpha gene polymorphisms in Iranian Azeri Turkish patients with Behcet's disease. Rheumatol Int. 2009;30(2):285–9.
9. Akman A, Sallakci N, Coskun M, Bacanli A, Yavuzer U, Alpsoy E, Yegin O. TNF-alpha gene 1031 T/C polymorphism in Turkish patients with Behcet's disease. Br J Dermatol. 2006;155(2):350–6.
10. Kamoun M, Chelbi H, Houman MH, Lacheb J, Hamzaoui K. Tumor necrosis factor gene polymorphisms in Tunisian patients with Behcet's disease. Hum Immunol. 2007;68(3):201–5.

11. Akman A, Sallakci N, Kacaroglu H, Tosun O, Yavuzer U, Alpsoy E, Yegin O. Relationship between periodontal findings and the TNF-alpha gene 1031T/C polymorphism in Turkish patients with Behcet's disease. J Eur Acad Dermatol Venereol. 2008;22(8):950–7.
12. Leng RX, Chen GM, Pan HF, Ye DQ. The role of IL-23/IL-17 axis in the etiopathogenesis of Behcet's disease. Clin Rheumatol. 2010;29(10):1209.
13. Ekinci NS, Alpsoy E, Karakas AA, Yilmaz SB, Yegin O. IL-17A has an important role in the acute attacks of Behcet's disease. J Invest Dermatol. 2010;130(8): 2136–8.
14. Yokota K, Hayashi S, Araki Y, Isogai E, Kotake S, Yoshikawa K, Fujii N, Hirai Y, Oguma K. Characterization of Streptococcus sanguis isolated from patients with Behcet's disease. Microbiol Immunol. 1995;39(9):729–32.
15. La Regina M, Orlandini F, Prisco D, Dentali F. Homocysteine in vascular Behcet disease: a meta-analysis. Arterioscler Thromb Vasc Biol. 2010;30(10): 2067–74.
16. Shanker J, Gasparyan AY, Kitas GD, Kakkar W. Platelet function and antiplatelet therapy in cardiovascular disease: implications of genetic polymorphisms. Curr Vasc Pharmacol. 2011;9(4):479–89.
17. Gasparyan AY, Ayvazyan L, Mikhailidis DP, Kitas GD. Mean platelet volume: a link between thrombosis and inflammation? Curr Pharm Des. 2011;17(1):47–58.
18. Belguendouz H, Messaoudene D, Lahmar K, Ahmedi L, Medjeber O, Hartani D, Lahlou-Boukoffa O, Touil-Boukoffa C. Interferon-gamma and nitric oxide production during Behcet uveitis: immunomodulatory effect of interleukin-10. J Interf Cytokine Res. 2011;31(9):643–51.
19. Ketari JS, Chaaba H, Ben DB, Boussema F, Kochbati S, Cherif O, Rokbani L. Arterial involvement in Behcet's disease: a series of 7 cases. Tunis Med. 2009;87(9):583–8.
20. Kojima N, Sakano Y, Ohki S, Misawa Y. Rapidly growing aortic arch aneurysm in Behcet's disease. Interact Cardiovasc Thorac Surg. 2011;12(3): 502–4.
21. Spiliotopoulos K, Yanagawa B, Crean A, Overgaard C, Brister SJ. Surgical management of a left anterior descending pseudoaneurysm related to Behcet's disease. Ann Thorac Surg. 2011;91(3):912–4.
22. Rico JV, Pedrajas FG, Gonzalez IC, Segura IR. Urgent endovascular treatment of a ruptured tibioperoneal pseudoaneurysm in Behcet's disease. Ann Vasc Surg. 2011;25(3):311–85.
23. Ullery BW, Pochettino A, Wang GJ, Jackson BM, Fairman RM, Woo EY. Celiac artery aneurysm repair in Behcet disease complicated by recurrent thoracoabdominal aortic aneurysms. Vasc Endovasc Surg. 2010;44(2):146–9.
24. Calguneri M, Kiraz S, Ertenli I, Benekli M, Karaarslan Y, Celik I. The effect of prophylactic penicillin treatment on the course of arthritis episodes in patients with Behcet's disease. A randomized clinical trial. Arthritis Rheum. 1996;39(12):2062–5.
25. Kim WH, Choi D, Kim JS, Ko YG, Jang Y, Shim WH. Effectiveness and safety of endovascular aneurysm treatment in patients with vasculo-Behcet disease. J Endovasc Ther. 2009;16(5):631–6.
26. Shen C, Li W, Zhang Y, Li Q, Jiao Y, Zhang T, Zhang X. Outcomes of surgery for patients with Behcet's disease causing aortic pseudoaneurysm: a shift from open surgery to endovascular repair. Clinics (Sao Paulo). 2016;71(6): 302–10.
27. Naganuma M, Iwao Y, Inoue N, Hisamatsu T, Imaeda H, Ishii H, Kanai T, Watanabe M, Hibi T. Analysis of clinical course and long-term prognosis of surgical and nonsurgical patients with intestinal Behçet's disease. Am J Gastroenterol. 2000;95(10):2848–51.
28. Kwon TW, Park SJ, Kim HK, Yoon HK, Kim GE, Yu B. Surgical treatment result of abdominal aortic aneurysm in Behcet's disease. Eur J Vasc Endovasc Surg. 2008;35(2):173–80.

Lipoprotein(a) and lipid profiles of patients awaiting coronary artery bypass graft

E. M. S. Bandara[1], S. Ekanayake[1*], C. A. Wanigatunge[2] and A. Kapuruge[3]

Abstract

Background: Lipoprotein(a) (Lp(a)) excess is an independent risk factor of coronary artery disease (CAD) and have shown wide ethnic variations. Further, lipid parameters used in the assessment and management of risk factors for CAD may not reflect accurately the disease or severity if the patients are on pharmacological interventions when compared to Lp(a). Lp(a) levels of Sri Lankan CAD patients awaiting coronary artery bypass graft are not documented.

Methods: A cross sectional study was carried out with patients ($n = 102$) awaiting coronary artery bypass graft at a tertiary healthcare institution in Sri Lanka. Lp(a) was determined by immunoturbidimetric method (Konelab 20XT) and information on risk factors collected using a standardized questionnaire. The severity of CAD was determined by Gensini score. Lipid parameters and pharmacological treatment data were obtained from the Medical Records. Data were analysed using independent sample t-test, Pearson and Spearman tests respectively.

Results: Total cholesterol (TC), LDL cholesterol (LDLc) and HDL cholesterol (HDLc) of the total study sample (average ± SD) were, 150 ± 36 mg/dL, 92 ± 36 mg/dL and 34 ± 9 mg/dL respectively with no significant difference irrespective of being on pharmacological treatment or not. All lipid parameters were significantly high ($p < 0.05$) in females. The average Lp(a) was 50 ± 38 (SD) mg/dL with no significant difference in males or females independent of being on treatment (50 ± 39 mg/dL) or not (49 ± 39 mg/dL) and above the cut off value (30 mg/dL).

Conclusions: Despite pharmacological interventions 27 % of the study population had high LDLc and majority low HDLc. Mean Lp(a) was in excess irrespective of risk factors or being on treatment or not and is confirmed as an independent, potential marker for assessing the susceptibility for CAD especially in those with other intermediate risk factors but considered non-hyperlipidemic by conventional methods.

Keywords: Lipoprotein(a), Coronary artery disease (CAD), Lipid profile, Risk factors, Sri Lankan CAD patients

Background

Cardio Vascular Disease (CVD) is a leading cause of death in the world. In Sri Lanka 40 % of proportional mortality is due to CVD [1]. South Asians are susceptible to Acute Myocardial Infarction (AMI) at an earlier age as they tend to develop higher risk-factor levels much earlier in life [2]. Sudden cardiac death (SCD) is estimated to account for 50 % of deaths from cardiovascular causes and about half of these deaths occur in subjects who were previously undiagnosed with heart disease [3, 4]. Coronary artery disease is the underlying cause in 80 % of SCDs, consequently, risk factors for coronary artery disease also predispose to SCD [3]. Risk factors for CVD comprise dyslipidemia, diabetes, hypertension, obesity, sedentary lifestyle, smoking, alcohol, family history, menopause and advancing age [1]. Further, homocysteine, fibrinogen, lipoprotein(a), low density lipoprotein particle size and c-reactive protein are the conditional risk

* Correspondence: sagarikae@hotmail.com
[1]Department of Biochemistry, Faculty of Medical Sciences, University of Sri Jayewardenepura, Nugegoda, Sri Lanka
Full list of author information is available at the end of the article

factors that contribute to CVD [1]. Recently it has been shown that factors associated with culprit plaque rupture (CPR) to be different depending on clinical presentation. Hypertension was the only clinical predictor for STEMI, while advanced age, diabetes mellitus and hyperlipidaemia were the predictors in NSTEMI and unstable angina with no clinical predictor for stable angina [5].

The prevalence of hypercholesterolemia, hypertriglyceridemia and low HDLc were 14.86, 8.46 and 11.18 % among Sri Lankan adults [6]. A subsequent study reported elevated triglyceride (TG) and low HDLc in 12.2 % of subjects of <16 years and 24.5 % of subjects >16 years with a high prevalence in males [7]. A more recent study indicate an increasing trend in risk factors for CAD among Sri Lankans with the prevalence of hypercholesterolemia (>5.2 mmol/l), high LDLc (>3.4 mmol/L), high TG (>1.7 mmol/L) and low HDLc (<1.0 mmol/L) being 53.6, 24.7, 22.7 and 53.1 % respectively [8]. Statins are the most effective drug therapy used in controlling LDL cholesterol levels.

Management of lipid levels as part of risk factor modification associated with CAD is usually based on lipid profiles. Several studies indicate elevated Lp(a) is independently and linearly predictive of future adverse coronary events [9, 10]. Lp(a) excess increase the risk of premature CAD 3–100 fold depending on the absence or presence of concomitant risk factors [11, 12]. The inter-individual variability in the concentration of Lp (a) is mainly due to genetic regulation of rate of apoprotein (a) production [13]. Lp(a) promote pro-atherogenic processes by many mechanisms ie; interacting with fibrin and tissue matrix components in vessel walls [14, 15], inhibiting activation of plasminogen to plasmin [16], inhibiting plasmin mediated activation of transforming growth factor β (TGF-β) leading to increased proliferation of smooth muscle cells [17] and promoting inflammatory process by inducing monocyte chemotactic activity of vascular endothelial cells [18]. Thus Lp(a) would be a better risk marker for management of those with CAD and also for prediction of CAD susceptibility.

Patients with chronic stable angina undergoing diagnostic coronary angiography had significantly high ($p = 0.002$) plasma Lp(a) concentration than those without CAD. A significantly higher Lp(a) concentrations in CAD patients with a history of myocardial infarction (MI) (52.5 mg/dL) was observed compared to patients without MI (25.2 mg/dL) [19]. A South Indian study confirms the positive correlation with Lp(a) and severity of CHD [12]. As Lp(a) levels have shown wide ethnic variations [20] the present study assessed Lp(a) and lipid profile parameters of patients with confirmed diagnosis of CAD to observe the association of Lp(a) levels and lipid parameters and to study the effect of lipid lowering drugs on these parameters in a Sri Lankan study sample as these data are currently unavailable.

Methods

Study design and sample calculation

The current research was conducted as a prospective cross sectional study during the years 2013 and 2014. Study sample consisted of consenting patients ($n = 102$) awaiting Coronary Artery Bypass Graft (CABG) at the Cardiothoracic Unit, Sri Jayewardenepura General Hospital, Sri Lanka. The required sample size with an estimated prevalence of 30 % CVD [21], at 95 % significance level and a 10 % margin of error was 81. Since some diagnosed as CVD may not be CAD a study sample of 102 was enrolled.

Lipoprotein(a) assay

Pre-operative blood samples were collected in to plain tubes. Serum was separated (3500 rpm, 5–10 min) and Lp(a) content was measured by immunoturbidimetric method (Thermo Scientific, Finland). Lipoprotein(a) calibrator and control (Thermo Scientific, Finland) were used for calibration. A specific anti serum (5 μL of anti-human Lp(a) from rabbit, NaN_3 and NaCl) was added to buffered (140 μL; phosphate buffer saline) serum (24 μL), mixed and incubated at 37 °C. The absorbance of the immune-complex, produced from Lp(a) and anti-serum was measured at 340 nm (Konelab 20XT). The absorbance was considered proportional to the concentration of Lp(a).

Lipid profile, risk factor data and severity of CAD

Data on total cholesterol (TC), low density lipoprotein cholesterol (LDLc), high density lipoprotein cholesterol (HDLc), triglyceride (TG) were collected from each patient's data records and TC:HDLc ratio calculated. A standardized interviewer administered questionnaire was used to collect data on risk factors related to development of CAD. The Gensini score system was used to evaluate the severity of CAD from coronary angiography [22]. The data on coronary angiography were gathered from the medical records. The Gensini score was computed by assigning a severity score according to the degree of luminal narrowing and geographical importance of each coronary stenosis. The sum severity score of all coronary arteries was expressed as the Gensini score.

Statistical analysis

The data are presented as mean ± 1 standard deviation (SD). *P* value of less than 0.05 ($p < 0.05$) was considered to be significant. Independent sample t-test and paired sample t-test were used for analysis of parametric variables. Correlations of parametric data were analysed by Spearman test.

Results

Demographic data and risk factors of the study sample are included in Table 1. The study sample comprised of 102 patients awaiting Coronary Artery Bypass Graft (CABG) at Sri Jayewardenepura General Hospital, Sri Lanka. Males constituted 65.7 % ($n = 67$) of the sample. Majority of the patients (43.1 %) were between 51 and 60 years with 4.9 % less than 40 years. The average age of male and female patients was 56.9 ± 10 and 57.8 ± 7. From the study sample 70.6 % ($n = 72$), 53.9 % ($n = 55$) and 87.3 % ($n = 89$) individuals had a history of hypertension, diabetes mellitus and dyslipidemia respectively. Dyslipidemia was the most frequent disease related risk factor among both males and females. Family history of CHD was a risk among 54 % of the sample with females having a higher frequency (77 %).

Lipid profile values (total cholesterol (TC), low density lipoprotein cholesterol (LDLc), high density lipoprotein cholesterol (HDLc), triglyceride (TG), TC:HDLc ratio), and (Lp(a)) of the study sample are stated in Table 2. The study sample consisted 87.3 % of patients on statins which comprised 83.6 % of males and 94.3 % females. The mean total cholesterol (<200 mg/dL) was well within the normal reference. LDLc of some females (36 %) on treatment were higher than recommended. Females on statins ($n = 33$) had significantly high TC ($p = 0.001$), LDLc ($p = 0.02$) and HDLc ($p = 0.02$) when compared to males on statins. From among 50 patients on statin therapy most patients ($n = 48$) were on atovastatin, either 20 mg (60 %) or 40 mg. However, the exact dose and the type of statin were not available for the other patients ($n = 39$). The TC:HDLc ratio was above 4.5 in majority of subjects.

Irrespective of statin therapy the Lp(a) concentration was not significantly different among males or females and was higher than 45 mg/dL. Variation of lipid profile values with high and low Lp(a) concentrations is stated in Table 3. The average TC and LDLc were within the normal range irrespective of Lp(a) being above 30 mg/dL (upper limit reagent kit) or more than 25 mg/dL as suggested cutoff for South Asians [12].

Discussion

The mean concentrations of TC, LDLc, TG of both males and females on statin therapy and without statins were within the recommended [23] concentrations with lower HDLc. However, even though the therapeutic target of LDLc is <100 mg/dL for a person with CHD, 26.7 % ($n = 27$) from the total sample had higher LDLc concentrations and 8.8 % ($n = 9$) of females had TC concentration >200 mg/dL indicating inadequate control despite treatment. Haddad et al. [24] also reported mean values of LDLc as 146.7 ± 50.9 mg/dL and 118.9 ± 45.9 mg/dL of patients confirmed as CHD and that of controls respectively. The prevalence of hypercholesterolemia and mean total cholesterol concentration in Sri Lankan adults were 53.6 % and 5.35 ± 1.13 mmol/L (206.5 ± 43.6 mg/dL) respectively [8]. According to non-fasting results of total cholesterol, the prevalence of high TC was 20–25.9 % [25]. These data are a clear indication of the necessity in controlling not only total cholesterol but also the LDLc.

Table 1 Demographic and risk factor data of the study sample

Variable		Total	Male ($n = 67$)	Female ($n = 35$)
Age		57 ± 9	56.9 ± 10	57.8 ± 7
Residency	Urban	59.8 %	55.2 %	68.6 %
	Rural	40.2 %	44.8 %	31.4 %
Monthly income (LKR)	<10 000	10.8 %	10.4 %	11.4 %
	11 000–30 000	72.5 %	70.1 %	77.1 %
	>31 000	16.7 %	19.4 %	11.5 %
Disease related risk factors				
Hypertension	Hypertensive	70.6 %	58.2 %	94.3 %
	Normotensive	29.4 %	41.8 %	5.7 %
Diabetes Mellitus	Diabetic	53.9 %	53.7 %	54.3 %
	Non Diabetic	46.1 %	46.3 %	45.7 %
Dyslipidemia	Dyslipidemic	87.3 %	83.6 %	94.3 %
	Non dyslipidemic	12.7 %	16.4 %	5.7 %
Family history of CAD	With family history	53.9 %	41 %	77 %
	No family history	46.1 %	59 %	23 %
Severity of CAD	Gensini score	48 ± 26	51 ± 25	44 ± 2

Table 2 Lipid test measurements

Test (Reference range- mg/dL)	Total ($n = 102$)	Total ($n = 102$)		Male ($n = 67$)	Male ($n = 67$)		Female ($n = 35$)	Female ($n = 35$)	
		A ($n = 89$)	B ($n = 13$)		A ($n = 56$)	B ($n = 11$)		A ($n = 33$)	B ($n = 2$)
[a]TC (< 200)	150 ± 36	152 ± 36	137 ± 31	142 ± 29	143 ± 28	135 ± 33	167 ± 43[#]	168 ± 44*	151 ± 19
[a]LDLc (< 100)	92 ± 36	94 ± 37	82 ± 27	85 ± 24	87 ± 24	80 ± 28	105 ± 49[#]	105 ± 50*	98 ± 4.2
[a]HDLc (> 40)	34 ± 9	34 ± 10	31 ± 8	32 ± 9	32 ± 10	31 ± 8	37 ± 8[#]	37 ± 9*	33 ± 5.6
[a]TG (<150)	133 ± 60	134 ± 60	124 ± 64	127 ± 53	127 ± 51	129 ± 67	143 ± 71	146 ± 72	98 ± 45
[c]TC:HDL (< 5)	4.6 ± 1.2	4.6 ± 1.3	4.5 ± 1.0	4.6 ± 1.1	4.6 ± 1.2	4.5 ± 1.1	4.7 ± 1.4	4.6 ± 1.4	4.6 ± 0.2
[b]Lp(a) (< 30)	50 ± 38	50 ± 39	49 ± 39	47 ± 37	47 ± 36	49 ± 40	54 ± 41	54 ± 42	56 ± 41

A; on statins, *B*; without statins, *TC*; total cholesterol, *LDLc*; low density lipoprotein cholesterol, *HDLc*; high density lipoprotein cholesterol, *TG*; triglyceride
[#]Significant differences ($p < 0.05$) between male and female total concentrations; *Significant difference ($p < 0.05$) between male and females on statins
[a]Third Report of the National Cholesterol Education Programme (Adult Treatment Panel III), 2002 (23)
[b]Reference range as per lipoprotein(a) kit

When considering the TG, 30.4 % males and females had triglyceride above 150 mg/dL. Correlating with above the waist to hip ratio of more than 90 % of the study sample indicated high risk [26]. HDLc concentrations of 77.5 % of patients were less than 40 mg/dL. The low HDLc correlated with the low physical activity level and the high prevalence of central obesity [26] in the present study sample. Majority of the patients [$n = 89$] in this study were on statins and mean concentrations of TC and LDLc were within the reference range [23]. However, since the exact dose and the statin are not available for some ($n = 39$) we are unable to make any inference on the dose and type correlations and lipid parameters. Notably, 45 % among the study sample was unaware that they were on statins and dyslipidemic despite good compliance. Thus the consumption of red meat, chicken, fish, egg with yolk and fast food was comparatively higher in the group who were not aware that they were dyslipidemic [26].

The above indicates that it is necessary to make the patients aware regarding usage of drugs which may reduce the adverse effects if any occur. Likewise, with prescription of drugs, information on lifestyle changes to maintain lipid parameters within normal ranges need to be imparted to these patients as above data shows this information is lacking.

TC:HDLc ratio of majority of patients was above 4.5. It clearly indicates that even though cholesterol was below the recommended value their HDLc need to be increased. Lifestyle changes are now being advocated to such patients. By and large a cut off of <5 for this ratio is being used in most Sri Lankan hospitals and thus it is necessary to evaluate the suitability of reducing the cut-off given the susceptibility of South Asians to Acute Myocardial Infarction (AMI) at an earlier age [2].

Lipoprotein(a) excess is an independent risk factor for coronary artery disease [9]. Lipoprotein (a) concentration of dyslipidemic (49.6 ± 38.5 mg/dL) and non dyslipidemic (51.1 ± 39.6 mg/dL) patients were not significantly different and 166 % higher than the cut-off (30 mg/dL) according to the present study and confirms its potential as an independent risk factor for CAD even among Sri Lankans. Despite the fact that male gender is a risk factor for CAD a non significant increase in Lp(a) in females was observed. This could be due to the lower samples size when compared to the males. A study where normolipidemic acute myocardial infarct (AMI) patients and controls of both Sri Lankan and Indian origin had been studied indicated a significantly high ($p = 0.0001$) concentration of Lp(a) [27] in the test group. This also clearly proves the importance of Lp(a) as an independent and an early marker for assessing the susceptibility for CAD especially in those with other intermediate risk factors such as hypertension, diabetes, overweight and obese with a family history but considered non-hyperlipidemic by conventional methods. However, around 2/3 of patients in this study samples had Lp(a) concentration >30 mg/dL, which is the upper limit of the reference suggested by the kit.

Table 3 Lipid profile results in patients with high (>30 mg/dL or >25 mg/dL) vs. low (<30 mg/dL or <25 mg/dL) Lp(a) levels

Lipid test	Lp(a) >30 mg/dL	Lp(a) <30 mg/dL	Lp(a) >25 mg/dL	Lp(a) <25 mg/dL
TC (< 200 mg/dL)	154.6 ± 32.2	143.3 ± 39.6	153.7 ± 34.3	142.0 ± 39.2
LDLc (< 100 mg/dL)	95.4 ± 28.9	84.4 ± 33.5	94.3 ± 30.1	83.8 ± 32.6
HDLc (> 40 mg/dL)	34.3 ± 7.4	33.0 ± 11.9	34.7 ± 9.8	31.7 ± 8.0
TG (<150)	128.7 ± 47.0	138.5 ± 77.0	131.2 ± 48.4	135.9 ± 82.6
TC:HDLc (< 5)	4.6 ± 1.2	4.6 ± 1.4	4.6 ± 1.2	4.6 ± 1.3

This percentage is further increased when considering the cut-off value (>25 mg/dL) suggested for the South Indian population [12]. Except one patient who had a Lp(a) concentration of 1.3 mg/dL and was hyperlipidemic, all others had Lp(a) concentration >10 mg/dL. Therefore, a Lp(a) lower than 30 mg/dL is suggested as the cutoff to determine susceptibility of Sri Lankans to CAD considering the reported ethnic variation in Lp(a) [20]. However, for this Lp(a) levels of a control group needs to be studied.

Over 90 % of patients had TC within the recommended level and most had LDLc also within the normal range due to being on statin therapy. This indicates even with normal TC and LDLc, Lp(a) would indicate the CAD risk and can be considered as a potential independent risk marker as all the patients enrolled in this study were to undergo CABG.

High fat intake may lead to higher plasma Lp(a) levels in patients [28]. This could be correlated to the >20 % of expatriate workers both male and female who informed of dietary pattern changes towards high fat intake while living outside Sri Lanka. When their family history was considered, 64 % with family history had Lp(a) >30 mg/dL. This indicates that other factors such as diet may also have contributed to the increase in Lp(a) and the development of CAD in these patients.

Female sex, family history of CHD, high concentrations of TC and LDLc were reported to be associated with high concentration of Lp(a) [12]. In the present study an association with female sex and Lp(a) was observed. Europe and Atherosclerosis Society Consensus Panel also recommends screening of Lp(a) in individuals with intermediate or high risk of cardiovascular diseases/CHD. Lp(a) concentration of <50 mg/dL was suggested as a desirable level as a function of global cardiovascular risk [29]. In the present sample 2/3 of patients had Lp(a) of >30 mg/dL indicating a lower cutoff for Sri Lankans can also be considered as Lp (a) levels have shown wide ethnic variations [20] and are susceptible to change with the dietary patterns [28]. Similarly a Lp(a) concentration of 25 mg/dL had been suggested as the cutoff as risk of CHD in a South Indian study [12]. It is also recommended Lp(a) to be considered an additional marker for screening for CAD in susceptible individuals.

Limitations

Comparison of data on Lp(a) and lipid profiles with an age and sex matched apparently healthy control group would have improved the study outcome.

A complete data set on the type and the intensity of statin therapy would have helped to find their effect on lipid parameters and the severity of the disease.

Conclusions

Notwithstanding pharmacological interventions 27 % of the study population had high LDLc with more among females. Majority of patients had low HDLc and a TC:HDLc ratio of <5 which is within the recommended range. This highlights the urgent need for considering a lower cut-off for Sri Lankan population as there is clear evidence of increasing prevalence of CAD among Sri Lankans according to reported data. Lp(a) could be considered as an independent, potential marker for assessing the susceptibility for CAD in Sri Lankans especially in those with other intermediate risk factors but considered non-hyperlipidemic by conventional methods.

Abbreviations

CABG: Coronary artery bypass graft; CAD: Coronary artery disease; CHD: Coronary heart disease; HDLc: High density lipoprotein cholesterol; LDLc: Low density lipoprotein cholesterol; Lp (a): Lipoprotein (a); TC: Total cholesterol; TG: Triglyceride

Acknowledgements

We would like to extend our gratitude to the patients who consented to be part of this study and staff and colleagues of the Cardiothoracic Unit, Sri Jayewardenepura General Hospital and Department of Biochemistry, University of Sri Jayewardenepura, Sri Lanka for their support.

Funding

This work was supported by a grant from the National Science Foundation (NSF/RG/2011/HS/18) Sri Lanka.

Authors' contributions

EMSB acquired data and analyzed the data, SE designed the study and drafted the manuscript for important intellectual content, CW designed the study and revised the manuscript critically, AK designed the study and revised the manuscript critically. All authors read and approved the final manuscript.

Competing interests

The authors declare that they have no competing interests.

Author details

[1]Department of Biochemistry, Faculty of Medical Sciences, University of Sri Jayewardenepura, Nugegoda, Sri Lanka. [2]Department of Pharmacology, Faculty of Medical Sciences, University of Sri Jayewardenepura, Nugegoda, Sri Lanka. [3]Cardiothoracic Unit, Sri Jayewardenepura General Hospital, Thalapathpitiya, Nugegoda, Sri Lanka.

References

1. World Health Organization. Noncommunicable diseases country profiles, Geneva. Geneva: WHO Document Production Services; 2014.
2. Joshi P, Islam S, Pais P, et al. Risk factors for early myocardial infarction in South Asians compared with individuals in other countries. JAMA. 2007;297(3):286–94.
3. Huikuri HV, Castellanos A, Myerburg RJ. Sudden death due to cardiac arrhythmias. N Engl J Med. 2001;345(20):1473–82.

4. Wellens HJ, Schwartz PJ, Lindemans FW, et al. Risk stratification for sudden cardiac death: current status and challenges for the future. Eur Heart J. 2014;35(25):1642–51.
5. Iannaccone M, Quadri G, Taha S, et al. Prevalence and predictors of culprit plaque rupture at OCT in patients with coronary artery disease: a meta-analysis. Eur Heart J Cardiovasc Imaging. 2015;17:1128–37.
6. Fernando DJ, Siribaddana SH, Silva DR, Perera SD. The prevalence of obesity and other coronary risk factors in a suburban Sri Lankan community. Asia Pac J Clin Nutr. 1994;3(4):155–9.
7. Wijesuriya M, Gulliford M, Charlton J, et al. High prevalence of cardio-metabolic risk factors in a young urban Sri-Lankan population. PLoS One. 2012;7(2):e31309.
8. Herath HRISI, Katulanda P, Matthews DR, et al. Prevalence and patterns of dyslipidemia among adult Sri Lankans. In: Sri Lanka Medical Association - 123rd Annual Scientific Sessions. 2010. p. 15.
9. Yusuf J, Yadav N, Mukhopadhyay S, et al. Relook at lipoprotein (A): Independent risk factor of coronary artery disease in North Indian population. Indian Heart J. 2014;66(3):272–9.
10. Erqou S, Kaptoge S, Perry PL, The emerging risk factors collaboration. Lipoprotein(a) concentration and the risk of coronary heart disease, stroke, and nonvascular mortality. JAMA. 2009;302:412–23.
11. Gambhir JK, Kaur H, Gambhir DS, Prabhu KM. Lipoprotein(a) as an independent risk factor for coronary artery disease in patients below 40 years of age. Indian Heart J. 2000;52(4):411–5 [PubMed].
12. Rajasekhar D, Saibaba KSS, Srinivasa Rao PVLN, Latheef SAA, Subramanyam G. Lipoprotein (A): better assessor of coronary heart disease risk in south Indian population. Indian J Clin Biochem. 2004;19(2):53–9.
13. Scanu M. Structural and functional polymorphism of Lipoprotein (a): biological and clinical implications. Clin Chem. 1995;41(1):170–2.
14. Scanu AM, Lawn RM, Berg K. Lipoprotein(a) and atherosclerosis. Ann Intern Med. 1991;115(3):209–18.
15. Scanu AM. Lipoprotein(a) and the atherothrombotic process: Mechanistic insights and clinical implications. Curr Atheroscler Rep. 2003;5(2):106–13.
16. Marcovina SM, Koschinsky ML. Lipoprotein(a) as a risk factor for coronary artery disease. Am J Cardiol. 1998;82(12):57U–66.
17. Grainger DJ, Kemp PR, Liu AC, Lawn RM. Activation of transforming growth factor-beta is inhibited in transgenic apolipoprotein(a) mice. Nature. 1994;370(6489):460–2.
18. Poon M, Zhang X, Dunsky KG, Taubman MB, Harpel PC. Apolipoprotein(a) induces monocyte chemotactic activity in human vascular endothelial cells. Circulation. 1997;96:2514–9.
19. Schwartzman RA, Cox ID, Poloniecki J, Crook R, Seymour CA, Kaski JC. Elevated plasma Lipoprotein (a) is associated with coronary artery disease in patients with chronic stable angina pectoris. J Am Coll Cardiol. 2011;31:1260–6.
20. Geethanjali FS, Luthra K, Lingenhel A, et al. Analysis of the apo(a) size polymorphism in Asian Indian populations: association with Lp(a) concentration and coronary heart disease. Atherosclerosis. 2003;169(1):121–30.
21. World Health Organization. Noncommunicable diseases country profiles. Geneva: WHO Document Production Services; 2011.
22. Gensini GG. A more meaningful scoring system for determining the severity of coronary heart disease. Am J Cardiol. 1983;51(3):606.
23. Expert Panel on Detection, Evaluation, and Treatment of High Blood Cholesterol in Adults. Executive Summary of the Third Report of the National Cholesterol Education Program (NCEP) Expert Panel on Detection, Evaluation, and Treatment of High Blood Cholesterol in Adults (Adult Treatment Panel III). JAMA. 2001;285(19):2486–97.
24. Haddad FH, Omari AA, Shamailah QM, et al. Lipid profile in patients with coronary artery disease. Saudi Med J. 2002;23(9):1054–8 [PubMed].
25. Tennakoon SUB, Kumar BN, Nugegoda DB, Meyer HE. Comparison of cardiovascular risk factors between Sri Lankans living in Kandy and Oslo. BMC Public Health. 2010;10(1):654.
26. Bandara EMS. Association of risk factors for development of coronary artery disease and nutritional and immune status on the recovery following coronary artery bypass surgery (2015), M Phil thesis; Faculty of Graduate Studies, University of Sri Jayewardenepura, Sri Lanka.
27. Kumar A, Sivakanesan R. Cardiovascular risk factors in normolipidemic acute myocardial infarct patients on admission - Do dietary fruits and vegetables offer any benefits? Online J Health Allied Scs. 2010;9(3):1–8.
28. Burman A, Jain K, Gulati R, Chopra V, Agarwal DP, Vasisht S. Lipoprotein(a) as a marker of coronary artery disease and its association with dietary fat. J Assoc Physicians India. 2004;52:99–102.
29. Nordestgaard BG, Chapman MJ, et al. Lipoprotein(a) as a cardiovascular risk factor: current status. Eur Heart J. 2010;31(23):2844–53.

25

Effects of the cardiac myosin activator Omecamtiv-mecarbil on severe chronic aortic regurgitation in Wistar rats

Bachar El-Oumeiri[1*], Kathleen Mc Entee[2], Filippo Annoni[3], Antoine Herpain[3], Frédéric Vanden Eynden[1], Pascal Jespers[2], Guido Van Nooten[1] and Philippe van de Borne[4]

Abstract

Background: Aortic regurgitation (AR) is a valvular disease that can lead to systolic heart failure. Treatment options besides cardiac surgery are limited and consequently severe AR is associated with higher mortality and morbidity when not operated. In this investigation, we examined the effects of a novel cardiac myosin activator, Omecamtiv-mecarbil (OM), in rats with chronic severe AR.

Methods: AR was created by retrograde puncture of the aortic valve leaflets in 20 adults Wistar rats. 12 animals survived the acute AR phase and were randomized 2 months thereafter into OM ($n = 7$) or placebo groups ($n = 5$). Two rats underwent a sham operation and served as controls. Equal volumes of OM or placebo (NaCl 0.9%) were perfused in the femoral vein by continuous infusion (1.2 mg/kg/hour) during 30 min. Doppler-echocardiography was performed before and at the end of the infusion periods.

Results: OM increased indices of global cardiac function (cardiac output, stroke volume), and increased systolic performance (fractional shortening, ejection fraction, left ventricular end systolic diameter) (all $p < 0.05$). These effects concurred with decreases in indices of LV preload (left atrial size, left ventricular end diastolic diameter) as well in the aortic pre-ejection period / left ventricular ejection time ratio (all $p < 0.05$). The severity score of the regurgitant AR jet did not change. Placebo infusion did not affect these parameters.

Conclusion: The cardiac myosin activator OM exerts favorable hemodynamic effects in rats with experimental chronic AR.

Keywords: Omecamtiv-mecarbil, Aortic regurgitation, Doppler-echocardiography, Wistar rat, Left ventricle

Background

Aortic regurgitation (AR) is a valvular disease that affects men more than women, and whose incidence increases with age [1]. Severe AR is associated with higher morbidity and mortality compared to the general population [2]. Chronic AR secondary to rheumatic fever is a frequent condition in developing countries and in populations having no adequate access to health care [3]. Chronic severe AR imposes a combined left ventricular (LV) volume and pressure overload. Volume increase is a direct consequence of the regurgitant volume itself, while pressure overload results from increased parietal stress and systolic hypertension [4]. AR is associated with a long asymptomatic period during which the LV progressively enlarges and hypertrophies in response to a chronic volume overload. The increased wall stress and LV volume/mass ratio can lead to impaired LV systolic function, clinical signs of heart failure and, finally, become irreversible and lethal [5]. So far, vasodilators are the only drugs indicated in asymptomatic AR, but their hemodynamic effects are inconsistent and their impact on clinical outcomes is largely uncertain [6, 7]. Rats are convenient animals to evaluate the response of the LV to severe AR as they develop LV abnormalities in a relatively short period of time (weeks). This is in contrast to humans, who can tolerate this condition without apparent LV dysfunction for decades [8]. The rats develop progressive LV dilatation and eccentric

* Correspondence: Bachar.El.Oumeiri@erasme.ulb.ac.be
[1]Department of Cardiac surgery, Erasme Hospital, ULB, 808 Lennik road, 1070, Brussels, Belgium
Full list of author information is available at the end of the article

hypertrophy, due to a chronic LV volume overload, as well as progressive irreversible LV systolic dysfunction, mimicking closely the evolution of the disease over a much larger time span in humans [9].

In chronic AR, indices of systolic function such as left ventricular ejection fraction (LVEF) are better prognostic indicators than indices of cardiac overload [2]. Moreover, markers of systolic function are useful for decision of a timely surgical valve replacement [10, 11]. Conventional medical treatment of congestive heart failure with altered ejection fraction is based on neuro-hormonal blockade, neuro-hormonal activation being considered responsible for aggravation of heart failure and loss of myocardial contractility [12]. Because of safety issues, conventional therapies that directly target cardiac contractility are sparsely used [13]. Heart failure (HF) remains a major public health problem worldwide. Existing drugs increase cardiac contractility indirectly through signaling cascades but are limited by their mechanism related adverse effects. To avoid this limitation Omecamtiv-mecarbil (OM) was developed. Omecamtiv-mecarbil, formerly called CK-1827452 (Cytokinetics Inc., San Francisco, CA, USA) is a novel drug which improves cardiac contractility by means of cardiac myosin activation. OM accelerated the transition of myosin from the weakly actin-bound to strongly actin-bound state measured by release of Hydrolazed Phosphate (Pi). OM appeared to shift the equilibrium towards myosin adenosine triphosphate (ATP) hydrolysis without affecting the rate of hydrolysis, in addition to accelerating the rate of Pi release. OM decreased the rate of Pi release when actin was removed. This decrease in actin-independent ATP hydrolysis potentially increases the overall energetic efficiency of the system by diminishing ATP use not associated with mechanical work [14]. Consequently, OM increases systolic ejection duration without changing the rate of left ventricular pressure development [15, 16].

In two different canine models of pacing-induced systolic heart failure (after myocardial infarction [15] and in the presence of left ventricular hypertrophy [15]), OM increased systolic wall thickness and fractional shortening (FS), leading to an improved global cardiac function and lowered heart rate (HR), while myocardial energetics and loading conditions did not change. Cardiac morphology alterations in tachycardia-induced cardiomyopathy include chamber dilatation and normal or reduced ventricular wall thickness, with little or no change in myocardial mass. These changes, together with myocardial energy depletion and impaired energy utilization, are reversible once HR normalizes [17].These characteristics differ completely from the chronic volume and pressure overload in severe AR, leading to LV dilatation and eccentric hypertrophy, an ultimately, to an irremediably compromised LV function. Favorable effects of OM in experimental pacing-induced cardiomyopathy may thus not apply to chronic severe AR. Consequently, the goal of the present study was to test the hypothesis that cardiac myosin activation with OM improved left ventricular function in a rat-model of chronic severe aortic regurgitation. The expanded goal of this study was to determine if OM affected AR severity.

Methods

Animals

Experiments were approved by the Institutional Animal Care and Use Committee of the Free University of Brussels. Studies were conducted in accordance with the Guide for the Care and Use of Laboratory Animals published by the National Institutes of Health (NIH Publication No. 85–23, revised 1996). Twenty-four male adult Wistar rats (401 ± 90 g body weight) were randomized to a sham intervention ($n = 4$) or to AR creation ($n = 20$). Rats that survived the acute phase ($n = 12$) were randomized into an OM group ($n = 7$) or a placebo group ($n = 5$). The 4 rats (two in the OM group and two in the placebo group) who underwent a sham operation served as controls for the effect of time and measurement repetition on the parameters investigated in the study.

Interventions

AR was created by retrograde puncture of the aortic valve leaflets under general anesthesia, as previously described [18]. Briefly, the animals were anesthetized with an intraperitoneal injection of 75 mg/kg of ketamine and 0.25 mg/kg of medetomidine. HR and rhythm were monitored via limb leads throughout the procedure. The right internal carotid artery was surgically exposed. A fixed core wire guide .025″ (COOK incorporated, IN, 47404, USA) was advanced toward the aortic valve in a retrograde manner to tear valve leaflets and induce AR. The following echocardiographic criteria with popping sensation at the time of surgery were used to include animals in the study: a jet extent above 30% of the length of the LV and color-Doppler ratio of regurgitant jet width to LV outflow tract diameter above 50% [19]. The 2 sham-operated animals had their right carotid artery cannulated without puncturing the aortic valve. Animals were closely observed during the first hours and days after surgery for any sign of respiratory distress suggestive of acute heart failure.

Measurements

Transthoracic 2D, M-mode and Doppler echocardiography were performed under general anesthesia with an ultrasound unit (Vivid-7, GE Healthcare, US) equipped with a 10Mhz surgical transducer. Rats were placed in the right and left lateral recumbent positions and their electrocardiogram was monitored via limb leads throughout the procedure. All measurements were made according to the recommendations of the American Society of Echocardiography currently applied to humans [19]. Standard right parasternal (long and short axis) and left apical parasternal views were used for data acquisition. Left atrial size was assessed in right parasternal short axis at the level of the aorta. Diastolic (d) and systolic (s), septal wall thickness (SWT), posterior wall thickness (PWT) and LV diameters (LVEDD, LVESD) were measured in M-mode from a LV short axis view at the level of chordae tendinae and fractional shortening (FS) was calculated. Ejection fraction (EF) were derived using the Teicholz formula. Left ventricle mass was calculated using the American Society of Echocardiography recommended formula: LV mass = 0.8 x $\{1.04[(LVEDD+PWTd + SWTd)^3-(LVEDD)^3]\}$ + 0.6 g. Aortic diameter was measured from the right long axis parasternal view. Aortic flow was measured from the left apical view to calculate forward stroke volume (SV) and cardiac output and to measure pre-ejection period (PEP: delay from Q wave of QRS to aortic opening, ms), LV ejection time (LVET: interval from beginning to termination of aortic flow, ms), and inter-beat interval (RR). Systolic time was determined as PEP + LVET (ms). Diastolic time (ms) consists in RR interval (ms) - systolic time (ms). PEP/LVET ratio was also calculated. PEP/LVET is a more useful index of overall LV performance [20]. This ratio is better correlated with other LV performance measurements than either PEP or LVET, and is considered independent of HR [21]. Severity of the regurgitant aortic jet was subjectively graded (1 to 4).

Experimental design

Doppler-echocardiography was performed before AR creation, during surgery to confirm the presence and the severity of AR, and 2 months thereafter, both before and after OM (1.2 mg/kg/hour) or placebo (NaCl 0.9%) infusion for 30 min, by means of a femoral vein perfusion. All animals received equal volumes (12 ml/kg) of placebo or OM. This achieved plasma concentration of nearly 400 ng of OM/ml in a previous study [22]. Doppler-Echocardiography was performed after 30 min infusion. All animals remained alive during these experimental sessions which could thus be completed in 5 rats with placebo and 7 rats with OM.

Statistical analysis

Results are expressed as means ± SD. A 2-factor ANOVA for repeated measures followed by post-hoc Bonferroni corrections for multiple comparisons was used to assess the effects of OM versus placebo, and any interaction between them, after 2 months of AR on the 16 animals. All other statistical analysis consisted of paired-t tests between variables. Significance was set at a p value less than 0.05. (SPSS 23.0, IBM, Chicago, Ill, USA).

Results

AR and LV measurements (Fig. 1)

AR was achieved in all 20 animals and confirmed by the presence of a regurgitant jet quantified as severe in all animals. Eight animals died of congestive heart failure within 2 months and were not included in the final analysis. After 2 months AR (graduated from 0 to 4) was achieved at 3.67 ± 0.44, and echocardiographic signs of volume overload and eccentric hypertrophy were present with increased left atrial diameter, LVEDD, LVEDV and LV mass (n = 12, all $p < 0.05$, paired t tests). Load dependent indices of LV systolic function (FS and EF) were unchanged but LVESD were increased. SV and cardiac output were decreased (n = 12, both $p < 0.01$, paired t tests). As expected, no AR was detected in sham operated rats (n = 4) with no modifications of LV function or dimension in the placebo group while only FS and EF increased after injection of OM ($p = 0.011$ and $p = 0.032$, respectively) (Table 1).

Effects of placebo in rats with AR (Table 2)

Before infusion, there was no difference in echocardiographic results between the 2 groups (placebo versus OM). NaCl infusion affected none of the echocardiographic parameters of global and systolic cardiac function neither the indices of LV preload (n = 5, $p > 0.06$, paired t tests).

Effects of OM in rats with AR (Table 3)

OM increased indices of global cardiac function (SV, cardiac output), decreased HR and increased systolic performance (FS, EF) (n = 7, all $p < 0.05$, paired t tests). These effects concurred with decreases in measures of LV preload (Left atrial diameter, LVEDD), and a decreased PEP/LVET ratio (n = 7, all $p < 0.05$, paired t tests). OM did not affect the severity score of the AR jet.

Effects of OM versus placebo after 2 months of AR (Table 4)

Two-way ANOVA with Bonferroni corrections for multiple comparisons after 2 months of AR were done on the effects of placebo versus OM. Only FS and EF increased after OM as compared to placebo ($p = 0.014$ and $p = 0.012$, respectively) (Fig. 2). None of the other hemodynamic changes investigated in this study achieved the level of significance in this analysis (none illustrated).

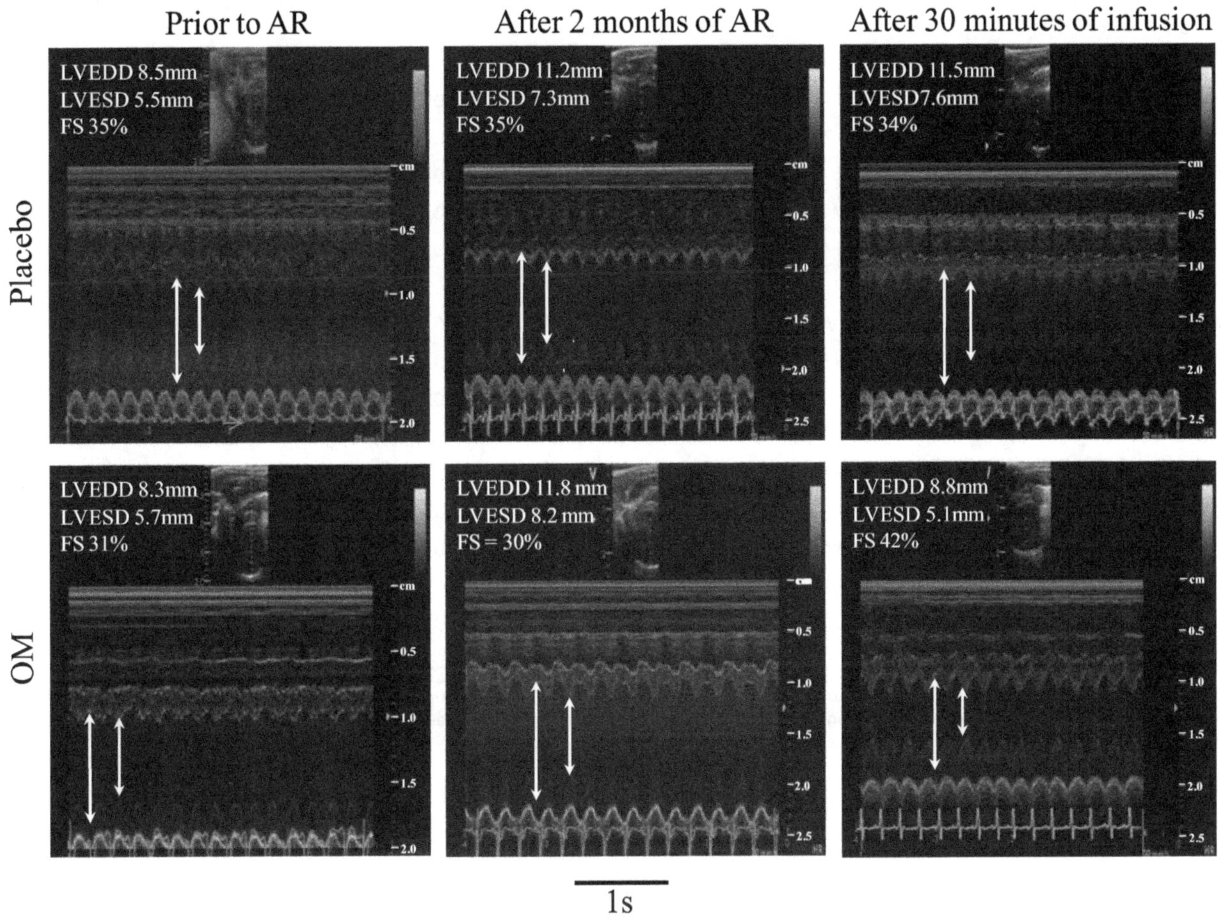

Fig. 1 Illustrative examples of M-mode echocardiography recordings in 2 Wistar rats during the entire study. The figure displays left ventricular end diastolic diameter (LVEDD, mm) and fractional shortening (FS, %) prior to AR (left tracings), after 2 months of AR (middle tracings) and after 30 min of placebo (upper tracings) and OM infusions (lower tracings)

Discussion

We investigated the effect of the cardiac myosin activator OM on severe chronic AR in an experimental rat-model. The main findings of our study are that OM decreases volume overload induced by chronic AR. As OM lessened LVEDD and LVESD and increased SWTs, we can assume that OM markedly decreased LV wall stress in the presence of a severe chronic AR. We are not aware of a previous similar placebo-controlled study.

Effects of OM on cardiac function

The central hemodynamic feature of chronic AR is a combined volume and pressure overload of the LV [4, 23]. The LV responds to volume overload with a series of compensatory mechanisms, including a LV dilatation, an increase in chamber compliance and a combination of eccentric and concentric hypertrophy. The ejection phase indexes of LV systolic function at rest remain normal. However, an enlarged chamber size with the associated increase in wall stress also results in a stimulus for further hypertrophy [24]. Despite the small number ($n = 4$) of sham animals, OM increase EF and FS in sham OM group ($n = 2$).

In our study OM decreased volume overload induced by AR during the whole cardiac cycle, by lowering LVEDD. Moreover, by decreasing LVEDD and LVESD and increasing SWTs, OM decreased wall stress in AR. This is of importance, since an increased wall stress may lead to overt LV systolic dysfunction [25]. Improving cardiac systolic function with a cardiac myosin activator could be favorable to ventricular remodeling [26].

In our study OM decreased the PEP/LVET ratio, a reliable index of LV performance. Acute reduction in afterload in patients with congestive heart failure improves LV systolic performance and decreases the PEP/LVET ratio, while an increase in preload will shorten PEP, prolong LVET and decrease PEP/LVET [27]. We found that despite preload reduction by OM, PEP was shortened and cardiac performance improved. This mechanism could explained the increase in stroke volume [28]. An improvement in cardiac function after infusion of OM in mongrel dogs, where heart failure was achieved by rapid ventricular

Table 1 Two-way ANOVA statistics with Bonferroni correction at base (T1), before injection (T2) and after injection (T3) for all sham animals ($n = 4$)

	T1	T2	*p*	T3	*p*
Heart Rate (beats/min)	258 ± 11	270 ± 7	0,756	193 ± 15	0,251
Left Atrium (mm)	4.6 ± 0.2	6.2 ± 0.3	0,872	5.5 ± 0.2	0,118
LVEDD (mm)	7.9 ± 0.5	11.1 ± 0.4	0,938	10.1 ± 0.5	0,209
LVESD (mm)	5.5 ± 0.4	7.6 ± 0.3	0,736	6.1 ± 0.4	0,072
FS (%)	31.5 ± 1.4	30.5 ± 1.0	0,937	35.4 ± 1.5	0,011
EF (%)	64.1 ± 2.0	63.9 ± 1.4	0,630	68.8 ± 2.5	0,032
Stroke Volume (ml)	0.34 ± 0.03	0.22 ± 0.18	0,448	0.30 ± 0.04	0,762
Cardiac Output (ml/min)	79.5 ± 9.3	52.0 ± 4.5	0,890	61.6 ± 8.6	0,393
SWTs (mm)	2.1 ± 0.1	2.3 ± 0.2	0,671	2.7 ± 0.2	0,457
SWTd (mm)	1.4 ± 0.1	1.7 ± 0.2	0,971	2.1 ± 0.2	0,092
Systolic time (ms)	126 ± 3.7	134 ± 2.6	0,245	135 ± 2.6	0,153
Diastolic time (ms)	139 ± 8.4	135 ± 8.3	0,207	157 ± 14.5	0,138
PEP (ms)	15.0 ± 1.6	25.4 ± 1.3	0,413	21.8 ± 1.0	0,308
LVET (ms)	110 ± 4.4	109 ± 2.8	0,310	113 ± 3.9	0,268
PEP/LVET	0.13 + 0.02	0.23 + 0.02	0,800	0.19 + 0.01	0,968
Systolic time/RR	0.48 + 0.02	0.50 + 0.02	0,344	0.47 + 0.02	0,370

Values are mean ± SD. *LVEDD* Left ventricle end-diastolic diameter, *LVEDV* Left ventricle end-diastolic volume, *LVESD* Left ventricle end-systolic diameter, *LVESD* Left ventricle end-systolic volume, *FS* Fractional shortening, *EF* Ejection fraction, *SV* stroke volume, *SWTs* septal wall thickness at end-systole, *SWTd* septal wall thickness at end-diastole, *PEP* aortic pre-ejection period, *LVET* Left ventricular ejection time, *RR* inter-beat interval

Table 2 Two-tailed T-test before and after Placebo infusion on LV function after 2 months of AR in a rat model ($n = 5$)

	Before infusion	After infusion	*p*-value
Heart Rate (beats/min)	249 ± 18	220 ± 41	0.437
Left Atrium (mm)	6.2 ± 0.8	5.8 ± 1.1	0.541
LVEDD (mm)	10.6 ± 0.8	12.24 ± 1.07	0.092
LVESD (mm)	7.5 ± 0.6	6.9 ± 0.84	0.341
FS (%)	28.8 ± 1.4	29.6 ± 5.2	0.706
EF (%)	60.8 ± 1.8	61.0 ± 8.4	0.968
Stroke Volume (ml)	0.24 ± 0.04	0.24 + 0.08	0.890
Cardiac Output (ml/min)	60 ± 8	60 ± 12	0.369
SWTs (mm)	3.0 ± 0.16	2.9 ± 0.47	0.122
SWTd (mm)	1.6 ± 0.17	1.7 ± 0.29	0.281
Systolic time (ms)	136 ± 5	123 ± 17	0.340
Diastolic time (ms)	144 ± 24	173 ± 41	0.054
PEP (ms)	25.8 ± 4.6	21.2 ± 6.2	0.125
LVET (ms)	110 ± 8	102 ± 14	0.490
PEP/LVET	0.24 ± 0.05	0.20 ± 0.05	0.182
Systolic time/RR	0.49 ± 0.05	0.42 ± 0.05	0.047

Values are mean ± SD. Left ventricle end-diastolic diameter; LVEDV: Left ventricle end-diastolic volume; LVESD: Left ventricle end-systolic diameter; LVESD: Left ventricle end-systolic volume; FS: Fractional shortening; EF: Ejection fraction; SV: stroke volume; SWTs: septal wall thickness at end-systole; SWTd: septal wall thickness at end-diastole PEP: aortic pre-ejection period; LVET: Left ventricular ejection time; RR: inter-beat interval

Table 3 Two-tailed T-test before and after OM infusion on LV function after 2 months of AR in a rat model ($n = 7$)

	Before infusion	After infusion	*p*-value
Heart Rate (beats/min)	253 ± 22	207 ± 35	0.091
Left Atrium (mm)	6.2 ± 0.8	5.5 ± 0.7	0.037
LVEDD (mm)	11.6 ± 1.09	9.0 ± 1.51	0.003
LVESD (mm)	7.8 ± 0.91	5.4 ± 1.30	0.009
FS (%)	32.1 ± 3.4	41.1 ± 5.3	0.004
EF (%)	65.0 ± 4.7	76.6 ± 5.8	0.002
Stroke Volume (ml)	0.19 ± 0.06	0.36 + 0.11	0.011
Cardiac Output (ml/min)	44 ± 16	76 ± 14	0.027
SWTs (mm)	2.67± 0.48	3.33 ± 0.51	0.390
SWTd (mm)	1.6 ± 0.17	2.4 ± 0.39	0.274
Systolic time (ms)	133 ± 7	147 ± 8	0.003
Diastolic time (ms)	127 ± 16	141 ± 33	0.384
PEP (ms)	25.0 ± 2.3	22.4 ± 1.8	0.042
LVET (ms)	108 ± 6	125 ± 9	0.002
PEP/LVET	0.23 ± 0.02	0.18 ± 0.02	0.007
Systolic time/RR	0.51 ± 0.04	0.52 ± 0.06	0.735

Values are mean ± SD. *LVEDD* Left ventricle end-diastolic diameter, *LVEDV* Left ventricle end-diastolic volume, *LVESD* Left ventricle end-systolic diameter, *LVESD* Left ventricle end systolic volume, *FS* Fractional shortening, *EF* Ejection fraction, *SV* stroke volume, *SWTs* septal wall thickness at end-systole, *SWTd* septal wall thickness at end-diastole, *PEP* aortic pre-ejection period, *LVET* Left ventricular ejection time, *RR* inter-beat interval

Table 4 Two-way ANOVA statistics with Bonferroni correction at base (T1), before injection (T2) and after injection (T3) for all animals ($n = 12$)

	T1	T2	p	T3	p
Heart Rate (beats/min)	226 ± 23	228 ± 21	0.890	208 ± 28	0.113
Left Atrium (mm)	4.6 ± 0.2	6.2 ± 0.3	0.966	5.5 ± 0.2	0.277
LVEDD (mm)	7.9 ± 0.5	11.1 ± 0.4	0.235	10.1 ± 0.5	0.066
LVESD (mm)	5.5 ± 0.4	7.6 ± 0.3	0.871	6.1 ± 0.4	0.092
FS (%)	31.5 ± 1.4	30.5 ± 1.0	0.144	35.4 ± 1.5	0.014
EF (%)	64.1 ± 2.0	63.9 ± 1.4	0.173	68.8 ± 2.5	0.012
Stroke Volume (ml)	0.34 ± 0.03	0.22 ± 0.18	0.129	0.30 ± 0.04	0.135
Cardiac Output (ml/min)	79.5 ± 9.3	52.0 ± 4.5	0.098	61.6 ± 8.6	0.203
SWTs (mm)	2.1 ± 0.1	2.3 ± 0.2	0.597	2.7 ± 0.2	0.652
SWTd (mm)	1.4 ± 0.1	1.7 ± 0.2	0.439	2.1 ± 0.2	0.040
Systolic time (ms)	126 ± 3.7	134 ± 2.6	0.626	135 ± 2.6	0.293
Diastolic time (ms)	139 ± 8.4	135 ± 8.3	0.341	157 ± 14.5	0.293
PEP (ms)	15.0 ± 1.6	25.4 ± 1.3	0.771	21.8 ± 1.0	0.577
LVET (ms)	110 ± 4.4	109 ± 2.8	0.752	113 ± 3.9	0.180
PEP/LVET	0.13 + 0.02	0.23 + 0.02	0.811	0.19 + 0.01	0.378
Systolic time/RR	0.48 + 0.02	0.50 + 0.02	0.567	0.47 + 0.02	0.063

Values are mean ± SD. *LVEDD* Left ventricle end-diastolic diameter, *LVEDV* Left ventricle end-diastolic volume, *LVESD* Left ventricle end-systolic diameter, *LVESD* Left ventricle end-systolic volume, *FS* Fractional shortening, *EF* Ejection fraction, *SV* stroke volume, *SWTs* septal wall thickness at end-systole, *SWTd* septal wall thickness at end-diastole, *PEP* aortic pre-ejection period, *LVET* Left ventricular ejection time, *RR* inter-beat interval

pacing-induced energy depletion, has also been reported, because OM decreased LV end-diastolic pressure without affecting LV systolic pressure [15].

In contrast to our initial hypothesis, we found that OM did not affect the severity of the aortic leakage since the diastolic time-span remained unchanged, as a result of a reduction in HR. In mitigation, however, excessive prolongation the duration of systole might compromise myocardial blood flow, and thereby aggravate ischemia; even if studies with OM in patients with angina and ischemic cardiomyopathy seem reassuring in this regard [29]. This stands in contrast with inotropic drugs that enhance the risk of ischemia, arrhythmias and death. Hence forth those risks have limited their utility in treating acute and chronic heart failure [30].

Ketamine is a dissociative anesthetic agent that has cardiovascular effect resembling sympathetic nervous system stimulation,increase heart rate and cardiac output [31]. Medetomidine improves muscle relaxation, potentiates anesthetic action of ketamine and compensates the cardiac stimulating effect of ketamine by decreasing heart rate and cardiac output. Dexmedetomidine had no direct myocardial depressant effect in the rat heart in doses that are similar to those encountered under clinical conditions [32]. As animals were all anesthetized at the same regime, the decrease in heart rate observed in the OM group can be attributed to OM. However, we cannot predict if this bradycardic effect of OM had also been highlighted in conscious non-sedated animals.

Possible differential effects of OM as compared to other inotropic agents in AR

Dobutamine infusion, in patients with chronic aortic regurgitation and depressed LV ejection fraction, decreased LVEDD, LVEDV, LVESD and LVESV, while FS and EF improved [33]. In conscious dogs with heart failure, systemic and pulmonary systolic wall stress remained unchanged while HR, LV systolic pressure and LV dP/dt increased with Dobutamine [34]. Dobutamine also shortened LVET in healthy dogs [35]. On the opposite, in our study OM decreased HR and increased LVET, while others, in conscious dogs with systolic heart failure induced by rapid pacing, reported that OM did not affect LV dP/dt [15]. When a comparable concentration of OM than in our study was administrated in normal humans (400 ng/ml) [36], blood pressure did not change. Thus OM and Dobutamine tend to enhance LV contractility by increasing wall thickening and fractional shortening, but in the presence of unchanged afterload conditions with OM [37], while arterial pressure and total vascular resistance increase with Dobutamine.

Currently available inotropes Dobutamin, Dopamin, Milrinone and Levosimendan have demonstrated proarrhythmic effects linked to increased mortality that can limit their clinical utility [38]. Most inotropic agents modify calcium cellular homeostasis. This is important, as intracellular calcium plays an important role in myocardial oxygen demand [39]. The well-known and widely used sympathomimetic drug dobutamine increases calcium

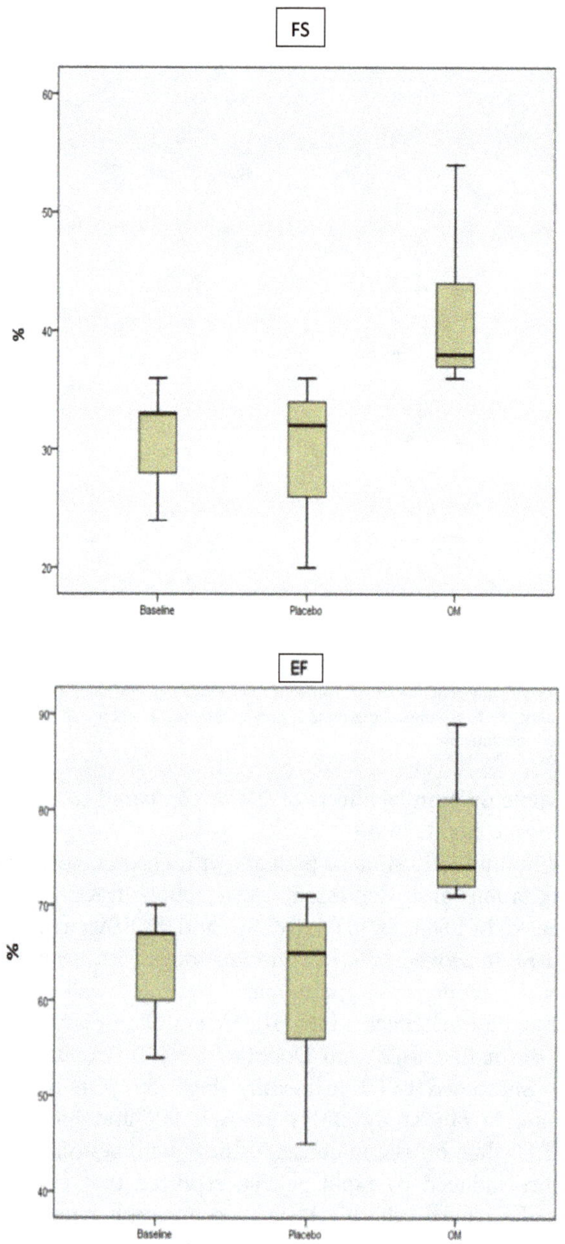

Fig. 2 Two-way ANOVA with Bonferroni corrections for multiple comparisons on the effects of OM versus placebo on FS ($p = 0.014$) and EF ($p = 0.012$) after 2 months of AR. Box and Whisker plots before infusion, and after infusion of OM vs. placebo (median: horizontal band within the box, box top and bottom: upper and lower first quartiles, top and bottom whiskers: highest and lowest quartiles; $n = 12$)

channels accessibility [40]. Other medications, such as levosimendan, enhance the sensitivity of troponin-c towards calcium, not at the expense of an increase in intracellular calcium concentration [22]. Levosimendan increases contractility by enhancing cross-bridge formation between actin and myosin [22, 41]. The side effect of these increases in contractility is that they raise also myocardial oxygen consumption which is also pro arrhythmic. The molecules may also alter the expression of genes and promote the apoptosis of myocardial cells elicited by the increased intracellular calcium [39, 41]. OM inhibits non-actin dependent cardiac myosin adenosine triphosphate [16] and does not raise myocardial oxygen consumption [15]. A recent study in anesthetized animals suggested the opposite, namely that OM increased myocardial oxygen consumption [42], and however this was apparently undermined by methodological limitations [43]. These favorable characteristics of OM could prove useful in patients with AR.

Effects of OM dose on the observed changes

In our study we administrated 1.2 mg/kg/h of OM during 30 min. This was expected to raise plasma concentrations of OM to nearly 400 ng/ml [44]. In rats with heart failure induced by a ligation of the left coronary artery, infusion of OM resulted in comparable increases in FS than in our study, starting at plasma concentrations of approximately 200 ng/ml [44]. Administration of less than 0.48 mg/kg/h of OM yield plasma levels < 160 ng/ml, where no LV functional improvements where observed [36]. In healthy human improvements in EF began at a dose of 0.5 mg/kg/h, while improvements in FS, LVET and SV began at an infusion rate of 0.125 mg/kg/h [36]. No change in orthostatic vital signs was noted in this study [45]. In patients with heart failure [45], LVET increased at OM concentrations > 100 ng/ml, while SV and FS raised at plasma levels > 200 ng/ml. EF increased only beginning concentrations > 300 ng/ml. Supine and standing systolic blood pressure decreased at > 400 and > 500 ng/ml, respectively. Last, in the ATOMIC-AHF study [46], patients with acute heart failure treated with OM disclosed a concentration-dependent reduction in HR at a concentration > 200 ng/ml while blood pressure increased at a concentration > 300 ng/ml, as compared to placebo. There was also a concentration-related decrease in LVESD and increase in LVET. OM concentrations > 400 ng/ml achieved a better dyspnea response. Thus the dose administered in our study seems in the upper range of the concentrations where favorable hemodynamic modifications of OM are clear-cut, without being harmful. Adverse effects of OM consist in an excessive prolongation of systolic ejection time > 110 ms [36]. This was observed with supra therapeutic concentrations of OM (~ 1200 ng/ml) which may induce myocardial ischemia by reducing the time during which diastolic coronary blood flow can occur [46]. A drug overdose in a patient with heart failure, with a predicted concentration of 1750 ng/ml at the time of infusion termination, resulted in chest pain, sweating, hypotension, and ECG changes suggestive of ischemia [45]. It is not known, however, that the angina symptoms, observed at supra-therapeutic concentrations of OM, are related - or not - to the presently recognized ryanodine receptors activating effect of OM [47].

Study limitations

The tested animal group was small because many rats did not recover from the acute AR procedure. Another striking limitation of our study resides in the fact that we could not achieve ventricular blood pressure measurement during the study. As such, our assessment of ventricular loading conditions remains incomplete. Several studies suggest however that systemic blood pressure is not affected at the OM concentrations we achieved in our study [36, 37]. Our study did also not assess whether OM has dose-dependent hemodynamic effects in our model of AR. Lower doses of OM may still exert favorable hemodynamic effects, while even further reducing the risk of excessive prolongations in LVET. This will require additional studies. Moreover, as already discussed, a direct comparison of the effects of different inotropic agents in AR-related heart failure would also provide further insights in the differential hemodynamic effects of OM, as compared to other inotropic agents. Last, the effects of OM on animals who might otherwise not survive the decompensation period after an acute AR should be also studied. This is a very poorly tolerated condition in humans [48], which could benefit from further studies on the best hemodynamic support while awaiting cardiac surgery [48]. Last, the sham group in our study comprised only 2 animals in the OM group and 2 animals in the placebo group.

Another limitation of the study, the possible fistula with left atrium created during aortic valve leaflets puncture, this fistula can explain the decrease of stroke volume and cardiac output after the creation of the aortic regurgitation.

Conclusion

The present placebo-controlled study shows improvements in cardiac function after infusion of OM. Our investigations demonstrate these effects for the first time in the rat-model with chronic severe AR. We observed a decrease in volume overload and an increase in cardiac output and wall thickness. Moreover OM enhanced EF and FS, while coincidently lowering the HR and wall stress. On the other hand, OM did not affect the duration of diastole and the severity of AR.

Abbreviations

AR: Aortic regurgitation; ATP: Adenosin triphosphate; EF: Ejection fraction; FS: Fractional shortening; HR: Heart rate; LV: Left ventricle; LVEDD: Left ventricle end-diastolic diameter; LVESD: Left ventricle end-systolic diameter; LVET: Left ventricular ejection time; OM: Omecamtiv-mecarbil; PEP: Pre-ejection period; Pi: Hydrolazed phosphate; RR: Inter-beat interval; SV: Stroke volume

Funding

This study was supported and funded by the for Cardiac Surgery Foundation of the Free University of Brussels (B. El Oumeiri), the Saucez-Van Pouke Foundation (B. El Oumeiri, K. Mc Entee, and P. Van de Borne).

Authors' contributions

BE carried out the experiments, performed the statistical analysis and drafted the manuscript and participated in the design of the study. KME coordinated the study and participated in its design.
FA and AH carried out the echocardiography. FVD participated in the coordination of the study. PJ did the technical assistance GVN performed the statistical analysis and reviewed the manuscript. PVB conceived the study and participated in the drafting of the manuscript. All authors read and approved the final manuscript.

Competing interests

The authors declare that they have no competing interests.

Author details

[1]Department of Cardiac surgery, Erasme Hospital, ULB, 808 Lennik road, 1070, Brussels, Belgium. [2]Laboratory of Physiology and Pharmacology, ULB, Brussels, Belgium. [3]Department of intensive care, Erasme Hospital, ULB, Brussels, Belgium. [4]Department of Cardiology, Erasme Hospital, ULB, Brussels, Belgium.

References

1. Maurer G. Aortic regurgitation. Heart. 2006 Jul;92(7):994–1000.
2. Dujardin KS, Enriquez-Sarano M, Schaff HV, Bailey KR, Seward JB, Tajik AJ. Mortality and morbidity of aortic regurgitation in clinical practice. A long-term follow-up study. Circulation. 1999 Apr 13;99(14):1851–7.
3. Chockalingam A, Gnanavelu G, Elangovan S, Chockalingam V. Current profile of acute rheumatic fever and valvulitis in southern India. J Heart Valve Dis. 2003 Sep;12(5):573–6.
4. Carabello BA. Aortic regurgitation. A lesion with similarities to both aortic stenosis and mitral regurgitation. Circulation. 1990 Sep;82(3):1051–3.
5. Bonow RO. Aortic Regurgitation. Curr Treat Options Cardiovasc Med. 2000 Apr;2(2):125–32.
6. Evangelista A, Tornos P, Sambola A, Permanyer-Miralda G, Soler-Soler J. Long-term vasodilator therapy in patients with severe aortic regurgitation. N Engl J Med. 2005 Sep 29;353(13):1342–9.
7. Mahajerin A, Gurm HS, Tsai TT, Chan PS, Nallamothu BK. Vasodilator therapy in patients with aortic insufficiency: a systematic review. Am Heart J. 2007 Apr;153(4):454–61.
8. Magid NM, Opio G, Wallerson DC, Young MS, Borer JS. Heart failure due to chronic experimental aortic regurgitation. Am J Physiol. 1994 Aug;267(2 Pt 2):H556–62.
9. Plante E, Couet J, Gaudreau M, Dumas MP, Drolet MC, Arsenault M. Left ventricular response to sustained volume overload from chronic aortic valve regurgitation in rats. J Card Fail. 2003 Apr;9(2):128–40.
10. Borer JS, Hochreiter C, Herrold EM, et al. Prediction of indications for valve replacement among asymptomatic or minimally symptomatic patients with chronic aortic regurgitation and normal left ventricular performance. Circulation. 1998;97:525–34.
11. Borow KM. Surgical outcome in chronic aortic regurgitation: a physiologic framework for assessing preoperative predictors. J Am Coll Cardiol. 1987 Nov;10(5):1165–70.
12. Weber KT, Brilla CG. Pathological hypertrophy and cardiac interstitium. Fibrosis and renin-angiotensin-aldosterone system. Circulation. 1991 Jun;83(6):1849–65.
13. Krum H, Teerlink JR. Medical therapy for chronic heart failure. Lancet. 2011 Aug 20;378(9792):713–21.
14. Psotka MA, Teerlink JR. Direct myosin activation by Omecamtiv Mecarbil for heart failure with reduced ejection fraction. Handb Exp Pharmacol. 2017; 243:465–90.

15. Shen YT, Malik FI, Zhao X, Depre C, Dhar SK, Abarzúa P, Morgans DJ, Vatner SF. Improvement of cardiac function by a cardiac myosin activator in conscious dogs with systolic heart failure. Circ Heart Fail. 2010 Jul;3(4):522–7.
16. Malik FI, Hartman JJ, Elias KA, Morgan BP, Rodriguez H, Brejc K, et al. Cardiac myosin activation: a potential therapeutic approach for systolic heart failure. Science. 2011 Mar 18;331(6023):1439–43.
17. Umana E, Solares CA, Alpert MA. Tachycardia-induced cardiomyopathy. Am J Med. 2003 Jan;114(1):51–5.
18. Arsenault M, Plante E, Drolet MC, Couet J. Experimental aortic regurgitation in rats under echocardiographic guidance. J Heart Valve Dis. 2002 Jan;11(1): 128–34.
19. Zoghbi WA, Enriquez-Sarano M, Foster E, Grayburn PA, Kraft CD, Levine RA, et al. Recommendations for evaluation of the severity of native valvular regurgitation with two-dimensional and Doppler echocardiography. J Am Soc Echocardiogr. 2003 Jul;16(7):777–802.
20. Lewis RP, Rittogers SE, Froester WF, Boudoulas H. A critical review of the systolic time intervals. Circulation. 1977 Aug;56(2):146–58.
21. Spodick DH, Doi YL, Bishop RL, Hashimoto T. Systolic time intervals reconsidered. Reevaluation of the preejection period: absence of relation to heart rate. Am J Cardiol. 1984 Jun 1;53(11):1667–70.
22. Stevenson LW. Clinical use of inotropic therapy for heart failure: looking backward or forward? Part II: chronic inotropic therapy. Circulation. 2003 Jul 29;108(4):492–7.
23. Wisenbaugh T, Allen P, Cooper G 4th, O'Connor WN, Mezaros L, Streter F, Bahinski A, Houser S, Spann JF. Hypertrophy without contractile dysfunction after reversal of pressure overload in the cat. Am J Phys. 1984 Jul;247(1 Pt 2): H146–54.
24. Bekeredjian R, Grayburn PA. Valvular heart disease: aortic regurgitation. Circulation. 2005 Jul 5;112(1):125–34.
25. Boudoulas H. Systolic time intervals. Eur Heart J. 1990 Dec;11 Suppl I:93–104.
26. Teerlink JR, Felker GM, McMurray JJ, Solomon SD, Adams KF Jr, Cleland JG, Ezekowitz JA, Goudev A, Macdonald P, Metra M, Mitrovic V, Ponikowski P, Serpytis P, Spinar J, Tomcsányi J, Vandekerckhove HJ, Voors AA, Monsalvo ML, Johnston J, Malik FI. Honarpour N; COSMIC-HF investigators. Chronic oral study of myosin activation to increase contractility in heart failure (COSMIC-HF): a phase 2, pharmacokinetic, randomised, placebo-controlled trial. Lancet. 2016 Dec 10;388(10062):2895–903.
27. Wallace AG, Mitchell JH, Skinner NS, Sarnoff SJ. Duration of the phases of left ventricular systole. Circ Res. 1963 Jun;12:611–9.
28. Greenberg BH, Chou W, Saikali KG, Escandón R, Lee JH, Chen MM, Treshkur T, Megreladze I, Wasserman SM, Eisenberg P, Malik FI, Wolff AA, Shaburishvili T. Safety and tolerability of omecamtiv mecarbil during exercise in patients with ischemic cardiomyopathy and angina. JACC Heart Fail. 2015 Jan;3(1):22–9.
29. Petersen JW, Felker GM. Inotropes in the management of acute heart failure. Crit Care Med. 2008 Jan;36(1 Suppl):S106–11.
30. Espinola-Zavaleta N, Gómez-Núñez N, Chávez PY, Sahagun-Sánchez G, Keirns C, Casanova JM, Romero-Cárdenas A, Roldán FJ, Vargas-Barrón J. Evaluation of the response to pharmacological stress in chronic aortic regurgitation. Echocardiography. 2001 Aug;18(6):491–6.
31. Levänen J, Mäkelä ML, Scheinin H. Dexmedetomidine premedication attenuates ketamine-induced cardio-stimulatory effects and post-anesthetic delirium. Anesthesiology. 1995 May;82(5):1117–25.
32. Lee K, Hwang HJ, Kim OS, Oh YJ. Assessment of dexmedetomidine effects on left ventricular function using pressure-volume loops in rats. J Anesth. 2017 Feb;31(1):18–24.
33. Asai K, Uechi M, Sato N, Shen W, Meguro T, Mathier MA, Shannon RP, Vatner SF. Lack of desensitization and enhanced efficiency of calcium channel promoter in conscious dogs with heart failure. Am J Phys. 1998 Dec;275(6 Pt 2):H2219–26.
34. Banfor PN, Preusser LC, Campbell TJ, Marsh KC, Polakowski JS, Reinhart GA, Cox BF, Fryer RM. Comparative effects of levosimendan, OR-1896, OR-1855, dobutamine, and milrinone on vascular resistance, indexes of cardiac function, and O2 consumption in dogs. Am J Physiol Heart Circ Physiol. 2008 Jan;294(1):H238–48.
35. Anderson RL, Sueoka SH, Lee KH, Rodriguez HM, Kawas RF, Godinez G, Morgan BP, Sakowicz R, Morgans DJ, Malik F, Elias KA. In vitro and in vivo characterization of CK-1827452, a selective cardiac myosin activator. J Card Fail. 2006;12:S86.
36. Teerlink JR, Clarke CP, Saikali KG, Lee JH, Chen MM, Escandon RD, Elliott L, Bee R, Habibzadeh MR, Goldman JH, Schiller NB, Malik FI, Wolff AA. Dose-dependent augmentation of cardiac systolic function with the selective cardiac myosin activator, omecamtiv mecarbil: a first-in-man study. Lancet. 2011 Aug 20;378(9792):667–75.
37. Tariq S, Aronow WS. Use of inotropic agents in treatment of systolic heart failure. Int J Mol Sci. 2015 Dec 4;16(12):29060–8.
38. Kojima S, Wu ST, Parmley WW, Wikman-Coffelt J. Relationship between intracellular calcium and oxygen consumption: effects of perfusion pressure, extracellular calcium, dobutamine, and nifedipine. Am Heart J. 1994 Feb; 127(2):386–91.
39. Tsien RW, Bean BP, Hess P, Lansman JB, Nilius B, Nowycky MC. Mechanisms of calcium channel modulation by beta-adrenergic agents and dihydropyridine calcium agonists. J Mol Cell Cardiol. 1986 Jul;18(7):691–710.
40. \Hasenfuss G, Pieske B, Castell M, Kretschmann B, Maier LS, Just H. Influence of the novel inotropic agent levosimendan on isometric tension and calcium cycling in failing human myocardium. Circulation. 1998 Nov 17;98(20):2141–7.
41. Moin DS, Sackheim J, Hamo CE, Butler J. Cardiac Myosin Activators in Systolic Heart Failure: More Friend than Foe? Curr Cardiol Rep. 2016 Oct;18(10):100.
42. Bakkehaug JP, Kildal AB, Engstad ET, Boardman N, Næsheim T, Rønning L, Aasum E, Larsen TS, Myrmel T, How OJ. Myosin Activator Omecamtiv Mecarbil Increases Myocardial Oxygen Consumption and Impairs Cardiac Efficiency Mediated by Resting Myosin ATPase Activity. Circ Heart Fail. 2015 Jul;8(4):766–75.
43. Teerlink JR, Malik FI, Kass DA. Letter by Teerlink et al regarding article, "myosin activator Omecamtiv Mecarbil increases myocardial oxygen consumption and impairs cardiac efficiency mediated by resting myosin ATPase activity". Circ Heart Fail. 2015 Nov;8(6):1141.
44. Anderson RL, Sueoka SH, Rodriguez HM, Lee KH, Cox DR, Kawas R, Morgan BP, Sakowicz R, Morgans DJ, Malik F, Elias KA. In vitro and in vivo efficacy of the cardiac myosin activator CK-1827452. Mol bio cell. 2005;16(abstract #1728). https://cytokinetics.com/wp-content/uploads/2015/10/ASCB_1728.pdf.
45. Cleland JG, Teerlink JR, Senior R, Nifontov EM, Mc Murray JJ, Lang CC, et al. The effects of the cardiac myosin activator, omecamtiv mecarbil, on cardiac function in systolic heart failure: a double-blind, placebo-controlled, crossover, dose-ranging phase 2 trial. Lancet. 2011 Aug 20;378(9792):676–83.
46. Teerlink JR, Felker GM, McMurray JJ, Ponikowski P, Metra M, Filippatos GS. ATOMIC-AHF investigators. Acute treatment with Omecamtiv Mecarbil to increase contractility in acute heart failure: the ATOMIC-AHF study. J Am Coll Cardiol. 2016 Mar 29;67(12):1444–55.
47. Nánási P Jr, Gaburjakova M, Gaburjakova J, Almássy J. Omecamtiv mecarbil activates ryanodine receptors from canine cardiac but not skeletal muscle. Eur J Pharmacol. 2017 Aug 15;809:73–9.
48. Dervan J, Goldberg S. Acute aortic regurgitation: pathophysiology and management. Cardiovasc Clin. 1986;16(2):281–8.

Permissions

All chapters in this book were first published in CD, by BioMed Central; hereby published with permission under the Creative Commons Attribution License or equivalent. Every chapter published in this book has been scrutinized by our experts. Their significance has been extensively debated. The topics covered herein carry significant findings which will fuel the growth of the discipline. They may even be implemented as practical applications or may be referred to as a beginning point for another development.

The contributors of this book come from diverse backgrounds, making this book a truly international effort. This book will bring forth new frontiers with its revolutionizing research information and detailed analysis of the nascent developments around the world.

We would like to thank all the contributing authors for lending their expertise to make the book truly unique. They have played a crucial role in the development of this book. Without their invaluable contributions this book wouldn't have been possible. They have made vital efforts to compile up to date information on the varied aspects of this subject to make this book a valuable addition to the collection of many professionals and students.

This book was conceptualized with the vision of imparting up-to-date information and advanced data in this field. To ensure the same, a matchless editorial board was set up. Every individual on the board went through rigorous rounds of assessment to prove their worth. After which they invested a large part of their time researching and compiling the most relevant data for our readers.

The editorial board has been involved in producing this book since its inception. They have spent rigorous hours researching and exploring the diverse topics which have resulted in the successful publishing of this book. They have passed on their knowledge of decades through this book. To expedite this challenging task, the publisher supported the team at every step. A small team of assistant editors was also appointed to further simplify the editing procedure and attain best results for the readers.

Apart from the editorial board, the designing team has also invested a significant amount of their time in understanding the subject and creating the most relevant covers. They scrutinized every image to scout for the most suitable representation of the subject and create an appropriate cover for the book.

The publishing team has been an ardent support to the editorial, designing and production team. Their endless efforts to recruit the best for this project, has resulted in the accomplishment of this book. They are a veteran in the field of academics and their pool of knowledge is as vast as their experience in printing. Their expertise and guidance has proved useful at every step. Their uncompromising quality standards have made this book an exceptional effort. Their encouragement from time to time has been an inspiration for everyone.

The publisher and the editorial board hope that this book will prove to be a valuable piece of knowledge for researchers, students, practitioners and scholars across the globe.

List of Contributors

Mehmet Oezkur, Armin Gorski, Jennifer Peltz, Maria Lazariotou, Christoph Schimmer and Rainer G Leyh
Department of Cardiovascular Surgery, University Hospital Würzburg, Würzburg, Germany

Martin Wagner and Peter U Heuschmann
Institute of Clinical Epidemiology and Biometry, Comprehensive Heart Failure Center, University of Würzburg, Würzburg, Germany

Peter U Heuschmann
Clinical Trial Center Würzburg, University Hospital Würzburg, Würzburg, Germany

Yaron Arbel, Nevena Zivkovic, Dhruven Mehta, Sam Radhakrishnan, Stephen E. Fremes and Harindra C. Wijeysundera
Schulich Heart Centre, Division of Cardiology and Cardiac surgery, Sunnybrook Health Sciences Centre, Toronto, ON, Canada

Yaron Arbel, Nevena Zivkovic, Dhruven Mehta, Sam Radhakrishnan, Stephen E. Fremes, Effat Rezaei, Asim N. Cheema, Sami Al-Nasser and Harindra C. Wijeysundera
University of Toronto, Toronto, ON, Canada

Harindra C. Wijeysundera
Institute for Clinical Evaluative Sciences (ICES), 2075 Bayview Avenue, Suite A202, Toronto, ON M4N 3M5, Canada
Sunnybrook Research Institute (SRI), Dept. of Medicine & Institute of Health Policy, Management and Evaluation, University of Toronto, Toronto, ON, Canada

Effat Rezaei and Asim N. Cheema
St. Michael's Hospital, Toronto, ON, Canada

Yaron Arbel and Ariel Finkelstein
Department of Cardiology, Tel Aviv Medical Center, Tel Aviv, affiliated to the Sackler School of Medicine, Tel Aviv University, Tel Aviv, Israel

Ryoto Hourai, Koichi Sohmiya, Yohei Yamauchi, Shu-ichi Fujita, Masaaki Hoshiga and Nobukazu Ishizaka
Department of Cardiology, Osaka Medical College, Daigaku-machi 2-7, Takatsuki, Osaka 569-8686, Japan

Satomi Kasashima
Department of Pathology, National Hospital Organization, Kanazawa Medical Center, Kanazawa, Japan

Hideki Ozawa, Takahiro Katsumata and Masahiro Daimon
Department of Thoracic and Cardiovascular Surgery, Osaka Medical College, Osaka, Japan

Yoshinobu Hirose and Yasuhiro Ogino
Department of Pathology Osaka Medical College, Osaka, Japan

Maria Elena Soto, Ricardo Marquez and Rafael Bojalil-Parra
Immunology Department, Instituto Nacional de Cardiología "Ignacio Chávez", Juan Badiano número 1, Colonia Sección XVI, Delegación Tlalpan, Mexico CP 14080, Mexico

Jose Luis Salas
Echocardiography Department, Instituto Nacional de Cardiología "Ignacio Chávez", Mexico, Mexico

Jesus Vargas-Barron
Investigation Department, Instituto Nacional de Cardiología "Ignacio Chávez", Mexico, Mexico

Alejandra Rodriguez-Hernandez
Intensive care Department, Instituto Nacional de Cardiología "Ignacio Chavez", Mexico, Mexico

Israel Pérez-Torres
Department of Pathology, Instituto Nacional de Cardiología "Ignacio Chavez", Mexico, Mexico

Veronica Guarner-Lans
Department of Physiology, Instituto Nacional de Cardiología "Ignacio Chávez", Mexico, Mexico

Qi Jin, Steen Pehrson, Peter Karl Jacobsen and Xu Chen
Department of Cardiology, The Heart Centre, Rigshospitalet, University of Copenhagen, Copenhagen, Denmark

Qi Jin
Department of Cardiology, Shanghai Ruijin Hospital, Shanghai Jiao Tong University School of Medicine, Shanghai, China

Ahmed Elmaraezy, Ammar Ismail and Ammar M. AlSafadi
Faculty of Medicine, Al-Azhar University, Cairo, Egypt

Ahmed Elmaraezy, Ammar Ismail, Abdelrahman Ibrahim Abushouk and Ammar M. AlSafadi
NovaMed Medical Research Association, Cairo, Egypt

Abdelrahman Ibrahim Abushouk
Faculty of Medicine, Ain Shams University, Cairo, Egypt

Moutaz Eltoomy
Genetic Engineering & Biotechnology Research Institute (GEBRI), University of Sadat City, Sadat City, Egypt

Soha Saad
Faculty of Medicine, Tanta University, Tanta, Egypt

Ahmed Negida
Faculty of Medicine, Zagazig University, Zagazig, Egypt

Osama Mahmoud Abdelaty
Ahmed Maher Teaching Hospital, Cairo, Egypt

Ahmed Ramadan Abdallah and Ahmed Magdy Aboelfotoh
Faculty of Medicine, Benha University, Benha, Egypt

Hossam Mahmoud Hassan
Faculty of Medicine, Beni Suef University, Beni suef, Egypt

Aya Gamal Elmaraezy and Mahmoud Morsi
Faculty of Medicine, Minoufia University, Shebin El-Kom, Egypt

Farah Althaher and Moath Althaher
Faculty of Medicine, Misr University for science and technology (MUST), 6th of October City, Giza, Egypt

Ammar M. AlSafadi
Faculty of Medicine, Damascus University, Damascus, Syria

Anthony Alozie, Bernd Westphal, Alexander Kaminski, Magnus Sindt and Gustav Steinhoff
Department of Cardiac Surgery, Heart Center Rostock, Schillingallee 35, 18057 Rostock, Germany

Liliya Paranskaya, Mohammad Sherif, Alper Öner and Hüseyin Ince
Department of Cardiology, Heart Center Rostock, Ernst-Heydemannstrasse 6, 18057 Rostock, Germany

Jochen Schubert
Department of Anesthesiology and Intensive Care Medicine, Heart Center Rostock, Schillingallee 35, 18057 Rostock, Germany

Stephan Kische
Kardiologie und Konservative Intensivmedizin, Landsbergerallee 49, 10249 Berlin, Germany

Doreen Diedrich
Institute For Biostatistics and Informatics in Medicine And Ageing Research, Ernst Heydemanstr. 8, 18057 Rostock, Germany

Ye Zhu and Xiang Gu
Clinical Medical College, Yangzhou University, Yangzhou, Jiangsu 225001, China

Ye Zhu and Xiang Gu
Department of Cardiology, Northern Jiangsu Province Hospital, Yangzhou, Jiangsu 225001, China

Chao Xu
Department of Global Biostatistics and Data Science, School of Public Health and Tropical Medicine, Tulane University, New Orleans, LA 70112, USA

Mads Phillip Kofoed Grabas, Christian Torp-Pedersen, Henrik Bøggild, Line Rosenkilde Ullits, Ulrik Deding and Charlotte Overgaard
Department of Health Science and Technology, Public Health and Epidemiology Group, Aalborg University, Niels Jernes Vej 14, 9220 Aalborg Øst, Denmark

Steen Møller Hansen, Christian Torp-Pedersen and Berit Jamie Nielsen
Department of Clinical Epidemiology, Aalborg University Hospital, Sdr. Skovvej 15, DK-9000 Aalborg, Denmark

Per Føge Jensen
Department of Anaesthesiology, Næstved Hospital, Ringstedgade 61, DK-4700 Næstved, Denmark

Zsuzsanna Cserép and Roland Tóth
The School of Ph.D. Studies, Semmelweis University, Budapest, Hungary

Zsuzsanna Cserép, János Gál and Andrea Székely
The Department of Anesthesia and Intensive Care, Semmelweis University, Budapest, Hungary

Eszter Losoncz, Attila Tóth and Andrea Székely
The Department of Anesthesia and Intensive Care, Gottsegen György Hungarian Institute of Cardiology, Budapest, Hungary

Roland Tóth and Boglárka Juhász
The Department of Cardiac Surgery of Gottsegen György Hungarian Institute of Cardiology, Budapest, Hungary

Piroska Balog
The Institute of Behavioral Sciences, Semmelweis University, Budapest, Hungary

Péter Vargha
The Hungary Heart Center, Semmelweis University, Budapest, Hungary

Richard J Contrada
The Department of Psychology, Rutgers the State University of New Jersey, New Brunswick, New Jersey, USA

Paul RJ Falger
Department of Psychiatry and Neuropsychiatry, Faculty of Health Medicine and Life Sciences, Maastricht University, Maastricht, The Netherlands

Jae Young Cho, Soon Jun Hong and Do-Sun Lim
Department of Cardiology, Korea University Anam Hospital, Inchon-ro 73, Seongbuk-gu, Seoul, South Korea

Wei-Chieh Lee, Huang-Chung Chen, Yung-Lung Chen, Tzu-Hsien Tsai and Mien-Cheng Chen
Division of Cardiology, Department of Internal Medicine, Kaohsiung Chang Gung Memorial Hospital, Chang Gung University College of Medicine, 123 Ta Pei Road, Niao Sung District, Kaohsiung City 83301, Taiwan

Kuo-Li Pan and Yu-Sheng Lin
Division of Cardiology, Chang Gung Memorial Hospital, Chiayi, Taiwan

Pravesh Kumar Bundhun, Tao Qin and Meng-Hua Chen
Institute of Cardiovascular Diseases, the First Affiliated Hospital of Guangxi Medical University, Nanning, Guangxi 530027, P. R. China

Ru-Wen Chang
Department of Physiology, College of Medicine, National Taiwan University, No. 1, Sec. 1, Ren'ai Rd., Zhongzheng Dist., Taipei 10051, Taiwan

Chien-Ming Luo, Hsi-Yu Yu and Chih-Hsien Wang
Department of Surgery, National Taiwan University Hospital, Hsin-Chu Branch, NO. 25, Lane 442, Sec. 1, Jingguo Rd., Hsin-Chu 30059, Taiwan

Hsi-Yu Yu, Yih-Sharng Chen and Chih-Hsien Wang
Cardiovascular Surgery, Department of Surgery, National Taiwan University Hospital, No. 7, Zhongshan S. Rd., Zhongzheng Dist., Taipei 10002, Taiwan

Jochen Reinöhl, Klaus Kaier, Anja Gutmann, Constantin von zur Mühlen, Martin Moser, Annette Geibel, Andreas Zirlik, Christoph Bode and Manfred Zehender
Department of Cardiology and Angiology I, Heart Center Freiburg University, Hugstetter Str. 55, 79106 Freiburg, Germany

Stefan Sorg, Matthias Siepe and Friedhelm Beyersdorf
Department of Cardiovascular Surgery, Heart Center Freiburg University, Freiburg, Germany

Philipp Blanke
Department of Diagnostic Radiology, Medical Center-University of Freiburg, Freiburg, Germany

Hardy Baumbach
Department of Cardiovascular Surgery, Robert-Bosch-Krankenhaus Stuttgart, Stuttgart, Germany

Klaus Kaier and Werner Vach
Center for Medical Biometry and Medical Informatics, Medical Center-University of Freiburg, Freiburg, Germany

Regina Maria de Aquino Xavier, Vitor Manuel Pereira Azevedo, Arn Migowski, Antonio, Rogério Brant Martins Chaves, Marcelo Goulart Correia and Clara Weksler
Hospital School, National Institute of Cardiology (INC), Ministry of Health, Rua das Laranjeiras 374, Laranjeiras, Rio de Janeiro, RJ, Brazil

Paulo Henrique Godoy
Hospital Naval Marcílio Dias, Rio de Janeiro, Brazil

Luiz Pinho Ribeiro
University Hospital and School of Medicine - Universidade Federal de Minas Gerais (UFMG), Minas Gerais, Brazil

Carolina de Aquino Xavier
University Hospital and School of Medicine, Federal University of Rio de Janeiro (UFRJ), Rio de Janeiro, Brazil

Lucas de Aquino Hashimoto and Nelson Albuquerque Souza e Silva
Hospital Municipal Salgado Filho, Rio de Janeiro, Brazil

Zhouping Zou, Bo Shen, Jiarui Xu, Wuhua Jiang, Jie Teng and Xiaoqiang Ding
Department of Nephrology, Zhongshan Hospital, Shanghai Medical College, Fudan University, No 180 Fenglin Road, Shanghai 200032, China

Zhouping Zou, Bo Shen, Jie Teng and Xiaoqiang Ding
Shanghai Medical Center of Kidney, No 180 Fenglin Road, Shanghai 200032, China

Zhouping Zou, Bo Shen, Jiarui Xu, Wuhua Jiang, Jie Teng and Xiaoqiang Ding
Shanghai Institute for Kidney and Dialysis, No 180 Fenglin Road, Shanghai 200032, China

Zhouping Zou, Bo Shen, Jiarui Xu, Wuhua Jiang, Jie Teng and Xiaoqiang Ding
Shanghai Key Laboratory of Kidney and Blood Purification, No 180 Fenglin Road, Shanghai 200032, China

Zhe Luo, Yamin Zhuang and Lan Liu
Department of Critical Care Medicine, Zhongshan Hospital, Shanghai Medical College, Fudan University, No 180 Fenglin Road, Shanghai 200032, China

Jie Teng and Xiaoqiang Ding
Hemodialysis Quality of Control Center of Shanghai, No 180 Fenglin Road, Shanghai 200032, China
Department of Nephrology, Xiamen Branch, Zhongshan Hospital, Fudan University, No 668 Jinhu Road, Xiamen 361015, Fujian, China

Chunsheng Wang
Department of Cardiovascular Surgery, Zhongshan Hospital, Shanghai Medical College, Fudan University, No 180 Fenglin Road, Shanghai 200032, China

Cheng Zheng, Wei-Qian Lin, Yuan-Zheng Lin, Hao Lian, Zhi-Rui Liu and Jia-Feng Lin
Department of Cardiology, Second Affiliated Hospital and Yuying Children's Hospital of Wenzhou Medical University, 109 Xueyuan Road, Wenzhou, Zhejiang 325000, China

Jia-Hui Chen
Department of Cardiology, Taishun general hospital, Wenzhou 325000, China

Yue Wang, Yue Wang, Mengru Liu and Xiaofan Wu
Department of Cardiology, Beijing Anzhen Hospital, Capital Medical University, Beijing 100029, China

Gary S. Mintz
Cardiovascular Research Foundation, New York, NY, USA

Zhichun Gu
Department of Pharmacy, Renji Hospital, School of Medicine, Shanghai Jiao Tong University, Shanghai 200127, China

Yue Qi
Department of Epidemiology, The Key Laboratory of Remodeling-Related Cardiovascular Diseases, Ministry of Education, Beijing Institute of Heart, Lung and Blood Vessel Diseases, Beijing Anzhen Hospital, Capital Medical University, Beijing, China

Marlena V. Habal, Kumaraswamy Nanthakumar, Peter C. Austin and Douglas S. Lee
University of Toronto, Toronto, ON, Canada

Kumaraswamy Nanthakumar, Cassandra Freitas and Douglas S. Lee
Peter Munk Cardiac Centre, University Health Network, Toronto, ON, Canada

Peter C. Austin, Christopher Labos and Douglas S. Lee
Institute for Clinical Evaluative Sciences, Toronto, ON, Canada

Cassandra Freitas and Douglas S. Lee
Ted Rogers Centre for Heart Research, Toronto, ON, Canada

Douglas S. Lee
University Health Network, Toronto General Hospital, 200 Elizabeth Street, 4NU-482, Toronto, ON M5G 2C4, Canada

Yoshito Kadoya, Kan Zen and Satoaki Matoba
Department of Cardiovascular Medicine, Graduate School of Medical Science, Kyoto Prefectural University of Medicine, 465 Kajii-cho, Kawaramachi-Hirokoji, Kamigyo-ku, Kyoto 602-8566, Japan

Xiao-Fei Gao, Zhi-Mei Wang, Feng Wang, Shao-Liang Chen and Jun-Jie Zhang
Department of Cardiology, Nanjing First Hospital, Nanjing Medical University, No. 68 Changle Road, Nanjing 210006, China

Shu Lu
Department of Cardiology, The First People's Hospital of Taicang, Suzhou, China

Zhen Ge, Guang-Feng Zuo, Xiang-Quan Kong, Shao-Liang Chen and Jun-Jie Zhang
Department of Cardiology, Nanjing Heart Center, Nanjing, China

Fang Jiang, Hui Xiang and Zhi-Yong Peng
Department of Critical Care Medicine, Zhongnan Hospital of Wuhan University, 169 Dong'hu Road, Wuhan 430071, Hubei, People's Republic of China

E. M. S. Bandara and S. Ekanayake
Department of Biochemistry, Faculty of Medical Sciences, University of Sri Jayewardenepura, Nugegoda, Sri Lanka

C. A. Wanigatunge
Department of Pharmacology, Faculty of Medical Sciences, University of Sri Jayewardenepura, Nugegoda, Sri Lanka

A. Kapuruge
Cardiothoracic Unit, Sri Jayewardenepura General Hospital, Thalapathpitiya, Nugegoda, Sri Lanka

Bachar El-Oumeiri, Frédéric Vanden Eynden and Guido Van Nooten
Department of Cardiac surgery, Erasme Hospital, ULB, 808 Lennik road, 1070, Brussels, Belgium

Kathleen Mc Entee and Pascal Jespers
Laboratory of Physiology and Pharmacology, ULB, Brussels, Belgium

Filippo Annoni and Antoine Herpain
Department of intensive care, Erasme Hospital, ULB, Brussels, Belgium

Philippe van de Borne
Department of Cardiology, Erasme Hospital, ULB, Brussels, Belgium

Index

A

Abdominal Aortic Pseudoaneurysm, 180

Anastomotic Pseudoaneurysms, 180

Angina, 62, 80-82, 139, 157, 163-165, 171, 187, 191, 197, 199-200

Angiotensin Receptor Blockers, 80, 83, 87

Annular Repair, 124

Anterior Interventricular Vein, 141-142, 144

Anti-tachycardia Pacing, 56, 58-59, 89

Antiplatelet Therapy, 96-97, 106-107, 145, 156, 170, 176, 178-179, 185

Aortic Aneurysm, 16-18, 20-23, 184-185

Aortic Cross-clamp, 135-139

Aortic Regurgitation, 9, 16, 18, 36-37, 42, 45, 127-128, 192-193, 197, 199-200

Aortic Valve Stenosis, 14, 23, 30, 37, 45-46, 48, 115, 121-123

Asphyxial Cardiac Arrest, 108-109, 111-113

Atherosclerosis, 25, 30, 84, 86-87, 114, 157, 163, 190-191

Atrial Arrhythmias, 32-34

Atrial Flutter, 32, 34-35

Atrial Septum Puncture, 141, 143

Atrial Tachycardia, 32, 34-35

B

Behcet's Disease, 180, 184-185

Beta-blockers, 98, 157-159, 161, 178

Binary Restenosis, 80, 85

C

Cardiac Resynchronization Therapy Pacemaker, 141, 144

Cardiac Valve, 30, 124-125, 133

Cardiovascular Organs, 16

Cavotricuspid Isthmus, 32

Cilostazol, 96-98, 101, 103-107, 177, 179

Clopidogrel, 83, 96-97, 101, 103, 106-107, 170-179

Conscious Sedation, 7, 9-10, 12

Coronary Fistula, 62

Coronary Stents Implantation, 96-97, 101

Coronary Thromboendarterectomy, 62

D

Diverticular Disease, 64

Doppler-echocardiography, 192, 194

Drug-eluting Stent Implantation, 80-81, 87, 107, 148, 156, 178

Dyslipidemia, 10, 12, 159, 186, 188, 191

Dyspnea, 142, 164-165, 198

E

Electrolyte Disorders, 59

Endovascular Treatment, 164-165, 167-168, 185

Extracorporeal Life Support, 108, 110-114

F

Fatty Acid Binding Protein, 1, 5

H

Homocysteine, 185-186

I

Interleukin 1, 24, 30

Intracoronary Stenting, 96-97, 102-104, 106

L

Late Lumen Loss, 80, 82-83, 85

Left Atrial Appendage, 47

Left Ventricular Remodeling, 30, 89, 95

Leg Edema, 164-165

Leukoaraiosis, 134

Lipoprotein, 68-69, 186-191

Lymphoplasmacytic Infiltration, 16-17, 20, 22

M

Mean Corpuscular Volume, 134, 139

Metabolic Syndrome, 1, 3-6

Mitraclip, 47-51, 53-55

Mitral Regurgitation, 9, 17-18, 47-48, 55, 127-129, 199

Mitral Stenosis, 16-18, 51, 124, 126-129, 132

Myocardial Infarction, 5, 9, 13, 36-37, 42-44, 46, 51-52, 55, 59-62, 66-67, 69-70, 72-74, 79, 81, 85, 95-96, 99, 107, 117, 132, 134, 138-140, 146-147, 163, 170-171, 177-178, 189, 191, 193

N

Narrow Qrs, 141-142

Neointima, 80-81, 84, 86

O

Obliterating Phlebitis, 16, 18, 20

Omecamtiv-mecarbil, 192-193, 199

Optical Coherence Tomography, 80-81, 85-87

P

Pacemaker Implantation, 36-37, 42, 51, 123, 141-144

Paravalvular Aortic Regurgitation, 36-37, 42

Phlebitis, 16, 18, 20-21, 180

Platelet Reactivity Index, 96-97, 99

Preoperative Serum H-fabp, 1

Primary Biliary Cirrhosis, 134, 139

Proinflammatory Cytokine, 24

Pulmonary Embolism, 134, 140

Pulmonary Vein Ablation, 47, 49-50

Pulmonary Venous Flow, 89

R

Renal Arteriography, 164, 167-168

Rheumatic Heart Disease, 56, 59, 124, 126-129, 132-133, 141, 143

S

Stent Thrombosis, 86-87, 96-97, 99, 101, 106-107, 146-147, 152-156, 170-172, 174-176, 178

Storiform Fibrosis, 16, 18, 20-21

Subclavian, 9-10, 12-13, 142

T

Target Lesion Revascularization, 81, 86, 96-97, 99, 146-147, 152-155, 171, 174, 177

Thoracoabdominal Aorta, 63

Transplant Renal Artery Stenosis, 164-165, 168-169

Tricuspid Regurgitation, 26, 48, 53, 55

Triple Valve Replacement, 141-142

Tumoral Necrosis, 24

V

Valvular Disease, 25, 192

Vasodilators, 192

Vasopressors, 108-109

Ventricular Arrhythmia, 56, 60, 95

Ventricular Dyssynchronization, 141

www.ingramcontent.com/pod-product-compliance
Lightning Source LLC
LaVergne TN
LVHW080651210926
848485LV00003B/360